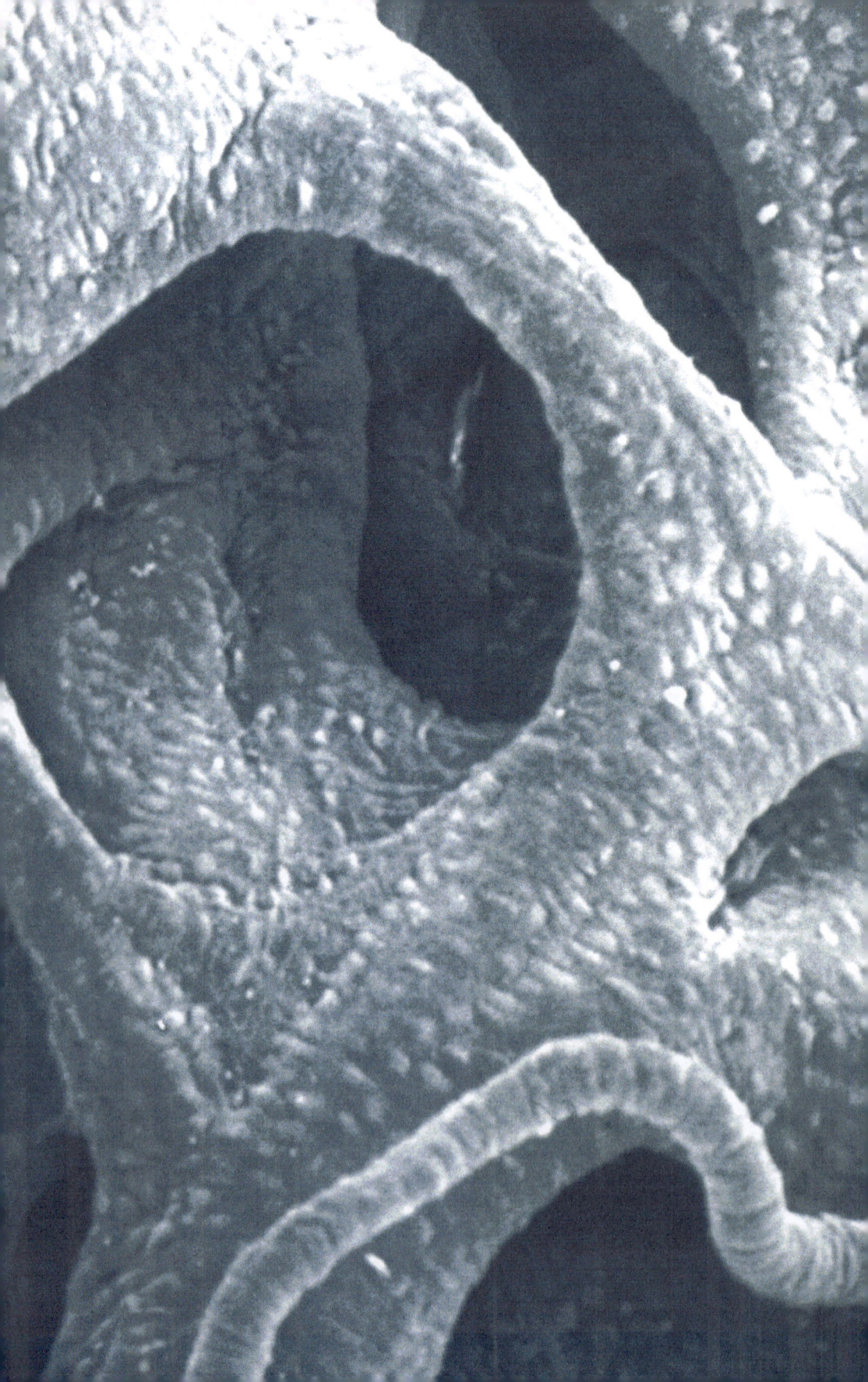

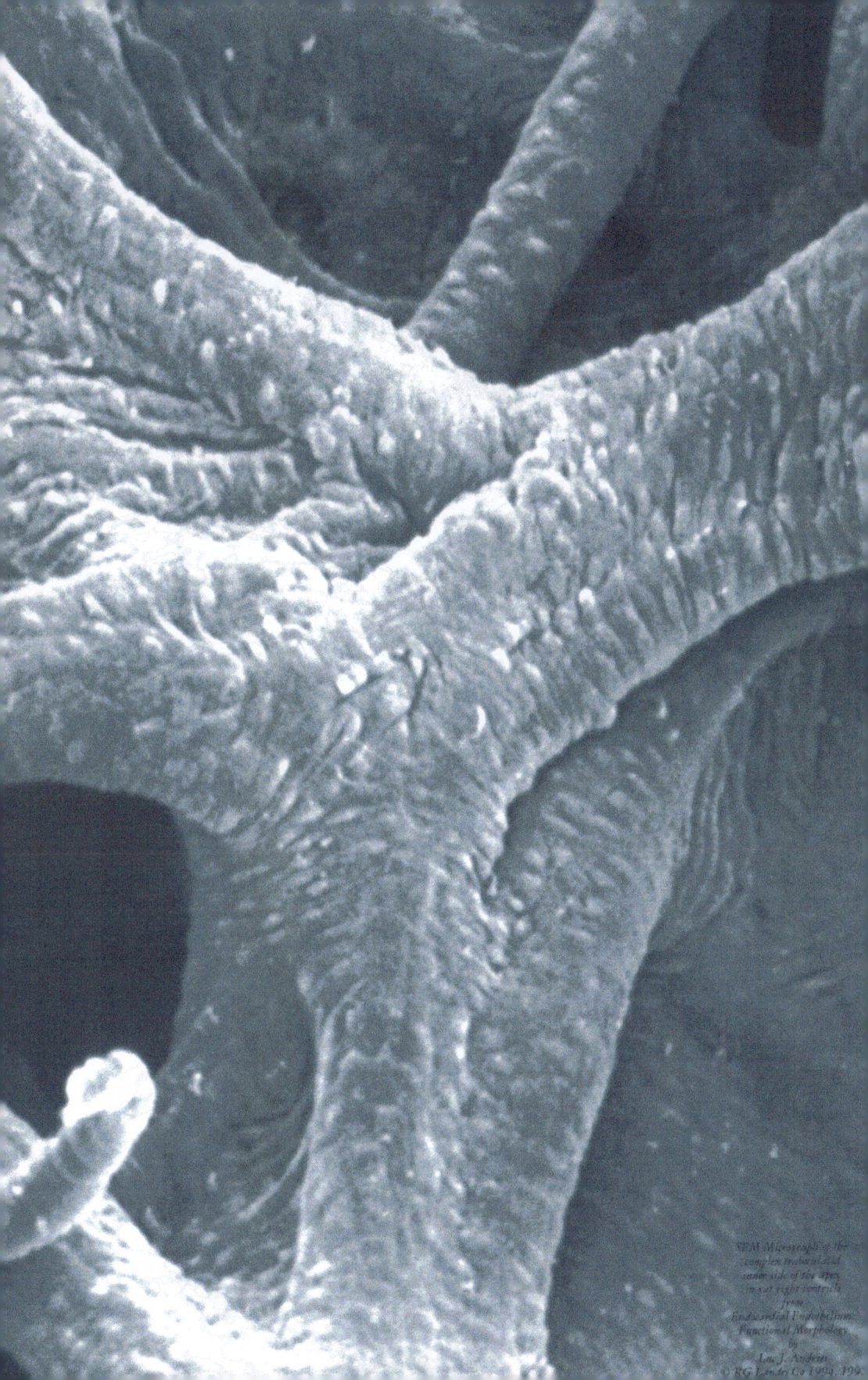

MEDICAL
INTELLIGENCE
UNIT

CLINICAL BENEFITS OF LEUKODEPLETED BLOOD PRODUCTS

Joseph Sweeney, M.D.

The Miriam and Roger Williams Hospitals
Providence, Rhode Island, U.S.A.

Andrew Heaton, M.D.

Irwin Memorial Blood Center
San Francisco, California, U.S.A.

R.G. LANDES COMPANY
AUSTIN

MEDICAL INTELLIGENCE UNIT

CLINICAL BENEFITS OF LEUKODEPLETED BLOOD PRODUCTS

R.G. LANDES COMPANY
Austin, Texas, U.S.A.

Submitted: September 1994
Published: January 1995

ISBN 978-1-57059-122-8   ISBN 978-3-662-26538-3 (eBook)
DOI 10.1007/978-3-662-26538-3

While the authors, editors and publisher believe that drug selection and dosage and the specifications and usage of equipment and devices, as set forth in this book, are in accord with current recommendations and practice at the time of publication, they make no warranty, expressed or implied, with respect to material described in this book. In view of the ongoing research, equipment development, changes in governmental regulations and the rapid accumulation of information relating to the biomedical sciences, the reader is urged to carefully review and evaluate the information provided herein.

Publisher's Note

R.G. Landes Company publishes five book series: *Medical Intelligence Unit, Molecular Biology Intelligence Unit, Neuroscience Intelligence Unit, Tissue Engineering Intelligence Unit* and *Biotechnology Intelligence Unit*. The authors of our books are acknowledged leaders in their fields and the topics are unique. Almost without exception, no other similar books exist on these topics.

Our goal is to publish books in important and rapidly changing areas of medicine for sophisticated researchers and clinicians. To achieve this goal, we have accelerated our publishing program to conform to the fast pace in which information grows in biomedical science. Most of our books are published within 90 to 120 days of receipt of the manuscript. We would like to thank our readers for their continuing interest and welcome any comments or suggestions they may have for future books.

Deborah Muir Molsberry
Publications Director
R.G. Landes Company

CONTENTS

EDITORS

Joseph Sweeney, M.D.
Medical Director, Blood Bank, The Miriam and Roger William Hospitals
Providence, Rhode Island, U.S.A.
Chapter 1

Andrew Heaton, M.D.
President, Irwin Memorial Blood Center
San Francisco, California, U.S.A.
Chapter 1

CONTRIBUTORS

Maren D. Anderson, M.P.P.
Vice President
Health Technology Associates
Washington, D.C., U.S.A.
Chapter 14

Neil Blumberg, M.D.
Blood Bank Director
Strong Memorial Hospital
Rochester, New York, U.S.A.
Chapter 9

Michael P. Busch, M.D., Ph.D.
Vice President, Scientific Services
    and Research
Irwin Memorial Blood Center
San Francisco, California, U.S.A.
Chapter 8

Louis DePalma, M.D.
Chief, Hematopathology
Associate Professor of Pathology
    and of Anatomy
Division of Clinical Pathology
George Washington University
    Medical Center
Washington D.C., U.S.A.
Chapter 12

John M. Forbes, M.B.A.
Vice President of Marketing
Northfield Laboratories Inc.
Evanston, Illinois, U.S.A.
Chapter 14

Steven A. Gould, M.D.
Professor of Surgery
University of Illinois College of Medicine
President
Northfield Laboratories Inc.
Evanston, Illinois, U.S.A.
Chapter 14

Mr. Terry Gourlay
Department of Cardiac Surgery
Royal Postgraduate Medical School
Hammersmith Hospital
London, United Kingdom
Chapter 11

Stein Holme, Ph.D.
Scientific Director, American Red Cross
Associate Research Professor
Eastern Virginia Medical School
Norfolk, Virginia, U.S.A.
Chapter 5

Tzong-Hae Lee, M.D., Ph.D.
Irwin Memorial Blood Center
San Francisco, California, U.S.A.
Chapter 8

Naomi L.C. Luban, M.D.
Director, Transfusion Medicine
    and Hematology
Professor of Pediatrics and Pathology
George Washington University
    Medical Center
Washington D.C., U.S.A.
Chapter 12

CONTRIBUTORS

John P. Miller, M.D., Ph.D.
Blood Bank Fellow
University of Virginia
Health Sciences Center
Charlottesville, Virginia, U.S.A.
Chapter 13

Paul D. Mintz, M.D.
Professor of Pathology
    and Internal Medicine
Director, Blood Bank
    and Transfusion Services
University of Virginia
Health Sciences Center
Charlottesville, Virginia, U.S.A.
Chapter 13

Ruby N.I. Pietersz, M.D., Ph.D.
Deputive Director
Rode Kruis Bloedbank Amsterdam
    en Omstreken
Amsterdam, The Netherlands
Chapter 4

Mark A. Popovsky, M.D.
Medical Director
ARC Northeast Region
Dedham, Massachusetts, U.S.A.
Chapter 10

Paolo Rebulla, M.D.
Senior Assistant
Centro Trasfusionale e di Immunologia
    dei Trapianti
Ospedale Maggiore Policlinico
Milano, Italy
Chapter 3

Henk W. Reesink, M.D., Ph.D.
Medical Director
Rode Kruis Bloedbank Amsterdam
    en Omstreken
Amsterdam, The Netherlands
Chapter 4

Girolamo Sirchia, M.D.
Director
Centro Trasfusionale e di Immunologia
    dei Trapianti
Ospedale Maggiore Policlinico
Milano, Italy
Chapter 3

Edward Snyder, M.D.
Director, Transfusion Service
Yale-New Haven Hospital
New Haven, Connecticut, U.S.A.
Chapter 6

Irena Sniecinski, M.D.
Director, Department of Transfusion
    Medicine
City of Hope National Medical Center
Duarte, California, U.S.A.
Chapter 7

Gary Stack, M.D., Ph.D.
Chief, Pathology & Laboratory Medicine
    Service/113
West Haven VA Medical Center
West Haven, Connecticut, U.S.A.
Chapter 6

Ingeborg Steneker, Ph.D.
Quality Assurance Officer
Rode Kruis Bloedbank Amsterdam
    en Omstreken
Amsterdam, The Netherlands
Chapter 4

Professor Kenneth M. Taylor
Head of Cardiothoracic Surgery
RPMS Hammersmith Hospital
London, United Kingdom
Chapter 11

Darrell J. Triulzi, M.D.
Medical Director
Centralized Transfusion Service
Institute for Transfusion Medicine
Pittsburgh, Pennsylvania, U.S.A.
Chapter 9

Barry Wenz, M.D.
Director–Clinical Pathology
Bronx Municipal Hospital Center
Bronx, New York, U.S.A.
Chapter 2

INTRODUCTION

Joseph Sweeney, Andrew Heaton

The presence of allogeneic leukocytes in blood products received little attention until the mid-1950s when these "passenger" cells were implicated in the etiology of febrile transfusion reactions, and early strategies based on centrifugation were developed to effect their removal. In recent decades and, particularly in the past five years, there has been an accumulation of literature implicating leukocytes in a wide variety of undesirable reactions to blood transfusion.

White cells are the least numerous of the cellular elements in blood and ratios of white cells to platelets and white cells to red cells are approximately 1:15 to 1:1000 respectively. This ratio is maintained in whole blood, but may be altered slightly in the process of component preparation. Any production or processing step which intentionally decreases this ratio will result in a product which can be described as white cell depleted. It has, however, become more common to define the outcome as a residual white cell content, rather than a decrease in cellular ratios, although the latter makes more sense on theoretical grounds, since depletion of white cells needs to be put in the context of any unintentional loss of red cells or platelets. The end result of this intentional processing step, therefore, is generally expressed as the residual absolute number of white cells or as the degree of difference in white cell content, the latter expressed as either a percentage change or as a logarithmic reduction.

Several terms are in common use to describe these production changes or processing steps and these are listed in Table 1.1. There is no universal agreement as to the definition of any of these terms. For the purpose of this book, we chose to use the term, leukodepleted or leukocyte depleted (literally a product from which the white cells have been partly or wholly emptied) because of common usage and because it serves as an attractive, descriptive adjective with its associated verb (to leukodeplete or leukocytedeplete) and noun (leukodepletion or leukocytedepletion). We recognize that the term leukocyte-reduced conveys a similar notion, but this term has already been enshrined in the 16th Edition of the AABB Standards (D2.400) and carries the burden of being defined in terms of, and therefore associated with, absolute numbers. The term leukopoor

Clinical Benefits of Leukodepleted Blood Products, edited by Joseph Sweeney, M.D. and Andrew Heaton, M.D. © 1995 R.G. Landes Company.

Table 1.1. Confusing terminology, some in general use and some suggested candidate terms, used to describe blood products in which the ratio of white cells to other cellular elements is intentionally decreased in component production or processing

Leuko (cyte) depleted	Leukodeprived
Leuko (cyte) reduced	Leukoremoved
Leuko (cyte) poor	Leukoattenuated
Leuko (cyte) free	Deleukocytized (DLC)
Buffy coat depleted	Buffy (coat) poor

presents an impoverished image with possible connotations of impaired quality and leuko-free an unrealistic, if indeed measurable, goal. Neither term would appear to have an advantage over leukodepleted.

If leukodepletion can be used therefore, to describe this process, what then is the extent of the problem? Table 1.2 lists some of the commonly available end-blood components in current use and ranges of associated white cell content. Great variation is evident, this being determined by donor characteristics, volume of blood drawn or processed, devices used, and intermediate manufacturing steps. It is evident that the efficiency of the process expressed as a percentage reduction is unsatisfactory as it may yield products with widely differing absolute residual white cell contents. Residual white cell contents therefore, must be the essential defining feature of the leukodepleted product, but the efficiency of the production change must require definition of both the residual white cell as

well as the degree of reaction in the component intended for manufacture. Leukodepleted blood products must be judged by the impact of such products on quality, safety and cost. Quality, or product potency, is the ability to produce a measurable effect in the recipient: it is thus a measure of *benefit*. Safety relates to adverse effects and is thus, a measure of *risk*. Cost is the additional or *unique expense* incurred which improves the benefit or reduces the risk: The value of the expense incurred is a function of the gain in benefit or the reduction in risk and the cost benefit ratio is only evaluable when all appropriate information can be captured and quantitated.

The organization of each chapter is that it is preceded by a summary which captures the material content at the beginning and at the end itemized conclusions which define current status and indications for future work. Readers wishing to grasp salient points should read each summary and the itemized conclusions. For further in depth information, the main content should be read in detail. This format allows a reader to rapidly scan the whole area within a brief reading period, and the capability to explore an area of interest in greater depth at any point. The organization of the book is that an overview is initially presented with emphasis on methods (Dr. Wenz). It is suggested that this chapter be read at first. The success of these latter processing steps has resulted in the recognition of a new problem, i.e., the difficulty in counting low concentrations of white cells (Professor Sirchia and Dr. Rebulla). Due to the importance of filtration, a separate chapter is devoted to this

Table 1.2. Ranges of intact white cell content of various blood components at the time of manufacture

Red Blood Cells	$8 \times 10^8 - 5 \times 10^9$
Platelet Concentrates from Platelet Rich Plasma	$5 \times 10^7 - 1 \times 10^9$
Platelet Concentrates from Buffy Coat Fraction	$5 \times 10^6 - 1 \times 10^8$
Platelets, Pheresis	$5 \times 10^5 - 1 \times 10^9$
Prestorage Leukocyte depleted platelet concentrates	$1 \times 10^4 - 1 \times 10^6$

technique (Drs. Steneker, Reesink and Pietersz). Second, the impact of this process on the potency of the desired blood component will be discussed in order to attempt to define any apparent benefit (Drs. Sweeney, Heaton, and Holme). Third, a reduction in risk such as attenuation of cytokine mediated reactions or bacterial contamination, (Drs. Stack and Snyder), allosensitization (Dr. Sniecinski), viral disease attenuation (Drs. Busch and Lee), immunomodulation (Drs. Blumberg and Triulzi), transfusion-related acute lung injury (Dr. Popovsky) and reperfusion injury (Professor Taylor and Mr. Gourlay) will be discussed. Fourth, certain specific areas are discussed, such as neonatal transfusion (Drs. Luban and DePalma) and the transfusion support of patients undergoing stem cell reconstitution therapy (Dr. Miller and Mintz) where physicians with interest in this area can directly access information. Last, if leukodepleted products are to come into more widespread use, the cost benefit analysis of this approach needs to be firmly based (Mr. Forbes, Ms. Anderson, Dr. Gould).

The purpose of this book is to provide an up-to-date, state-of-the-art description of the status of leukodepleted blood products. It is so structured that each chapter can be read as an single unit. It is hoped to be of value to practicing surgeons, internists, pediatricians, in addition to pathologists, hematologists, oncologists as well as transfusion medicine specialists. It is hoped that each reader will read critically in order to develop an opinion as to the potential value of these products in their own practice.

CHAPTER 2

METHODS OF LEUKODEPLETION

Barry Wenz

SUMMARY

This chapter reviews methods of production of leukocyte-depleted blood components, comments concerning the procedures used in the quality control of these products and a discussion of the proved and potential clinical benefits derived from the transfusion of these products in lieu of conventional white blood cell containing components. The advantages documented for the use of these products include a reduced incidence of nonhemolytic febrile transfusion reactions, a minimized rate of sensitization to HLA antigens and the accompanying immunological refractoriness to platelet transfusions and the provision of and a means to provide "cytomegalovirus" safe blood other than the traditional search for seronegative donors. The benefit of leukodepleted blood products in curtailing transfusion induced HTLV-I transmission, avoiding the immunomodulation which follows the receipt of blood and decreasing the rate of infection and tumor metastases which may be statistically associated with allogeneic blood transfusion are interesting possibilities that require prospective study. During the past three decades the technologies for the production of leukodepleted blood products have evolved from primitive procedures capable of removing less than 90% of the products' native leukocytes to those that currently deplete -4 $\log_{10}$ of the white cells. These techniques include sedimentation, centrifugation, cell washing, red cell freezing followed by deglycerolization, top and bottom component preparation systems and the use of laboratory and bedside filters. Although by definition not a leukocyte-depletion technique, ultraviolet irradiation of platelet concentrate has been recently shown to hold potential for reducing transfusion induced HLA sensitization. As the technologies to remove leukocytes from blood improve, so must the methods to qualify and monitor the production methods and products. At present the lower standard for leukodepleted components has been set at units containing no more than 10^6 white cells (U.S. standard, 5×10^6). Clinical studies may change these standards. Prototype filters are capable of now providing product containing as few as 10^3 leukocytes. The virtual elimination of all white cells from

Clinical Benefits of Leukodepleted Blood Products, edited by Joseph Sweeney, M.D. and Andrew Heaton, M.D. © 1995 R.G. Landes Company.

a blood component could conceivably justify new applications, such as products that lack the potential to elicit graft versus host disease.

The clinical use of leukocyte-depleted blood products (LDBP), specifically red cell (RCC) and platelet concentrates (PC), has dramatically increased in the past 10 years. A recent survey conducted by the College of American Pathologists (1993 CAP Surveys Set J-A) found approximately two-thirds of all facilities provide WBC reduced components to their clinical services and one-third of the responding institutions transfuse more than 10% of their cellular components as LDBP. The survey also confirmed that the majority of WBC reduced products are produced by filtration techniques. Improved efficiency and simplified production account for the increased use of LDBP. Increased use has led to numerous studies which confirm the clinical benefits derived from the use of these products.

INDICATIONS

The most widely published indication for the use of LDBP is for the prevention of non-hemolytic febrile transfusion reactions (NHFTR).[1] The frequency of NHFTR ranges from 0.5% to 5.0% of all RCC transfusions.[2] This number is several orders of magnitude greater for transfusions of PC. Most of reactions are immunologically mediated and represent the clinical manifestation of reactions between allogeneic white blood cell (WBC) borne antigens and alloantibodies formed as a result of previous antigenic exposure. Previously transfused patients and multiparous women experience the majority of such reactions. People with hemoglobinopathies such as B° thalassemia are among the most consistently transfused patients. Cohorts of these patients are reported to have NHFTR rates in excess of 50% of all transfusions[3,4] (see chapter 6).

A more controversial issue is the use of LDBP to minimize the frequency of the transfusion related Adult Respiratory Distress Syndrome (ARDS).[5] A wide variety of clinical insults has been statistically associated with this syndrome.[6] Among these is

the massive transfusion of blood.[7] These products contain microaggregates, particles consisting of WBC and platelets which form in a spontaneous and progressive fashion in stored red cells. The formation of microaggregates is minimized in blood that has been leukodepleted prior to storage. A similar syndrome dubbed "transfusion related acute lung injury" (TRALI) has been described.[8] This problem is caused by the sequestration of the recipient's own WBC in his/her pulmonary vasculature as a result of the infusion of allogeneic plasma containing antibodies directed against cell surface determinants on the recipients cells. For the most part, WBC depletion and the use of LDBP do not prevent this reaction, however, exceptions to this statement and details of the TRALI syndrome are dealt with elsewhere in this text (see chapter 10).

Reducing the incidence of alloimmunization to HLA class I antigens is a major indication for the use of LDBP.[9,10] HLA antigens are traditionally divided into class I (A, B and C loci) and class II antigens (D loci). Class I HLA antigens are present on all cells of endothelial derivation, however, the class II antigens are present on dendritic cells, B lymphocytes, monocytes and macrophages. The class I antigen remains the target for antibodies directed against the HLA system. Class I antigens, however, are incapable of eliciting a primary immune response without assistance from those cells bearing class II antigens. In the absence of such cells, antigen presentation does not occur, cytokines are not liberated and the chance of alloimmunization is minimized.[11] Since it is only the WBC in a blood product that express class II antigens, removal of these cells from RCC and PC reduces the rate of alloimmunization and its clinical sequelae; specifically immunological refractoriness to platelet transfusions (see chapter 7).

Viral disease is transmitted by the transfusion of both cellular and acellular allogeneic blood products. Two transfusion transmitted viral infections, however, are mediated solely by the transfusion of infected WBC. Transmission of the cytomegalovirus (CMV) can be eliminated by reducing the white cell load of the transfused blood product.[12] The incidence of CMV seropositivity exceeds 50% in the USA, as well as in most developed countries. In donors over the age of sixty, seropositivity is as high as 85%.[13] CMV, a Herpes virus, achieves latency following the acute infection. This is an asymptomatic and lifelong period. Past studies prove that the rate of CMV seroconversion in recipients of unscreened blood is dramatically reduced when WBC are removed from the blood product prior to transfusion.[14] It is assumed that similar data prevail for transfusion induced HTLV-1 viral infection, since this virus is also confined to WBC in blood products[15] (see chapter 8).

Immunomodulation, specifically immune suppression, is associated with the transfusion of allogeneic blood. This observation has been capitalized on to enhance renal allograft survival. The mechanism(s) behind this association is not totally understood, however, it is recognized that at least in part, immunosuppression is achieved by the transfusion of leukocyte containing blood components and possibly plasma containing soluble white blood cell antigens.[16] Blajchman et al using an animal model demonstrated that use of LDBP minimizes the ability of allogeneic blood transfusion to enhance malignant tumor growth and metastasis.[17] Individuals exchanged transfused at birth have been shown to retain features of immunosuppression for many years and possibly for their entire lives. This is highly undesirable since loss of immune surveillance has been associated with increased rates of malignancy. Waymack has demonstrated impaired host defense mechanisms in mice following transfusion.[18] In his studies, mice are inflicted with burn wounds that are subsequently colonized with bacteria and the animals are observed for sepsis. The cohort of mice transfused with allogeneic blood experience higher rates of sepsis and death than do their liter mates who are subjected to the same protocol but receive syngeneic transfusions. Many authors, most prominently Jensen,[19]

Tartter[20] and Blumberg[21] have proved the clinical importance of these observations. In their studies, data collected from patients recovering from elective surgery prove a definitive correlation between the likelihood of postoperative infection and/or sepsis and the transfusion of allogeneic blood products (see chapter 9).

Based on the foregoing considerations, the use of LDBP is advisable for a significant number of transfusion recipients.[22] In deciding which method(s) should be used to provide LDBP, the maximum allowable concentration of WBC in these products must first be determined. The mean concentration of WBC in units of freshly donated, conventionally anticoagulated whole blood ranges from 2 to 3 x 10^9 leukocytes per 500 mL WBC. Individual units of PC average 1-2 $\log_{10}$ fewer, i.e., the standard random donor pool of platelets contains 10^8 leukocytes. Single donor apheresis platelets collected by 'non-leukocyte depleting technology' also contain an excess of 10^8 leukocytes. It is this concentration of WBC that are responsible for the majority of leukocyte associated adverse transfusion reactions.

It has been conclusively demonstrated that more than 75% of NHFTR are successfully avoided by use of red cell products which contain -1 $\log_{10}$ fewer WBC.[23] This number targets a residual WBC concentration of ~10^8 leukocytes per red cell product. A definitive number to achieve the same goal for PC has not as yet been established. This concentration of leukocytes, 10^8/unit transfused, has been defined as the critical antigenic leukocyte load (CALL),[24] representing the quantity of WBC necessary to elicit symptoms in a host who is already sensitized. The CALL number contrasts with another numerical term, the critical immunogenic leukocyte load (CILL)[25] which is defined as the concentration of WBC required to cause a primary immune response in a previously non-sensitized patient. The CILL is believed to be no higher than 10^6 WBC.[26] Accordingly, a reduction of at least -3 $\log_{10}$ is required to produce blood products that will not initiate such responses.

Achieving a reduction in the incidence of transfusion associated CMV infection by use of LDBP is possible as demonstrated by work published by Bowden et al.[27] These authors found that it is necessary for this purpose to use blood products which are leukodepleted by approximately -3$\log_{10}$ of their native WBC. The effect of leukodepletion on transfusion induced immunomodulation in humans has not been proved, however, previously cited work published by Blajchman and colleagues[17] in animal models, again suggests a minimal -3$\log_{10}$ depletion of WBC in transfused products.

These data create a strong bias in favor of defining a LDBP as a component which is minimally depleted of its original WBC concentration by -3 $\log_{10}$ (99.9%), resulting in a residual quantity of leukocytes no greater than 1-5 x 10^6 cells. The assurance that any technique used to produce LDBP yields components at this level of depletion is a demanding task. Monitoring the results of historical leukocyte depleting procedures which were comparatively inefficient was easily performed with the assistance of automated cell counters and low volume hemocytometers. These procedures yield precise and accurate data for WBC reductions of 90% or less. However, technologies which remove -3 $\log_{10}$ or more of WBC from blood products defy monitoring by conventional cell counting techniques.[28] Low volume chamber counts are inaccurate at a level of 10 cells/μL, due to a lack of precision in this range. The automated blood cell counters lose linearity below 100 cells/μL. Of promise is the use of fluorescence-activated cell sorters. Preliminary studies suggest these instruments are capable of monitoring a WBC reduction as great as -6 $\log_{10}$.[29] Gaining in popularity is use of chambers with volumes of 50 μL, such as the Nageotte chamber, a procedure recommended by the Biomedical Excellence for Safer Transfusion (BEST) party of the International Society of Blood Transfusion. These chambers accurately monitor concentrations of leukocytes at levels which approximate 1 cell/μL (see chapter 3).

There are seven procedures that are or have been employed to remove WBC from either RCC, PC or both. These include sedimentation, centrifugation, cell washing, freeze-thaw deglycerolization, laboratory filtration, bedside filtration and the use of the "top and bottom" system of component preparation. Additionally, ultraviolet (UV) irradiation of platelet concentrates (PC) and the use of apheresis procedures which yield PC with low residual WBC contamination must be added to the list of techniques which hold potential for reducing some of the risks associated with the transfusion of homologous leukocytes (Table 2.1).

SEDIMENTATION

Red cells remain suspended in physiological diluents for an indefinite period a result of the negatively charged cells' inability to form rouleaux. Rouleaux formation is a prerequisite to sedimentation. The red cell charge at the level of sheer is defined as the zeta potential and must be overcome if rouleaux are to form and sedimentation is to occur.[30] Zeta potentials can be minimized by the addition of bipolar, macromolecules to the blood product. These compounds such as dextran, polyvinylpyrrolidone and hydroxyethyl starch, reduce the repulsive forces between the red cells, thereby facilitating the process of sedimentation.[31] Formed elements in whole blood sediment in respect to their individual densities. The result is their separation into visibly distinct layers of red cells, white cells/platelets and plasma. Obviously these layers are merely enriched for the various components and the procedure resists any attempt at process control. The features which accounted for the previous popularity of the sedimentation technique were the need for minimal supplies and no capital equipment. The procedure causes a small loss of red cells, approximately 5%, and a single volume sedimentation roughly results in an 80% reduction of WBC.[32] The results can be enhanced by use of a double sedimentation procedure which requires two to three hours and removes 95% (-1.5 $\log_{10}$) of the native leukocyte load.[33]

Table 2.1. Techniques which result in leukocyte attenuation of red cell products

Technique	WBC Removal %(Log_{10})	Red Cell Loss	Comments
Sedimentation			
- single	80% (~0.9 Log_{10})	5%	Obsolete
- double	95% (~1.5 Log_{10})	15%	
Centrifugation	70-80% (0.9 Log_{10})	15%	Widespread use worldwide
Washed Red Cells	70-95% (0.8-1.5 Log_{10})	15%	Useful if plasma removal required
Frozen-Thawed Washed Red Cells	95% (~1.5 Log_{10})	20%	Expensive, Time consuming
Laboratory Filtration	99-99.99% (2-4 Log_{10})	5-10%	
Bedside Filtration:			
Microaggregate	85-95% (0.9-1.5 Log_{10})	5-15%	
Leukoabsorbent	99-99.99% (2-4 Log_{10})		
UV Irradiation	N/A	N/A	Unproven
Top and Bottom Systems	~80%	15%	

Sedimentation is a time consuming procedure which is performed by "open processing." Its product falls short of the target value of 10^6 residual leukocytes. Its time demanding requirements and shortcomings have made this technique obsolete.

CENTRIFUGATION

World-wide, the most common technique used for the production of leukodepleted blood products is centrifugation. This yields a product referred to as "buffy coat" poor red cell concentrate. The centrifugal process is influenced and limited by most of the factors that govern the sedimentation process. Centrifugation relies on an increase in gravitational force instead of the use of macromolecules to enhance rouleaux formation. Like sedimentation, it visibly segregates the various blood components from one another. The popularity of blood component production makes the separation of blood by centrifugation a readily available and desirable adjunct. Removal of the buffy coat imposes little burden beyond the routine procedure. In some laboratories, the ability to sell the buffy coat to commercial firms for the production of interferons serves as a source of revenue. The technique is simple, per-formed within a closed-bag multiple pack system, and does not prematurely accelerate the expiration date of the processed unit. In spite of all of these desirable features, the technique produces a LDBP with a WBC residual too high to provide the majority of previously cited clinical advantages. At best, only 70-80% of the native leukocytes are removed from a unit of red cells by the centrifugation and buffy coat extraction process. Poorer results are obtained if the process is applied to platelet concentrates. Twenty percent of the red cells are lost during this procedure, which ultimately exposes the recipient to a greater number of donor products.[34] As with products produced by the sedimentation procedure, buffy coat reduced blood requires further processing to serve as a true LDBP.

RED BLOOD CELL WASHING

Automated red blood cell washers employ the same principles described for centrifugation, adding the dimension of a continuous introduction of physiological saline wash fluid. The technique is a "spin-off" from technology developed to remove cryopreservatives from red cell concentrates stored by freezing. The centrifugation process is carried out in uniquely shaped bowls or containers designed to allow the various blood components to be removed at will in order of their specific densities. This is accomplished by a "spill over" effect through ports that are strategically positioned in the container. One outstanding feature of the cell washing procedures is its ability to remove the majority of plasma from a unit of whole blood or concentrate. The efficiency of this method approaches a plasma removal of 95%.[35] The removal of WBC is less dramatic. Depending on the protocol and equipment used, the range of leukocyte depletion varies from 70-95%, and red cell loss approximates 15%.[36] The technique is time consuming and despite the automated procedure requires the operator's total attention. Since the anticoagulant/nutritive solution is removed from the product and the system is exposed to the environment, the shelf-life of the product is reduced to 24 hours. Use of this procedure currently has few advocates and has been replaced by the logistical ease and effectiveness of filtration procedures.

FROZEN-THAWED WASHED RED BLOOD CELLS

Until the availability of filtration procedures which are discussed in following sections, the "industrial standard" for leukocyte depleted red cell products was accepted as frozen deglycerolized red cells. Leukocyte depleted platelet concentrate had no similar standard prior to the advent of filters, since the deglycerolization procedure is not applicable to PC. To preserve red blood cells by freezing it is first necessary to add a cryoprotective agent to the concentrate. This agent is generally glycerol. The cryoprotectant is avidly taken up by the red cells, displacing the majority of their intracellular water in the process. The cryoprotectant is not effectively incorporated by WBC and platelets and these cells maintain their normal state of hydration.[37] Formation of intracellular ice crystals during the freezing process causes the WBC and platelet membranes to rupture and form stromal debris. The centrifugation-saline wash procedure which is used to re-move the glycerol from the thawed product, first aggregates the stroma and then removes it. The efficiency of this technique in removing WBC and platelets from red cell concentrate averages -1.5 $\log_{10}$ (95%).[38] Some concern has been raised regarding the unremoved stroma and its potential to be immunogenic.[39] For the most part, this is a mute point since the level to which the WBC themselves are reduced by the procedure does not fulfill the CILL criterion. The technique continues to be used for the preservation of red cells of rare phenotypes which can be stored in frozen state for as long as 10 years prior to use.

LABORATORY FILTRATION

The current widespread use of LDBP is directly related to the commercial production of efficient leukocyte depletion filters. These filters have evolved through multiple generations of improved function and currently are capable of producing a unit of red cells, pooled platelet concentrate or single donor apheresis platelets which contain fewer than 500,000 WBC. In fact, newly developed experimental filters are capable of producing LDBP with a total leukocyte content below 5,000 cells. Clearly the filtration method is the only procedure which produces products which consistently meet the defined criterion for leukodepleted blood. Filters are available in two configurations, those suitable for production of LDBP in the laboratory and those intended for use at the bedside during transfusion. The removal of WBC by filtration depends on the selective adsorption characteristics of the medium employed. It is also influenced by the medium's critical surface tension. Currently available filters are composed of cellulose acetate, cotton wool and polyester fiber. Cellulose acetate adsorbs polymorphonuclear leukocytes more tenaciously than lymphocytes.[40,41] Up to 25% of the red blood cell mass may be lost with the cellulose acetate filters. As with centrifugation, this loss can ultimately increase the recipient's exposure to the number of allogeneic donor products transfused. Cotton wool filters and polyester fibers adsorb mononuclear cells and granulocytes with the same degree of efficiency.[42] Proprietary geometry and fiber modifications are essential to the function of the filters. The older cotton wool and cellulose acetate filters effectively reduce the WBC concentration of blood products by approximately -2 $\log_{10}$, whereas some of the polyester filters function at a level of -4 $\log_{10}$.[43] A newly available product incorporates a polyester red cell depletion filter as an integral component of the collection system (Leukotrap RC System, Cutter/Miles West Haven, CT), which eliminates the need to sterile-dock the device to the container.

BEDSIDE FILTRATION

The removal of leukocytes from blood products by the use of bedside filters began with the use of devices designed to remove microaggregates from stored blood. As previously stated, microaggregates are particles composed of platelets and WBC which form in a spontaneous and progressive fashion in stored red blood cells.[44,45] It follows therefore, that a technique that maximizes microaggregate formation and removal, effectively produces a LDBP. Centrifugation of refrigerated blood increases the mass and frequency of these aggregates. However, these particles are friable and easily broken apart. An additional period of refrigeration increases the cohesive strength of the particles and prevents their disruption by filtration.[46] This phenomenon is possibly the result of the incorporation of fibronectin into the aggregates. The entire technique of centrifugation, refrigeration and microaggregate filtration is referred to as "spin, cool and filter" (SCF). The WBC removal efficacy of the technique does not exceed -1.5 $\log_{10}$ and preferentially removes granulocytes. However, SCF proved that bedside leukocyte depletion of blood was feasible and desirable. Such proof ultimately led to the development of specific leukocyte depleting filters. Currently, the leukocyte depleting filters available for bedside use in the U.S. are composed of polyester fibers. Cellulose ac-

etate filters are available in other countries. The most efficient polyester filters remove -4 $\log_{10}$ WBC from blood products, leaving a residual cell concentration of 10^5 leukocytes in the RCC or PC component.[47] The average final WBC concentration of units of blood filtered at the bedside approximates 5 WBC/μL. Unlike the SCF method, bedside filters require no special processing of the unit and are not influenced by the age of the blood.

The mechanism(s) which allows fibers made of cellulose acetate, cotton wool and polyester to selectively remove WBC from blood components is not known. All of the available devices are depth filters whose function traditionally involves adsorption phenomena. Steneker and her colleagues[48] (see chapter 4) using direct visualization techniques conclude that red cell leukodepletion filters remove lymphocytes and monocytes by direct interception, i.e., capturing them within the pores of the fiber matrix. On the other hand the authors conclude that granulocyte depletion is dependent on platelets first being adsorbed to the fiber which allows for a platelet-granulocyte interaction. The mechanism cited by these authors for the binding of granulocytes to platelets involves calcium dependent phenomena which presumbly are minimized in a unit of chelated RCC or PC. Callaberts et al[49] using leukocyte depleting platelet filters concluded that platelet retention did not correlate with WBC retention. A major problem with the quantitative data in both studies involves the WBC counting procedures employed. Both groups used methods known to be imprecise and inaccurate at the cell concentrations which were detected.[50]

UV IRRADIATION

By definition, UV irradiation of blood products is not a leukodepletion technique. However, it may hold promise for reducing the alloimmunization and immunological refractoriness associated with the transfusion of platelet products. Lindahl-Kiessling and Safwenberg originally reported that UV irradiated WBC did not proliferate nor stimulate allogeneic responder cells in mixed lymphocyte cultures.[51] Subsequently, the clinical correlate of this effect was demonstrated by exposing skin to UV irradiation. The ability of Langerhan's cells to function as antigen-presenting-cells is blocked[52] in irradiated skin and graft survival is prolonged.[53] Studies in canine models have demonstrated that UV irradiation can be used successfully to block transfusion-induced bone morrow graft rejection[54] and refractoriness to random donor platelet transfusions.[55] Few trials have been published using UV treated blood components in people. However, existing feasibility studies suggest that irradiation protocols and plastic storage containers can be formulated to provide adequate function of the UV modified product.[56] Factors such as energy source, wavelength and storage time appear to be key determinants in the viability and function of the treated product.[57] Enthusiasm for the routine use of UV irradiated blood products must be tempered by their currently unproved efficacy, the requirement that they be irradiated in containers with specific light transmission characteristics, and the difficulty involved in effectively irradiating red cell products. Questions have also been raised regarding the ability of UV irradiation to activate latent viruses[58] and concern remains about its mutagenic potential.[59]

The mechanism(s) involved in the process which allows UV light to inactivate antigen presentation and lymphocyte response has not been elucidated. Among the possible candidates are loss of Ia antigen due to shedding,[60] interference with the internalization and re-expression of HLA antigens by antigen presenting cells,[61] alteration of the dendritic cells ability to mobilize calcium and cytokines[54] and a reduction in the surface expression of the intracellular adhesion molecule ICAM-1.[57]

LEUKOCYTE DEPLETED APHERESIS PLATELETS

Alternative technologies such as apheresis procedures which harvest platelets with a reduced concentration of WBC are available. The WBC content of single donor platelets (SDP) harvested by apheresis is determined by a variety of factors such as the equipment and protocol, the type and amount of anticoagulant used and whether a "single or double arm" harvesting technique is employed.[62] As a consequence, the concentration of white blood cells in SDP has been reported to range from 0-28 x 10^6 (Baxter CS-3000 with and without the TNX6 chamber),[63] to 2.6-16 x 10^6 (Cobe Spectra)[64,65] and even as high as 210-400 x 10^6 (Haemonetics V50).[66,67] By extrapolating from the data in the cited studies, it is apparent that the V50 and CS-3000 without the TNX6 chamber fail to provide leukodepleted SDP within the recommended concentration of WBC. The Spectra and CS-3000 Plus fail to meet this criterion 15% of the time. Clinical studies as to their efficacy are lacking and extrapolated from other methodologies. It remains advisable to filter these products at the present time.

TOP AND BOTTOM SYSTEM

In 1988, Hogman and colleagues described the use of a modified blood collection bag which has outlet ports on both ends, the top and bottom.[68] Although this container has not gained popularity in North America, it is in use in Europe. The two ports allow for the simultaneous expression of plasma from above and red cells from below, after the whole blood is centrifuged. This leaves the buffy coat behind in the original container from which platelet concentrate can be made by use of a clamp device. A modification of the original procedure was evaluated by Pietersz et al[69] who found that the WBC concentration in RCC produced by this method was roughly one-fifth that of conventionally prepared RCC but still averaged 1.4 x 10^8, two logs greater than the leukocyte depletion target suggested by the Council of Europe. On the other hand, the concentration of WBC in platelet concentrates was three times greater in "top and bottom" prepared components than in the conventionally prepared product.

CONCLUSIONS

1. It is clear that most of the procedures previously used to provide leukocyte-depleted blood products had little clinical benefit other than reduction of the NHFTR. Intensive therapeutic protocols and transplantation procedures require LDBP which contain the least WBC residual possible.

2. Filtration is currently the only method that consistently achieves the target value of 10^6 residual WBC in leukodepleted blood components.

3. Leukodepleted PC obtained by apheresis procedures can only be used when a commitment to quality control all products by a qualified counting procedure has been made.

4. Qualified counting procedures include the use of Nageotte chambers and flow cytometry techniques.

5. UV irradiation of blood products has yet to be proved a useful clinical adjunct.

6. The clinical benefits derived from the use of adequately leukodepleted blood products include reductions in the rate of NHFTR, CMV seroconversion and alloimmunization.

7. The utility of leukodepleted components in influencing transfusion induced immunomodulation and GVHD has yet to be proved.

REFERENCES

1. Perkins HA, Payne R, Ferguson J, Wood M. Nonhemolytic febrile transfusion reactions. Vox Sang 11:578, 1966.

2. Kevy SV, Schmidt PJ, McGiniss MH, Workman WG. Febrile, nonhemolytic transfusion reactions and the limited role of leukoagglutinins in their etiology. Transfusion 2:7, 1962.

3. Sirchia G, Parravicini A, Rebulla P, Fattori L, Milani S. Evaluation of three procedures for the preparation of leukocyte-poor and leukocyte-free red blood cells for transfusion. Vox Sang 38:197, 1980.

4. Miner LV, Butcher K. Transfusion reactions reported after transfusion of red blood cells and of whole blood. Transfusion 18:493, 1978.

5. Barret J, deLongh DC, Miller E, Litwin MS. Microaggregate formation in stored human red cells. Ann Surg 183:109, 1976.

6. Swank RL. Alteration of blood on storage: measurement of adhesiveness of "aging" platelets and leucocytes and their removal by filtration. N Engl J Med 265:728, 1970.

7. Solis RT, Gibbs MB. Filtration of the microaggregates in stored blood. Transfusion 25:245, 1972.

8. Popovsky MA, Chaplin HC, Moore SB. Transfusion-related acute lung injury: a neglected, serious complication of hemotherapy. Transfusion 32:589, 1992.

9. Doan CA. The recognition of a biological differentiation in the white blood cell. JAMA 86:1593, 1926.

10. Kyger ER, Salyer KE. The role of donor passenger leukocytes in rat skin allograft rejection. Transplant 16:53, 1973.

11. Perkins HA. HLA antigens and blood transfusion: effect on renal transplants. Transplant Proc 9(Suppl 1):229, 1977.

12. Meyers JD. Infection in recipients of marrow transplants. In. Remington JS, Swartz MN eds. Current Clinical Topics In Infectious Disease. New York: Mc Graw Hill, 261, 1985.

13. Hersman J, Meyers JD, Thomas JD, Buckner CD, Clift R. The effect of granulocyte transfusions upon the incidence of cytomegalovirus infection after allogeneic marrow transplantation. Ann Intern Med 96:149, 1982.

14. Lang DJ, Ebert PA, Rodgers BM, Bogges HP, Rixse RS. Reduction of post transfusion cytomegalovirus infections following the use of leukocyte depleted blood. Transfusion 17:391, 1977.

15. Sato H, Okochi, K. Transmission of human T-cell leukemia virus (HTLV-I) by blood transfusion: demonstration of proviral DNA in recipients blood lymphocytes. Int J Cancer 37:395, 1986.

16. Baird MA, Bradley MP, Helsop BF. Prolonged survival of cardiac allografts in rats following the administration of heat treated donor lymphocytes. Transplant 42:1, 1986.

17. Blajchman MA, Bardossy L, Carmen R, Sastry A, Dharam PS. Allogeneic blood transfusion-induced enhancement of tumor

growth: two animal models showing amelioration by leukodepletion and passive transfer using spleen cells. Blood 81:1880, 1993.

18. Waymack JP, Robb E, Alexander JW. Effects of transfusion on immune function in a traumatized animal model. Arch Surg 122:935, 1987.

19. Jensen LS, Andersen AJ, Christansen PM, Hokland P, Juhl CO, Madsen G, Mortensen J, Maller-Nielsen C, Hanberg-Sorensen F, Hokland M. Postoprative infection and natural killer cell function following blood transfusion in patients undergoing elective colorectal surgery. Br J Surg 79:513, 1992.

20. Tartter PI. Blood transfusion and infectious complications following colorectal cancer surgery. Br J Surg 75:789, 1988.

21. Blumberg N, Triulzi DJ, Heal JM. Transfusion-induced immunomodulation and its clinical consequences. Transf Med Rev 4:24, 1990.

22. Wenz B. Leukocyte-poor blood. CRC critical reviews in laboratory sciences 24:1, 1985.

23. Wenz B, Apuzzo J. Removal of microaggregates from blood using various filters. Transfusion 24:88, 1984.

24. Geerdink P. "Why filter blood?" Leukocyte Poor Blood-Recent Developments. Dublin, Ireland, April, 1984.

25. Lieden G, Hilden JO. Febrile transfusion reactions reduced by the use buffy-coat-poor erythrocyte concentrates.Vox Sang 43:263, 1982.

26. Wenz, B. Leukocyte free red cells: The evolution of a safer blood product. in. McCarthy L.J. and Baldwin ML, eds. Controversies of leukocyte poor blood. Arlington, VA. AABB, 1989.

27. Bowden RA, Slichter SJ, Sayers MH, Mori M, Cays MJ, Meyers JD. Use of leukocyte-depleted platelets and cytomegalovirus-seronegative red blood cells for prevention of primary cytomegalovirus infection after marrow transplant. Blood 78:246, 1991.

28. Wenz B, Besso N. Quality control and evaluation of leukocyte depleting filters. Int Workshop on the Role of Leucocyte Depletion in Blood Transfusion Practice. July 1988; London, U.K.

29. Wenz, B., Burns, E.R., Lee, V. and Miller, W.K. A rare event analysis model for quantifying white blood cells in leukocyte depleted blood. Transfusion 31:156, 1991.

30. Pollack W, Reckel RP. The zeta potential and hemagglutination with Rh antibodies. Int Arch Allergy 38::482, 1970.

31. Pollack W, Hager HJ, Hollenbeck LL. The specificity of anti- human gamma globulin reagents. Transfusion 2:17, 1962.

32. Cassel M, Phillips DR, Chaplin H Jr. Transfusions of buffy coat-poor suspensions prepared by Dextran sedimentation. Description of newly designed equipment and evaluation of its use. Transfusion 2:216, 1962.

33. Chapel H Jr, Brittingham TE, Cassel M. Methods for preparation of suspensions of buffy coat-poor red cells for transfusion. Am J Clin Path 31:373, 1959.

34. Polesky HF, McCullough J, Helgeson MA, Nelson C. Evaluation of methods for the preparation of HLA antigen poor blood. Transfusion 13:383, 1973.

35. Uda M, Naito S, Yamamoto K, Ishii A, Nishizaki T. Optimal protocol for preparation of leukocyte-poor red cells with a blood cell processor. Transfusion 24:120, 1984.

36. Bijou H, Brady MT, Fortes P, Hawkins EP. Inconsistent leukocyte removal by IBM 2991 blood cell processor. Transfusion 23:260, 1983.

37. Luyet BJ. Ultra rapid freezing as a possible method of blood preservation. in; Preservation of the formed elements and of the proteins of the blood. ARC. Wash DC. 141, 1959.

38. Meryman HT, Hornblower M. Quality control of deglyceolized red blood cells. Transfusion 21:235, 1981.

39. Crowley JP, Wade PH, Wish C, Valeri CR. The purification of red cells for transfusion by freeze-preservation and washing. V. Red cell recovery and residual leukocytes after freeze-preservation with high concentrations of glycerol and washing in various systems. Transfusion 17:1, 1977.

40. Diepenhorst P, Sprokholt R, Prins HK. Removal of leukocytes from whole blood and erythrocyte suspensions by filtration through cotton wool. I. filtration technique. Vox Sang. 23:308, 1972.

41. Reesink HW, Veldman H, Henrichs HJ, Prins HK, Loos JA. Removal of leukocytes from blood by fibre filtration. Vox Sang 42:281, 1982.

42. Wenz B, Burns ER. Phenotypic characterization of white cells in white cell-reduced red cell concentrate using flow cytometry. Transfusion 31:829, 1991.

43. Rebulla P, Porretti L, Bertolini F, Marangoni F, Prati D, Smacchia C, Pappalettera M, Parravicini A, Sirchia G. White cell-reduced red cells prepared by filtration: a critical evaluation of current filters and methods for counting residual white cells. Transfusion 33:128, 1993.

44. Barret J, deLongh DC, Miller E, Litwin MS. Microaggregate formation in stored human red cells. Ann Surg 183:109, 1976.

45. Wenz B. Microaggregate blood transfusion and the febrile transfusion reaction. A comparative study. Transfusion 23:95, 1983.

46. Parravicini AM, Rebulla P, Apuzzo J, Wenz B, Sirchia G. The preparation of leukocyte-poor red cell for transfusion by a simple, cost effective technique. Transfusion 24:508, 1984.

47. Sirchia G., Wenz B, Rebulla P, Parravicini A, Carnelli A and Bertolini F. Removal of leukocytes from red blood cells by transfusion through a new filter. Transfusion 30:30, 1990.

48. Steneker I, Prins HK, Florie M, Loos JA, Biewenga J. Mechanisms of white cell reduction in red cell concentrates by filtration: the effect of the cellular composition of the red cell concentrates. Transfusion 33:42, 1993.

49. Callaberts AJ, Gielis ML, Spengers ED, Muylle L. The mechanism of white cell reduction by synthetic fiber cell filters. Transfusion 33:134, 1993.

50. Wenz B. and Besso, N. Automated vs microscopic chamber counts for leukocyte depleted blood. International workshop on the role of leucocyte-depleted blood products.In. The role of leucocyte depletion in transfusion practice. Proceedings of the international workshop. Ed. Brozovic. Blackwell Scientific Publications. London, U.K.

51. Lindahl-Kiessling K, Safwenberg J. Inability of UV-irradiated lymphocytes to stimulate allogeneic cells in mixed lymphocyte culture.Int Arch Allergy Appl Immunol 41:670, 1971.

52. Stingl G, Gazze-Stingl LA, Aberer W, Wolff K. Antigen presentation by murine epidermal Langerhans cells and its alteration by ultraviolet light. J Immunol 127:1707, 1981.

53. Gruner S, Meffert H, Karasek E, Sonnichsen N. Prolongation of skin graft survival in mice by in vitro PUVA treatment and failure of induction of specific immunologic memory By PUVA treated grafts. Arch Dermatol Res 276:82, 1984.

54. Deeg HJ, Aprile J, Graham TC, Applebaum FR, Sorb R. Ultraviolet irradiation of blood prevents transfusion-induced sensitization and marrow graft rejection in dogs. Blood 67:537, 1986.

55. Slichter SJ, Deeg HJ, Kennedy MS. Prevention of platelet alloimmunization in dogs with systemic cyclosporine and by UV-irradiation of or cyclosporine-loading of donor platelets. Blood 69:414, 1987.

56. Sherman L, Menitove J. Kagen LR, Davisson W Lin A, Aster RH, Buchholz DH. Ultraviolet-B irradiation of platelets: a preliminary trial of efficacy. Transfusion 32:402, 1992.

57. Johnson RB, Napychank S, Murphy S, Snyder EL. In vitro changes in platelet function and metabolism following increasing doses of ultraviolet-B irradiation. Transfusion 33:249, 1993.

58. Valerie K, Delers A, Bruck C, et al. Activation of human immunodeficiency virus type 1 by DNA damage in human cells. Nature 333:78, 1988.

59. Cornforth MN, Bedford JS. On the nature of a defect in cells from individuals with ataxia-telangiectasia. Science 227:1589, 1985.

60. Emerson SG, Pretell G, Cone RE. Physical and pharmacologic inhibition of shedding of I-A antigens. Exp Clin Immunogenet 1:9, 1984.

61. Pernis B. Internalization of lymphocyte membrane components.Immunol Today 6:45, 1985.

62. Price TH, Ford SE, Northway MM. Alter-

nate collection protocols for plateletpheresis using the Cobe Spectra. American Soc Apheresis, April, 1989; A61.

63. Shanwell A, Gullickson H, Berg BK, et al. Evaluation of platelets prepared by apheresis and stored for 5 days. In vitro and in vivo studies. Transfusion 29:783, 1989.

64. Sniecinski I, Nowicki B, Park HS, et al. Platelet yields and leukocyte contamination of plateletpheresis concentrates: Comparison of three continuous flow systems. 4th Int Cong World Apheresis Assoc. Saporo, Japan. June A174, 1992.

65. Kretschmer V, Rossa W, Eisenhardt G. Plateletpheresis with the new Cobe-Spectra. American Soc for Apheresis. 11th Annual Meeting, San Francisco, CA. March A72, 1990.

66. Rock G, Senack E, Tittley P. 5-day storage of platelets collected on a blood cell separator. Transfusion 29:626, 1989.

67. Anderson NA, Wilkes A, Smith H, et al. Platelet collection using the Cobe Spectra and Haemonetics V50 Autosurge with identical donors. 3rd Int Cong World Apheresis Association, Amsterdam, Netherlands. April, 1990; WE-PO-E.

68. Hogman CF, Eriksson L, Hedlund K, Wallvik J. The top and bottom system: A new technique for blood component preparation and storage. Vox Sang 55:211, 1988.

69. Pietersz RNI, Dekker WJA, Reesink HW. Comparison of a conventional quadruple-bag system with a 'top-and-bottom' system for blood processing. Vox Sang 59:205, 1990.

CHAPTER 3

ENUMERATION OF LOW WHITE CELLS

Girolamo Sirchia, Paolo Rebulla

SUMMARY

White blood cells (WBC) present in blood and blood components can cause a number of posttransfusion complications. At present, filtration is the most popular method developed to prepare blood components depleted of WBC. Current filters are capable of removing more than 99.9% WBC (3 $\log_{10}$ removal). Consequently, filtered products can contain as few as 1-10 WBC/μL (300,000-3,000,000 in a 300 mL unit), or less. At these levels routine WBC counting methods are greatly inaccurate and imprecise, as supported by theoretical considerations already presented in the medical literature almost 50 years ago. These considerations indicate that: (1) the error of counting approximates the square root of the number of cells counted. As a consequence, counting methods should aim at examining large sample volumes, so as to collect the greatest possible number of cells; (2) rare events, such as WBC randomly distributed in a counting chamber, follow the Poisson distribution. This distribution can be used to determine the level of confidence one can have that a certain count is below a certain level (upper confidence limit of that count). In reporting the results of evaluations performed in leukodepleted blood components this level should be preferred to mean or median counts, since at the clinical level it is important that the recipient receives *less than* rather than an *average* number of WBC.

Methods specifically designed for counting residual WBC include: (1) microscopic methods performed with traditional or large volume counting chambers; (2) flow cytometry procedures which use light scatter and/or DNA staining techniques; (3) radioimmunoassays; (4) techniques based on leukocyte DNA amplification and (5) a qualitative method based on trapping residual leukocytes in 3 μm pore size polycarbonate filters. Of these, counting in large volume chambers such as the Nageotte chamber has been recommended as the method offering the best compromise of

Clinical Benefits of Leukodepleted Blood Products, edited by Joseph Sweeney, M.D. and Andrew Heaton, M.D. © 1995 R.G. Landes Company.

precision and feasibility for routine quality control. Flow cytometry, which requires access to expensive equipment, shows similar levels of precision and accuracy and slightly better sensitivity. In view of the continuous improvement of filters for leukodepletion, better counting methods should be developed. In addition, since the prevention of different complications seems to require the achievement of different levels of leukodepletion, specific protocols for quality assurance should be designed in relation to the type of complication to be prevented (e.g. non-hemolytic, febrile transfusion reaction, CMV transmission, etc).

Finally, efforts to develop improved methods for counting residual WBC in leukodepleted blood components should be accompanied by conclusive studies designed to increase our knowledge on the minimum number of residual WBC capable of inducing different posttransfusion complications.

INTRODUCTION

During the last three decades it has been recognized that white blood cells (WBC) present in blood and blood components can cause a number of important side effects in the recipients.[1-4] This favored the development of methods for removing WBC from red blood cells (RBC) and platelet concentrates (PC), and prompted the identification of conditions where the use of leukodepleted blood components (LDBC) is indicated.[5,6]

At present, filtration through disposable filters is the most popular technology used to prepare LDBC. Filters of the latest generation are so effective that the number of residual WBC is often below the lower limit of accurate detection of routine manual and automated WBC counting methods. As a consequence, more sensitive techniques have been developed, with the aim of allowing a more reliable quality control (QC) of LDBC. Most of these procedures are modifications of the traditional manual methods based on sample dilution with agents capable of lysing the red cells and staining the WBC, followed by counting WBC with a microscope in a

hemocytometer (Table 3.1) or by flow cytometry. In general, these modifications aim at increasing the absolute number of WBC detected in the counting procedure, so as to improve the accuracy and precision of the WBC count.

In this chapter we will present the theoretical background of low WBC counts and review published methods specifically developed for the enumeration of WBC in filtered RBC and PC. Finally, we will discuss QC of these products.

THEORETICAL BACKGROUND

In his elegant paper on blood cell counts published in 1945,[7] W.N. Berg reported a statistical study by Berkson et al,[8] who identified at least three causes of variation in WBC counts: (1) random cell streaming (distribution of WBC across the squares of the chamber grid); (2) variations in sizes of chambers; (3) variations in pipets. From their studies Berkson et al[8] derived a formula for calculating the extent to which these factors may influence the chamber count. Using the formula developed by Berkson et al, Berg estimated that random streaming of cells and errors related to inaccuracy of pipettes and blood cell counting chambers would produce a 12% coefficient of variation for counts based on 100 WBC.[7] This is in agreement with the theoretical considerations presented by Dacie and Lewis to describe the inherent distribution error of WBC counts, which corresponds to approximately the square root of the number of cells counted.[9] As a consequence, the error can be minimized by increasing the number of cells counted, which, in turn, can be achieved by increasing the sample size and/or decreasing the sample dilution. Conversely, error approaches 100% for counts where very few WBC can be detected.

Table 3.1 shows the characteristics of the different hemocytometers currently in use and Table 3.2 reports the number of WBC theoretically expected to be present in one grid of different hemocytometers after 1:10 or 1:5 dilution of samples containing different numbers of WBC/μL.

Table 3.3 reports typical values of WBC counts that can be found in blood components prepared with different procedures.

By the combined use of information provided in Tables 3.1, 3.2 and 3.3 it can be anticipated that not infrequently, even with

Table 3.1. Characteristics of some hemocytometers used for the evaluation of residual WBC in leukodepleted blood components

Hemocytometer	Area (sqmm)	Depth (mm)	Volume per grid (µL)
Bürker or Neubauer	9	0.1	0.9
Fuchs-Rosenthal	16	0.2	3.2
Nageotte	100	0.5	50

Table 3.2. Number of WBC theoretically expected to be present in one grid of different hemocytometers after 1:10 or 1:5 dilution of samples containing different numbers of WBC

WBC/µL in neat sample	0.1		1		5		10	
Total WBC in a 300 mL unit	30,000		300,000		1,500,000		3,000,000	
Sample dilution	1:10	1:5	1:10	1:5	1:10	1:5	1:10	1:5
No. of WBC/hemocytometer grid:								
Bürker or Neubauer	0	0	0	0	0	1	1	2
Fuchs-Rosenthal	0	0	0	0	1-2	3	3	6
Nageotte	0	1	5	10	25	50	50	100

Table 3.3. Typical WBC counts (mean or median) in blood components prepared with different methods. Data have been reported from or calculated from figures reported in the publications cited

Blood component	Unit's volume (mL)	Number of WBC per RBC unit (x 10⁶)	per µL or PC pool	Ref.
RBC	288	2260	7847	19
RBC with buffy-coat removal	247	840	3400	19
Washed RBC	411	650	1581	49
Deglycerolyzed RBC	250	40	160	50
Filtered RBC	269	0.187	0.7	33
Pool of 7 PC (platelet-rich-plasma method)	350	310	886	51
Pool of 7 PC (buffy-coat method)	350	21	60	52
PC pool leukodepleted by centrifugation	320	84	262	53
Filtered PC pool	320	7	7	22

the largest chamber one could find no or very few WBC per chamber grid in samples from LDBC prepared with current filters.

Another element of variability of the WBC count is not related to cell streaming but to the distribution of the WBC in the filtered unit. This aspect relates to the consideration that, if the filtered unit is considered as the sum of very small volumes, chance causes that the number of WBC present in each very small volume is not exactly the same. In the most extreme case, there will be some very small volume samples containing no WBC. Using the Poisson distribution, that is suitable for this purpose since the volume of the unit greatly exceeds the volume of the sample, one can calculate the probability (p) that a sample of a certain volume collected from a filtered unit does *not* contain WBC.[10] The calculation is performed with the formula:

$$p = e^{-nv/V}$$

where V is the unit's volume, v is the volume of the undiluted sample analyzed in the counting chamber and n is the total number of WBC contained in the filtered unit. In the following example, we consider a 300 mL unit containing 60,000 WBC. Assume that the sample is counted in a Nageotte chamber, which displays a volume of 50 μL, and that the sample is diluted 1:10. Thus, the volume of native sample actually present in the Nageotte chamber is 5 μL. Based on these data one can expect that the entire Nageotte grid contains 1 WBC. However, no WBC will be present in 37% of cases. In fact,

$$e^{-60,000 \times 5:300,000} = e^{-1} = 2.718^{-1} = 0.37.$$

Therefore, by chance 37% of WBC counts performed as described above with 300-mL leukodepleted units containing 60,000 WBC will score "zero" in spite of their WBC content. The practical implications of this is that quality control procedures based on single counts will miss a contamination of 60,000 WBC per unit more than one-third of the time.

Although all the above is clearly demostrable on theoretical grounds, the practical implications of these considerations may appear minimal. In fact, it could be argued that 60,000 WBC per unit is well below the frequently reported figure of $1-5 \times 10^6$ WBC that is commonly considered as a threshold for some complications caused by the transfusion of allogeneic WBC.[11,12] Accordingly, even a big error or uncertainty around such a small value as 60,000 WBC per unit is not expected to determine a real risk that the true WBC content exceeds $1-5 \times 10^6$ WBC. However, the error at the extreme level of 60,000 WBC per unit (or even less) may soon become practically relevant in view of the continuous improvement of the effectiveness of leukodepletion filters. This could open new possibilities to leukodepletion, such as prevention of secondary immunization to HLA or even transfusion associated graft versus host disease, that seem infeasible today considering the number of WBC still present in LDBC prepared with the most effective filters. To give a general view of the point presented above, Figure 3.1 reports the expected percentage of "zero" counts with a sample diluted 1:10 and counted in one grid of a Nageotte chamber, as a function of the number of WBC present in a 300-mL leukodepleted unit.

The theoretical considerations, which have been discussed by Dumont in great detailed and applied to several methods for counting WBC in LDBC,[13] are relevant also for methods based on flow cytometry. The main difference between hemocytometer-based methods and flow cytometry is that with the latter large numbers of "events" (i.e. WBC) can be collected more easily.

METHODS FOR COUNTING WBC IN LDBC

Before discussing the details of these methods, the reader is referred to Table 3.4, which reports a definition of the terms "sensitivity", "accuracy" and "precision", as they specifically relate to counting WBC in LDBC. As far as accuracy is concerned, it must be stressed that it is adversely influ-

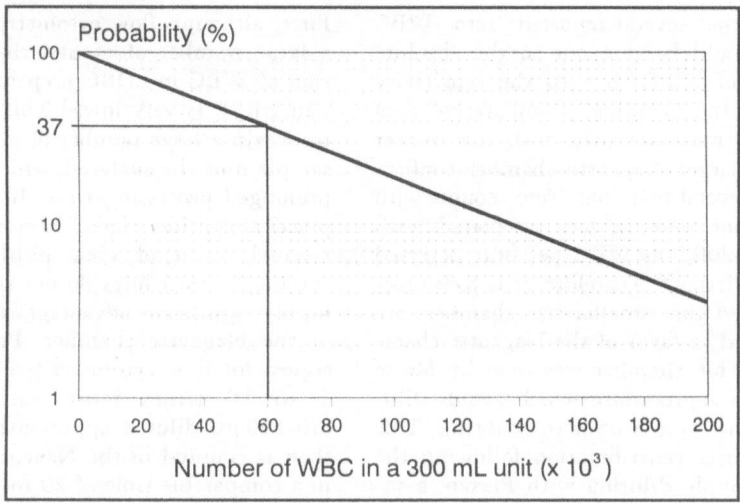

Fig 3.1. Probability for WBC to be absent in one grid (50 µL) of a Nageotte chamber as a function of the total number of WBC contained in a 300 ml leukodepleted unit if the sample to be counted is diluted 1:10.

enced by the content of degenerated WBC in LDBC, which can be a relevant proportion of the total number present in the unit, and that increases during storage.[14-16]

The available counting methods can be divided into five categories: (1) microscopic methods performed with traditional[9,12,17,18] or large volume counting chambers;[19,20] (2) flow cytometry methods which use light scatter[21] and/or DNA staining techniques;[22-26] (3) radioimmunoassays;[27,28] (4) methods based on leukocyte DNA amplification[29] and (5) a qualitative method based on trapping residual leukocytes in 3 µm pore size polycarbonate filters.[30]

Some methods use a diluted[9,12] or a concentrated[20] sample of LDBC. In other procedures, the target of decreasing the lower detection limit of the counting method requires that the whole unit is processed so as to concentrate residual WBC into a small volume through red cell lysis and unit centrifugation or by the use of gradients.[29,31] Besides the need to use the entire unit, which precludes applying these procedures to routine quality control, these methods suffer from variations in the yield of WBC. Lack of standardization at this level might outweigh the advantages offered by increased sensitivity. It is pos-

sible that refinements in Ficoll WBC purification techniques[32] could increase the validity of these methods, at least for research applications.

MICROSCOPIC CHAMBER COUNTS

Traditional methods for microscopic manual counting of WBC in peripheral blood involve 1:20 blood dilution and the use of a Bürker or a Neubauer chamber.[9] As shown in Table 3.1, both chambers contain grids with an individual volume of 0.9 µL. These chambers have been used for counting residual WBC in LDBC by a number of investigators,[12,17] but it was soon

---

Table 3.4. Definition of statistical terms used in the evaluation of methods for counting WBC

Term	Definition
Sensitivity	Smallest quantity statistically distinguishable from the background (zero). Better term is 'lower detection limit'
Precision	Concordance of replicate measures
Accuracy	Agreement of observed with true value

realized that several reported "zero" WBC counts could be due not to the absolute absence of WBC, but to the sensitivity limit of the chamber. Comparative data collected more recently with the Bürker and the larger Nageotte chamber confirm that on several occasions "zero" counts with the former were in fact associated with 100,000-200,000 WBC per unit detected with the latter.[33] Therefore, it is today recommended that smaller-size chambers are abandoned in favor of the Nageotte chamber.[19,34] This chamber was used by Masse et al[20] in a procedure which avoids dilution of the sample prior to counting. This method uses centrifugation following the initial sample dilution with Plaxan, a solution originally developed to count platelets in a hemocytometer. Centrifugation results in concentrating the residual WBC into the original sample volume, or even into half the original sample volume. These procedures are referred to as a "1:1 dilution" or a "2:1 concentration", respectively. The authors conclude that this approach allows for the precise detection of concentrations of WBC as low as 3×10^4 per unit. Other promising results have been obtained with samples concentrated by centrifugation into 1/20 of their original volume after initial 1:5 dilution with a paraformaldehyde solution. Preliminary results of this method, which uses a Nageotte chamber for the final count, support the expectation of being able to count reliably WBC at concentrations below 0.1/µL (D. Prati, unpublished observations).

FLOW CYTOMETRY

Flow cytometry generates data through a machine, and therefore is not subject to reader bias. In addition, it derives counts from a relatively high number of total events, e.g., 10,000-100,000 events per analysis. Several flow cytometry methods designed to count WBC in LDBC have been described.[21-26] Although these procedures can produce valuable information for research purposes, practical considerations make it difficult to "go with the flow" for the routine quality control of LDBC.[35]

First, although flow cytometry can detect a large number of events, the concentration of WBC in LDBC prepared with current filters is very low.[33] This means that to obtain a large number of events a large sample must be analyzed, which requires a prolonged processing time. In addition to practical considerations,[25] also from the statistical point of view published flow cytometry procedures do not seem to offer highly significant advantages over the use of the Nageotte chamber. Protocols designed for flow cytometry generally count 5 to 10 times more native sample (50-100 µL diluted approximately 1:10)[24] than is counted in the Nageotte chamber, in a comparable time of 20 to 30 minutes. Statistically, this decreases the variability of the count by a factor of 3 (i.e. square root of 10). At the concentration of WBC counted in LDBC, this advantage does not seem to justify the cost of the machine and effort. In addition, as stated above, advantages related to elimination of reader bias do not seem to be very important.[20,34] This notwithstanding, it is possible that refinements of flow cytometry methods mainly aimed at preventing autofluorescence and unwanted staining[36,37] or to determining the exact volume of sample examined[38] could greatly improve the ability of flow cytometry to detect very small numbers of residual WBC.

RADIOIMMUNOASSAYS

Procedures have been published which count WBC[28] as well as platelet fragments in leukodepleted RBC.[27] However, the use of radioimmunometric methods under routine conditions is impractical and generally discouraged for environmental reasons.

METHODS USING LEUKOCYTE DNA AMPLIFICATION

DNA amplification through the polymerase chain reaction (PCR) has been used in a method for counting WBC in LDBC. This method employs a technique to detect the HLA-DQ alpha gene.[29] Similarly to limiting dilution assays,[39,40] in this procedure the sample undergoes a series of dilutions, and PCR is performed on each diluted sample. The original number of copies (cells) in the undiluted sample is then calculated following the assumption, supported by data from a standard calibration curve, that the end point of the titration contains one DNA copy. This method requires thorough standardization and a statistical approach to the final evaluation of the results. As discussed above, approximately one-third of the assays will not contain DNA when one DNA copy per assay is expected. The original method which used liquid hybridization detection[29] has been recently modified to use enzyme immunoassay (EIA) to detect the amplified product. This EIA is based on a monoclonal antibody reacting only to double-helix DNA.[41] Although PCR is potentially more sensitive than current chamber methods, it is not likely that this method will be utilized for routine QA in the near future.

QUALITATIVE METHOD WITH POLYCARBONATE FILTERS

In this method filtered RBC are passed through a 3 µm polycarbonate filter. Residual WBC are trapped in the filter pores and their presence is detected by microscopic examination of the filters after May-Grunwald-Giemsa stain or immunocytochemistry using a monoclonal antibody to leukocyte common antigen.[30] Studies on the lower detection limit of this method are not available.

QUALITY CONTROL OF LDBC

Two critical aspects of QC regard the number of units that need to be controlled and the format of data presentation. As far as the number of units to be checked, different indications for the use of LDBC may require different approaches to QC. For example, NHFTR are easily prevented with RBC units containing less than 100 x 10^6 WBC. Therefore, if units are filtered through some of the currently available third generation filters for which extensive reports indicate that WBC residuals never exceed, for example, 10 x 10^6, it is probably sufficient to test a small (5-10?) num-

ber of filters in each new lot, whereas QC on each filtered unit is probably unnecessary. The case would be different if the indication of LDBC is the prevention of CMV transmission, which has been achieved by the transfusion of leukodepleted units containing less than approximately 10 x 10^6 WBC.[42-44] For this indication and for other more ambitious indications requiring more profound leukodepletion it is probably necessary to check all filtered units.[45]

Another important aspect regards the format of data presentation. Notwithstanding the great efforts to improve our ability to accurately determine the number of residual WBC in LDBC, variability of WBC counts performed in LDBC prepared with the most effective filters is still great. The main reason for this is that improvements in WBC counting methods have been paralleled by improvements in the efficiency in leukocyte depletion filters. Accordingly, the number of residual WBC detectable with any method has progressively become smaller and smaller. Thus, the recommendation made by Dumont seems particularly appropriate that WBC residuals are expressed not (or not only) as mean, median, or range values, but rather as the *level of confidence* one can have that the number of WBC is *below* a certain count.[13] This corresponds to the upper limit of the confidence interval for that count. It is difficult to give a recommendation about the most appropriate level of confidence. This probably differs with various indications to the use of LDBC, i.e., prevention of NHFTR, HLA alloimmunization, CMV transmission, etc. Although 95% confidence is generally considered sufficient, in some cases it may prove insufficient. In fact, at the 95% confidence interval, 2.5% of the components would contain more WBC than desired. Stated differently, 1 in every 40 units could be unacceptable, as that single unit could transmit, for example, CMV to a transplanted patient.

As far as the graphical presentation of data, the cumulative distribution format

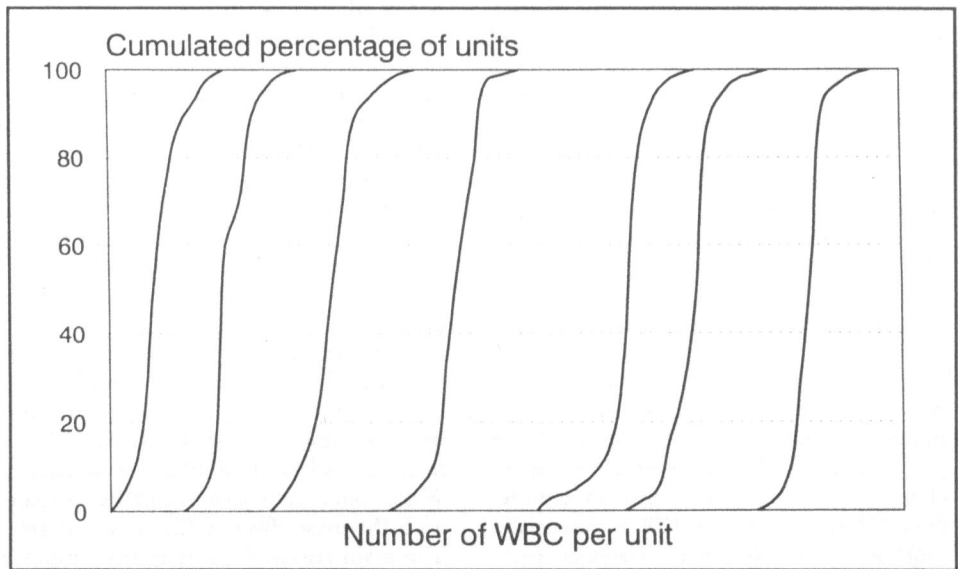

Fig 3.2. An example of graphic presentation of WBC residuals following the format used by Vakkila and Myllylä.[46] Each curve represents the cumulated percentage of leukodepleted units prepared with a certain method.

chosen by Vakkila and Myllylä[46] favors an easy comparison of LDBC prepared with different methods (Fig. 3.2).

QC of LDBC has been the object of recent work by 21 transfusion teams of the French Produits Sanguins Labiles (PSL) study group,[19] and by 20 laboratories of the BEST (Biomedical Excellence for Safer Transfusion) working party of the International Society of Blood Transfusion.[34]

The aim of the PSL study was to evaluate the performance of the Nageotte chamber method in about 1400 RBC units filtered through six commercial filters. The Nageotte method showed a 25% coefficient of variation for a concentration of 2.5 WBC/μL. In addition, for five of the six filters the median postfiltration WBC values in RBC units with and without buffy-coat depletion were 0.34 and 1.1 x 10[6] per unit respectively.[19]

The BEST group conducted two wet workshops aimed at: (1) determining the lower limit of WBC detection and balancing advantages and disadvantages of methods using flow cytometry and the Nageotte chamber; (2) evaluating three different pro-

tocols (1:10 vs 1:5 vs 1:1 dilution) using the Nageotte chamber. Workshop #1 showed that flow cytometry does not determine dramatic improvements in the detection of residual WBC versus the Nageotte chamber method. As expected, workshop #2 showed that the protocol involving the smallest dilution was associated with the most precise results. However, each of the three protocols produced valid counts at levels of ≥ 1 WBC/μL, while more precise methods are needed at counts below 1 WBC/μL.[34]

CONCLUSIONS

At the current level of technology, the following conclusions can be drawn on methods for enumerating low numbers of WBC in LDBC:

1. Methods for counting residual WBC in LDBC in routine QC procedures are available with sufficient precision down to 1 WBC/μL (300,000 WBC in a 300 mL unit). However, many of these procedures are time-consuming. In addition, it is expected that the production of more effective leukodepletion

filters will make soon these methods obsolete, thus requiring the development of new approaches to an accurate and precise quantitation of residual WBC.

2. Not only methods for counting should be improved but also QC protocols should be defined. It is likely that different indications to the use of LDBC need different QC protocols.

3. The greatest efforts of those interested in improving methods for the enumeration of low WBC in LDBC will be frustrated in the absence of conclusive studies aimed at improving our knowledge on the minimum number (and type[46-48] of residual WBC capable of inducing different posttransfusion complications.

REFERENCES

1. Brittingham TE, Chaplin H. Febrile transfusion reactions caused by sensitivity to donor leukocytes and platelets. JAMA 167:819, 1957.

2. Claas FHJ, Smeenk RJT, Schmidt R, et al. Alloimmunization against the MHC antigens after platelet transfusions is due to contaminating leukocytes in the platelet suspension. Exp Hematol 9:84, 1981.

3. Hersman J, Meyers JD, Thomas JD, et al. The effect of granulocyte transfusions upon the incidence of cytomegalovirus infection after allogeneic marrow transplantation. Ann Intern Med 96:49, 1982.

4. Sato H, Okochi K. Transmission of human t-cell leukemia virus (HTLV-I) by blood transfusion: demonstration of a proviral DNA in recipient's blood lymphocytes. Int J Cancer 37:395, 1986.

5. Lane TA, Anderson KC, Goodnough LT, et al. Leukocyte reduction in blood components therapy. Ann Int Med 117:151, 1992.

6. Consensus Conference. Leucocyte depletion of blood and blood components. The Royal College of Physicians of Edinburgh, 1993.

7. Berg WN. Blood cell counts. Their statistical interpretation. Am Rev Tuberc 52:179, 1945.

8. Berkson J, Magath TB, Hurn M. The error of estimate of the blood cell count as made

9. Dacie JV, Lewis SM. Practical haematology (7th ed.). Edinburgh: Churchill Livingstone, 1991.

10. Haight FA. Handbook of the Poisson Distribution. New York, John Wiley & Sons, 1967.

11. Fisher M, Chapman JR, Ting A, et al. Alloimmunization to HLA antigens following transfusion with leukocyte-poor and purified platelet suspensions. Vox Sang 49:331, 1985.

12. Sirchia G, Rebulla P, Mascaretti L, et al. The clinical importance of leukocyte depletion in regular erythrocyte transfusions. Vox Sang 51(suppl 1):2, 1986.

13. Dumont LJ. Sampling errors and the precision associated with counting very low numbers of white cells in blood components. Transfusion 31:428, 1991.

14. Turner JH, Hutchinson DL, Petricciani J. Cytogenetic and growth characteristics of human lymphocytes derived from stored donor blood packs. Scand J Haematol 8:169, 1971.

15. Skinnider L, Wrobel H, McSheffrey B. The nature of the leucocyte 'contamination' in platelet concentrates. Vox Sang 49:309, 1985.

16. Humbert JR, Fermin CD, Winsor EL. Early damage to granulocytes during storage. Sem Hematol 28(suppl 5):10, 1991.

17. Greenwalt TJ, Allen CM. A method for counting leukocytes in filtered components. Transfusion 30:377, 1990.

18. Kao KJ and Scornik JC. Accurate quantitation of the low number of white cells in white cell-depleted blood components. Transfusion 29:774, 1989.

19. Masse M, Andreu G, Angue M, et al. A multicenter study on the efficiency of white cell reduction by filtration of red cells. Transfusion 31:792, 1991.

20. Masse M, Neagelen C, Pellegrini N, et al. Validation of a simple method to count very low white cell concentrations in filtered red blood cells or platelets. Transfusion 32:565, 1992.

21. Al EJM, Visser SCE, Prins HK, et al. A flow cytometric method for determination

by the hemocytometer. Am J Physiol 128:309, 1940.

of white cell subpopulations in filtered red cells. Transfusion 31:835, 1991.

22. Bodensteiner BC. A flow cytometric technique to accurately measure post-filtration white blood cell counts. Transfusion 29:651, 1989.

23. Dzik WH, Ragosta A, Cusack WF. Flowcytometric method for counting very low numbers of leukocytes in platelet products. Vox Sang 59:153, 1990.

24. Wenz B, Burns ER, Lee V, Miller WK. A rare event analysis model for quantifying white cells in white cell-depleted blood. Transfusion 31:156, 1991.

25. Brecher ME, Harbaugh CA, Pineda AA. Accurate counting of low numbers of leukocytes. Am J Clin Pathol 97:872, 1992.

26. Lambrey Y, Creuzenet C, Bougy F, et al. Description et validation d'une méthode cytofluorimétrique d'estimation des leucocytes résiduels dans les concentrés globulaires deleucocytés. Rev Fr Transfus Hémobiol 36:375, 1993.

27. Vos JJE, Schoen C, Prins HK, et al. Use of radioimmunoassay detecting the platelet glycoprotein IIb-IIIa complex. Vox Sang 53:23, 1987.

28. Wester MR, Prins HK, Huisman JG. A new radioimmunoassay for the detection of small amounts of white cells and platelets in red cell concentrates: implications for blood transfusion. Transfusion 30:117, 1990.

29. Rawal BD, Schwadron R, Busch MP, et al. Evaluation of leukocyte removal filters modelled by use of HIV-infected cells and DNA amplification. Blood 76:2159, 1990.

30. Sivakumaran M, Norfolk DR, Major KE, et al. A new method to study the efficiency of third generation blood filters. Br J Haematol 84:175, 1993.

31. Sadoff BJ, Dooley DC, Kapoor V, et al. Methods for measuring a 6 log10 white cell depletion in red cells. Transfusion 31:150, 1991.

32. Boyum A, Lovhaug D, Tresland L, et al. Separation of leucocytes: improved cell purity by fine adjustments of gradient medium density and osmolality. Scand J Immunol 34:697, 1991.

33. Rebulla P, Porretti L, Bertolini F, et al.

White cell-reduced red cells prepared by filtration: a critical evaluation of current filters and methods for counting residual white cells. Transfusion 33:128, 1993.

34. Rebulla P, Dzik WH for the BEST Working Party of the International Society of Blood Transfusion. A multicenter evaluation of methods for counting residual white cells in leukocyte-depleted red blood cells. Vox Sanguinis 66:25, 1994.

35. Dzik WK. White cell-reduced blood components: should we go with the flow? Transfusion 31:789, 1991.

36. Schmid I, Krall WJ, Uittenbogaart CH, et al. Dead cell discrimination with 7-aminoactinomycic D in combination with dual color immunofluorescence in single laser flow cytometry. Cytometry 13:204, 1992.

37. Gross HJ, Verwer B, Houck D, et al. Detection of rare cells at a frequency of one per million by flow cytometry. Cytometry 14:519, 1993.

38. Schweppe F, Hausmann M, Hexel K, et al. An adapter for defined sample volumes makes it possible to count absolute particle numbers in flow cytometry. Anal Cell Pathol 4:325, 1992.

39. Taswell C. Limiting dilution assays for the determination of immunocompetent cell frequencies. I. Data analysis. J Immunol 126:1614, 1981.

40. Leftkovits I, Waldmann H. Limiting dilution analysis of the cells of immune system. I. The clonal basis of the immune response. Immunol Today 5:265, 1984.

41. Prati D, Rawal BD, Dang C, et al. DNA enzyme immunoassay using PCR-amplified HLA-DQ alpha gene applied to evaluate high efficiency leukocyte removal filters. Submitted for publication.

42. Gilbert GL, Hayes K, Hudson IL, et al. Prevention of transfusion-acquired cytomegalovirus infection in infants by blood filtration to remove leucocytes. Lancet 1:1228, 1989.

43. Bowden RA, Slichter SJ, Sayers MH, et al. Use of leukocyte-depleted platelets and cytomegalovirus-seronegative red blood cells for prevention of primary cytomegalovirus infection after marrow transplant. Blood 78:246, 1991.

44. Eisenfeld L, Silver H, McLaughlin J, et al. Prevention of transfusion-associated cytomegalovirus infection in neonatal patients by the removal of white cells from blood. Transfusion 32:205, 1992.

45. Perkins HA. Is white cell reduction cost-effective? Transfusion 33:626, 1993.

46. Vakkila J, Myllylä C. Amount and type of leukocytes in 'leukocyte-free' red cells and platelet concentrates. Vox Sang 53:76, 1987.

47. Wenz B, Burns ER. Phenotypic characterization of WBC in white cell-reduced red cell concentrate using flow cytometry. Transfusion 31:829, 1991.

48. Freedman J, Blanchette V, Hornstein A, et al. White cell depletion of red cell and pooled random-donor platelet concentrates by filtration and residual lymphocyte subset analysis. Transfusion 31:433, 1991.

49. Wenz B, Apuzzo JH, Ahuja KK. The preparation of leukocyte-poor red cells from liquid stored blood: an evaluation of the Haemonetics 102 cell washing system. Transfusion 20:306-310, 1980.

50. Valeri CR, Valeri DA, Anastasi J, Vecchione JJ, Dennis RC, Emerson CPO. Freezing in the primary polyvinylchloride plastic collection bag: a new system for preparing and freezing nonrejuvenated and rejuvenated red blood cells. Transfusion 21:138-149, 1981.

51. Champion AB, Carmen RA. Factors affecting white cell content in platelet concentrates. Transfusion 25:334-338, 1985.

52. Bertolini F, Rebulla P, Riccardi D, Cortellaro M, Ranzi ML, Sirchia G. Evaluation of platelet concentrates prepared from buffy coats and stored in a glucose-free crystalloid medium. Transfusion 29:6105-609, 1989.

53. Schiffer CA, Dutcher JP, Aisner J, Hogge D, Wiernik PH, Reilly JP. A randomized trial of leukocyte-depleted platelet transfusion to modify alloimmunization in patients with leukemia. Blood 62:815-820, 1983.

CHAPTER 4

Mechanisms of Leukodepletion by Filtration

Ingeborg Steneker, Ruby N.I. Pietersz, Henk W. Reesink

SUMMARY

Filtration of cellular blood products is the most effective method for removing leukocytes from cellular blood products. Although filtration of blood has been available for many decades, the recent development of filters capable of achieving a 3-4 log reduction in white cell content has stimulated interest in the use of these filters to prevent adverse effects such as HLA sensitization and CMV transfusion.

Blood filters are classified as screen or depth filters, and may be composed of synthetic material such as nylon or polyester or natural material such as cellulose acetate or cotton wool. Screen filters remove particles (cells) based on size; depth filters remove particles by mechanical sieving or cell adhesion.

Most of the high efficiency filters are depth filters composed of layers of synthetic fibers, surface coated with organic material(s). The filtration mechanism in such filters may depend on: (1) filter type, packing of fibers, fiber surface chemistry; (2) the physical properties of the blood cells such as deformability and surface expression of adhesive protein receptors; (3) the liquid suspension (plasma colloid or crystalloid and equavalent ionic content) in which the cells are suspended and (4) temperature and flow rate of the filtration process.

In general, granulocytes are largely entrapped by surface adhesion in the upper filter layers and mononuclear cells by mechanical seizing in the lower layers. The existence of so many variables which may influence the outcome of the filtration process indicate that quality control of this process under uncontrolled conditions (bedside) will never be satisfactory.

Clinical Benefits of Leukodepleted Blood Products, edited by Joseph Sweeney, M.D. and Andrew Heaton, M.D. © 1995 R.G. Landes Company.

INTRODUCTION

The growing knowledge of transfusion medicine has caused an increasing interest in the possibilities of separating blood into its pure components. Blood is composed of plasma containing factors such as the coagulation and fibrinolytic proteins, red blood cells, leukocytes and platelets. To separate blood components differential centrifugation, sedimentation, washing, freezing and thawing and filtration have all been evaluated.[1-5] The application of filtration is attractive because it is relatively easy to perform under sterile conditions. Not only plasma but cellular components can be separated from the cells and purified from each other.

For decades, it has been required practice to transfuse blood using on line filters with a pore size of 170-265 µm in order to prevent clots and debris from entering the blood circulation of the recipient. More recently, filters with pores of 40 µm were introduced to prevent respiratory complications after (massive) transfusions of whole blood.[6] It was suggested that disintegrating leukocytes, together with platelets, fibrin and red cells formed microaggregates in stored blood. After transfusion the microaggregates obstruct pulmonary capillaries and thus induce respiratory distress.[6]

The adverse effects of leukocytes in blood components, such as febrile transfusion reactions,[7] HLA-immunization[8-9] and transmission of various viruses[10-14] have prompted investigators to evaluate selective removal of leukocytes from cellular blood components, i.e., red cell concentrates (RCC) and platelet concentrates (PC).

As early as 1928 Fleming[15] used cotton wool to remove leukocytes from small quantities of blood, this method however, was only applicable in the laboratory. In 1962 Greenwalt et al[16] showed the importance of fibers type in removing granulocytes from heparinized blood. The best results were obtained by filtration with nylon fibers.[16] Diepenhorst et al[17] in 1972 introduced the first commercially available filter to remove leukocytes from RCC. This filter consisted of a column filled with cotton wool skeins, tightly packed and sterilized. Since that time, various types of leukocyte depletion filters have been developed, differing in housing size, density of packing, fiber type and in the electrostatic charge due to chemical properties of the fiber surface.[18] It was clear that different filters were necessary to remove leukocytes from RCC or from PC. In order to understand the background leading to development of the different types of filter this chapter will describe some of the mechanisms of filtration and the possible implications for developing new filters for removal of leukocytes from blood products.

FILTRATION PROCESSES

Two filtration processes are clearly described: surface, or screen, filtration and depth filtration. The mechanism of screen- or depth filtration differ significantly.[19]

SCREEN FILTRATION

Screen filtration is a process in which separation of particles from a solution is restricted to the filter surface. Complete separation of particles will be obtained when the particles are larger than the pores in the filter membrane. The large particles cannot pass the filter surface and the solution will flow through it. However, the concentration of the particles should be low, otherwise the filter will rapidly clog. In some occasions the filtered particles form a porous layer (a gel or a "cake") on the surface of the filter. As long as the flow through the "cake" is possible, the layer itself will contribute to the retention of more particles (cake filtration). Screen or surface filters consist of membranes of solid surface interchanged with (usually equal sized) pores.

Membrane filters can be divided into membranes for: (1) hyperfiltration, for retarding small molecules of less than 0.001 µm; (2) ultrafiltration for macromolecules and viruses of 0.01-0.5 µm, (3) microfiltration for colloidal or cellular particles of 0.1-10 µm and (4) macrofiltration for particles of 5 µm and greater. The 170 µm transfusion set filters and

40 μm microaggregate filters are screen or surface filters.

DEPTH FILTRATION

In depth filtration the retention of particles is not restricted to the filter surface. Depth filters usually consist of tightly packed granular or fibrous material.[19] The porous structure which contains a wide distribution of pore sizes throughout the filter matrix, allows the retention of particles at any place inside the filter. Particles can be entrapped by mechanical sieving or by adhesion.

Mechanical entrapment can occur by various mechanisms: (a) a single particle can be blocked inside a pore; (b) two or more particles (aggregates) can be entrapped by bridging when the particles simultaneously reach a pore or (c) a particle can be intercepted in dead ends of the filter fibers.

Adhesion of the particles to the filter fibers can be induced by: (a) the adhering capacity of the particles (cells), (b) mechanical forces such as flow or gravity pushing particles firmly against fibers to which they then adhere or (c) different surface charges attracting particles towards the fibers.

During mechanical sieving and adhesion particles can be entrapped transiently or permanently.[20] If the entrapment or the adhesion is transient, particles might detach and nevertheless pass the filter. Depending on the particle size, type and concentration, flow through the filter, gravity and type of fibers the above mechanisms play a role in depth filtration.

Because of the different sizes and properties of the various blood cells, depth filtration is favored in separating blood cells from each other, whereas for the separation of blood cells from plasma, screen filtration can be used.

FACTORS INFLUENCING BLOOD CELL FILTRATION BY DEPTH FILTERS

The depletion of leukocytes from blood components by depth filtration may depend on: (1) the type of fibers (surface hydrophilicity, surface charge and surface chemistry),[21-22] (2) physical properties of blood cells,[23-26] (see Table 4.1), which could be influenced by cell-cell interactions,[27-29] temperature[24,30-31] and cell age,[6,32-33] (3) the composition of the blood components (plasma proteins,[34-36] divalent ions,[16,17,34] anticoagulant[16,17,35] and type of blood cells[37]) and (4) the filtration method (temperature,[38-40] flow and contact time[36,41]).

FIBER MATERIAL

The influence of the fiber material in leukocyte depletion by filtration depends

Table 4.1. Concentration and physical properties of blood cells

Blood cells	Conc 10⁹/l	SizeR(μm)[23]	Specific gravity g/ml[73]	Mass fg	Deform-ability*	Adhesion°
red cell	5000	2.7	1.090–1.110	96	+++	–
platelet	250	1.6	1.054–1.062	17	+/–	+++
monocyte	0.5	5.6	1.055–1.065	786	+/–	+
granulocyte	3.5	4.8	1.065–1.090	486	+	++
lymphocyte	1	3.8	1.060–1.072	246	+/–	+/–

* deformability = the ability of the blood cells to pass through 5 μm pores.[41]
° adhesion = the capacity of blood cells to adhere to "artificial" materials.

on the physico-chemical properties of the fibers; surface charge,[22] surface wettability,[22] surface chemistry[42] and surface free energy.[21] Most of the effects of the physico-chemical properties of fiber materials are described in biomaterial research. However, it is difficult to study the effect of one single parameter because all these factors are related.[43] For example, introduction of specific chemical groups at the surface does not only change the surface chemistry but may also influence the surface charge and wettability. Moreover, the physico-chemical properties of the fiber surface may readily alter during filtration by the adsorption of plasma proteins from the cell suspension medium. This may explain why the results of biomaterial studies not always agree.

Surface Charge

The deposition of cells to a surface depends on the presence and the height of an energy barrier induced by electrostatic interactions and London-van der Waals forces between the cells and the surface. The surface charge of leukocytes is usually negative because of anionic groups, particularly phosphate, sialic acid and carboxylic acid groups.[22,44] It is postulated that the chance for cells to adhere is smaller when the surface charge is more negative. However the adhesion of leukocytes is not necessarily inhibited by negatively charged surfaces because leukocytes may form pseudopods penetrating the double electrical layer of a negatively charged surface.[45] The pseudopods facilitate close approach and molecular contact.

Wettability

Surface wettability (hydrophilicity) is important for the optimal contact between blood cells and fibers and the adhesion of blood cells onto the fibers. Optimal contact between fibers and blood cells is physically only possible when all fibers in the filter bed are surrounded by the medium in which the cells are suspended. To improve contact, non-wettable (hydrophobic) fibers may be primed with the medium in which the blood cells are resuspended (e.g.

additive solution). Moreover, priming of the filters removes air and decomposition products or possible contaminants from the filter bed. Removing air from the filter bed is important, because air-blood interfaces promote foaming and may have a denaturating effect on proteins and cell membranes. Furthermore, air pockets in the filterbed may induce an uneven distribution of the blood flow through the filter, which will result in a lower leukocyte depletion capacity of the filter for, in particular, the first 100 ml of blood. Coating or chemical treatment of the fibers will increase the wettability of the fibers and allow self-priming of the filters with blood components.

It is a widely accepted concept that hydrophilic surfaces allow better adhesion of leukocytes compared to non-wettable (hydrophobic) surfaces.[22,46] However, several authors have shown that leukocytes also adhere onto hydrophobic surfaces.[42,47]

FIBER MATERIAL IN ROUTINE APPLICATIONS

Nylon Wool Filter

Greenwalt et al[16] used a column filter filled with nylon wool soaked in saline. With these commercially available nylon fibers, leukocytes were only partially removed from heparinized blood. Following removal of the coating of these nylon fibers it was observed that 100% granulocytes and about 45% of the platelets were removed from 1-2 hours old heparinized blood. Removal of leukocytes was impaired when the temperature at filtration was decreased to 4°C, the blood was older than 2 hours or when citrated blood was used. It was concluded that filtration of blood cells on nylon wool was temperature, age and Ca^{2+} and Mg^{2+} dependent.

Cotton Wool filter

Cotton wool tightly packed into a column as described by Diepenhorst et al[17] removed leukocytes from blood collected in either citrate or EDTA, but using heparinized blood leukocytes were not retained.

Moreover, in citrated blood granulocytes were more efficiently removed than were lymphocytes. They concluded that filtration on cotton wool was not Ca^{2+} or Mg^{2+} dependent but were in agreement with Greenwalt et al[16] that filtration was hematocrit and temperature dependent.

Cellulose Acetate Filter

Cellulose acetate column filters consist of a polycarbonate housing with three, tightly packed, identical skeins of cellulose acetate fibers, providing a network with equally distributed pores (Fig. 4.1). The fiber diameter is 17 µm. Cellulose acetate fibers showed a better filtration result than expected on basis of the fiber diameter.[48] This finding suggests that cellulose acetate fibers capture leukocytes both by mechanical entrapment and adhesion. Steneker at al[49] showed that indeed granulocytes were most prominently captured by direct adhesion and cell-cell interactions in the top (inlet) part of the filter, whereas lymphocytes were captured by mechanical sieving in the middle and bottom (outlet) part of the filter.

Polyester Filter

Synthetic fibers such as polyester, polyethylene, polypropylene, polymethacrylate, polysterene or polyfluoroethylene are most suitable for the preparation of micro-fibers with a diameter of 0.3 µm to 3 µm. Nonwoven fabrics of micro-fibers may be prepared by melt-blown, spin bound or wet and dry layed techniques. In addition heat compression or point-melting may be used to increase the fiber packing. The wettability of the fibers is in part defined by surface charges and may be increased by chemical treatment or ionization.

In the past decade various so called flat bed filters (because of the flat housing) consisting of non-woven synthetic fabric have become available.[18] These filters usually consist of various layers of fibers which can roughly be divided in a pre-filter and a main-filter (Fig. 4.2). The pre-filter is usually composed of layers with fibers of 3 to 100 µm and a distance between adjacent fibers of 7 to 300 µm. This pre-filter with "coarse" fibers is intended for removal of storage-generated microaggregates. The thickness of a pre-filter can vary from 0.1 to 3 mm. The main-filter is composed of layers of "middle coarse" to "fine" fibers. The number of these layers may vary, depending on the brand of filter.

Non-woven fabrics with fibers of 0.3 µm and a distance of 0.5 µm between the fibers have a low mechanical strength and are vulnerable. As a result of damage blood cells may be injured or activated. Moreover, pores of less than 0.5 µm are too small for red cells to pass through and the filter will clog. Homogeneous nonwoven fabric with fibers of 3 µm and a distance between the fibers of more than 7 µm will have strong fibers and pores that are large enough for red cells to pass but which may be too large to capture leukocytes.

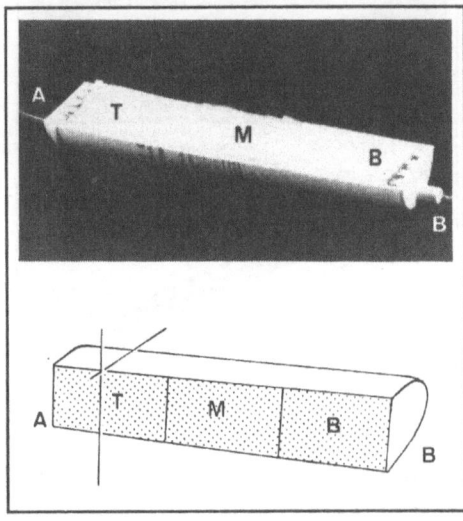

Fig 4.1. Photograph and schematic reproduction of a column filter. This filter consists of a tube with a length of 18 cm and an outer diameter of 5 cm at the top and 4 cm at the bottom. The polycarbonate tube is tightly filled with three identical skeins of cellulose-acetate fibers, providing a network with equally distributed pores. The fiber diameter is 17 µm. Each cellulose acetate skein has a length of 6 cm and a weight of about 18.5 gram. The total volume is about 150 ml. A = inlet; B = outlet; T = top; M = middle; Bo = bottom.

Therefore, in general, the non-woven layers of the main-filter in leukocyte depletion filters are composed of micro-fibers with a diameter of 1 to 5 μm and a distance between them of 3 to 15 μm.[18] The 'coarse' pre-filter is usually followed by a number of layers with "middle coarse" fibers and pores of 10 to 70 μm and then by several layers with 'fine' fibers and pores of 3 to 15 μm. The packing of the layers upon each other may also vary.

Summarizing flat bed filters differ in fiber material, number of "coarse" pre-filter layers, number of main-filter layers both "middle coarse" and "fine'" thickness of fibers, distance between adjacent fibers (i.e.

pores), thickness of the filter bed and available surface area. Moreover, the method of packing the layers and the insertion inside the housing may vary because the flow of the filtered material should be directed first through the pre-filter and subsequently through the main filter. Steneker et al[37,50,51] concluded that filtration of RCC on polyester filters depends on cell-cell interactions, adhesion and mechanical entrapment.

Polyurethane (PU) Membrane Filter

Preparation of membranes of porous material offer the possibility to adjust the pore size distribution, pore morphology, interconnectivity of the pores and porosity of the membranes.[52] Polyurethane polymers are well established in biomaterial research and have recently been investigated for preparation of leukocyte depletion filters.[52,53] However, the filters clogged very quickly due to red cells, although the leukocytes were adequately removed.[52] For the future this technique seems to be promising and needs further investigation.

FUNCTIONAL AND PHYSICAL PROPERTIES OF BLOOD CELLS

Based on the functional and physical properties of blood cells (Table 4.1) it could be expected that the retention of platelets and granulocytes in a filter differ from the retention of lymphocytes. This was confirmed by Steneker et al,[49-51] who showed that the depletion of leukocytes from fresh (16-24 hours old) RCC by filtration occurred by three mechanisms: (1) mechanical sieving, (2) direct adhesion and (3) cell-cell interactions. Platelets and granulocytes were mainly captured by direct adhesion or cell-cell interactions, whereas lymphocytes were prominently captured by mechanical sieving.[51]

Mechanical Sieving

The exact role of cell sieving in cell filtration processes is yet not known. In red cell filters, lymphocytes and a part of the granulocytes and monocytes were detected in small pores without cell-fiber contact.[37,49-51] These findings indicate that

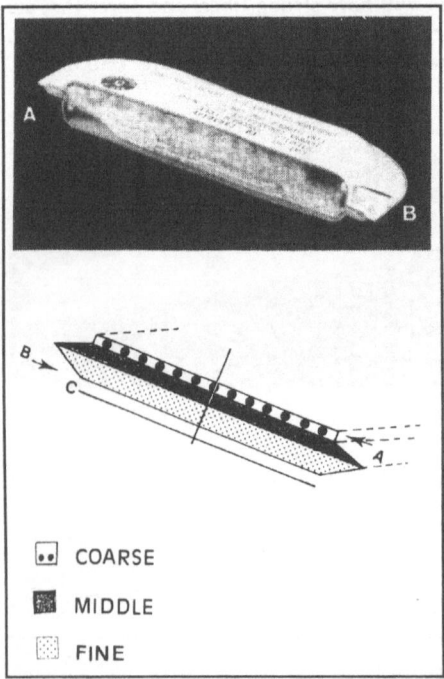

COARSE

MIDDLE

FINE

Fig 4.2. Photograph and schematic reproduction of a flat-bed filter. This filter consists of a flat PVC container of 1x13x8 cm. The filter is filled with 17 non-woven filter layers of polyethylene-terephthalate fibers. The first layer is a coarse layer with a pore size of 40-100 μm. The next 6 layers are medium coarse layers with a pore size of 10-70 μm. The remaining 10 layers contain fine fibers which provide a network with a pore size of 3-15 μm. The total volume is about 60 ml. A = inlet; B = outlet.

mechanical sieving of leukocytes occurred during filtration (Fig. 4.3A). Based on the deformability and adhesive capacity of granulocytes (Table 4.1) it is not expected that the cells would be trapped by cell sieving. Yet, it was found that a small number of granulocytes, due to cell swelling and morphologic alterations (Fig. 4.3D), was captured by this mechanism.[49-51] When red cells have their biconcave shape they can easily pass small pores.[41] However, histological examination of leukocyte depletion filters[50] revealed that a small part of the red cells, mostly spheroechinocytes, were also captured by mechanical sieving, which indicates that these red cells had lost their deformability probably due to aging.[32]

Direct Adhesion

The interaction of blood cells with artificial materials depends on the surface characteristics of these materials. In the previously mentioned filtration experiments,[49-51] leukocytes showed close contact with the fibers grading from contact through small pseudopods up to surrounding of the fibers with large pseudopods (Fig. 4.3C). These findings suggest that leukocytes adhered to the fibers by transient and by long lasting adhesion. In transient adhesion most cells will be round with small pseudopods and thus vulnerable for detachment. In long lasting adhesion the cells are flat, surrounding the fibers, which increases the adhesion tremendously.[20] A large proportion of the granulocytes as well as a small proportion of the monocytes in the small pores of a cellulose-acetate column filter as well as in flat bed polyester filters were captured by direct adhesion to the fibers.[51] Especially granulocytes directly adhered to the fibers showed morphologic features of activation, indicating that activation is needed for adhesion. The direct adhesion of granulocytes may be complement-mediated or adhesive protein-mediated.[54] Two observations suggest that direct adhesion of granulocytes during filtration is most likely complement-mediated. Firstly, a prelimi-

nary study showed that granulocytes, which were incubated with a monoclonal antibody (CD18) against the β-chain of the CR3 heterodimer (complement receptor 3), hardly adhered to the polyester fibers [personal observation]. The CR3 heterodimer

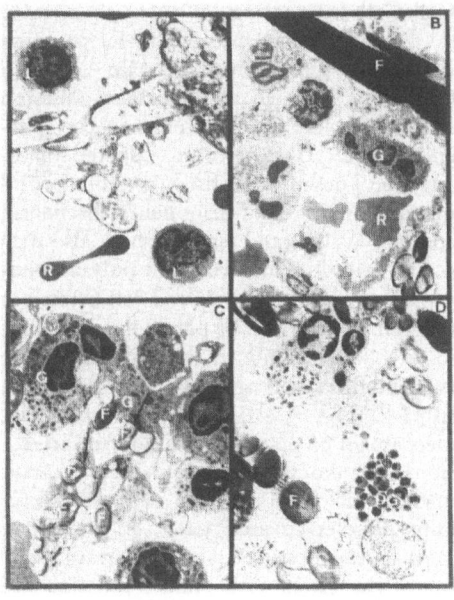

Fig. 4.3. TEM photomicrographs showing interactions between blood cells and fibers. A: Fibers in cross section (F) covered with platelets. Single non-activated lymfocytes (L) and red cells (R) were found in the pores (mechanical sieving). Magnification x 4700. B: Fiber (F) covered with platelets (P) in interaction with granulocytes (G) (indirect adhesion). Red cells (R) were found in the pores. Magnification x 4700. C: Fibers (F) surrounded (arrow) by granulocytes (G). (direct adhesion). Magnification x 7150. D: Fibers in cross section (F) covered with platelets (P). A disintegrated granulocyte (DG) was found in the pores (mechanical sieving). Magnification x 7150.

has been found to be the main molecule mediating both adherence and aggregation of granulocytes.[55] Secondly, artificial devices made of cellulose acetate are known to cause complement activation and subsequent granulocyte adhesion and aggregation.[54]

Cell-Cell Interactions

Activated and spread platelets have an increased expression of the selectin GMP-140,[28] which may mediate adhesion of granulocytes onto platelets in the presence of Ca^{2+}. Furthermore, adhered platelets are known to release granule-bound materials such as fibrinogen, fibronectin and von Willebrand factor, which also may act as bridging molecules to polymorphonuclear granulocytes.[56] In red cell filtrations cell-cell interactions of platelets and granulocytes were found in a cellulose acetate column filter and three polyester flat bed filters[37] (Fig. 4.3B). Although the exact mechanism of platelet-granulocyte interactions in leukocyte depletion filters remains unclear, efficient adhesion of granulocytes onto platelet-covered parts of the filters most likely occurred subsequent to coating of the fibers with plasma proteins and adherence and spreading of platelets.[56] This suggestion is in accordance with the results of Wester et al,[57] who showed that granulocytes and platelets can be found especially in the first 100 ml fraction of red cell filtrates from a cellulose acetate column filter.

Influence of Cell Age and Storage History

The functional and physical properties of blood cells will change during storage conditions.[24,31-33]

Granulocytes examined after 24 hour storage under blood bank conditions already show signs of dysfunction, with profound alterations of their bactericidal activity, chemotaxis, aggregation and superoxide production.[58-59] Moreover, transfused granulocytes stored at 4°C for 8 hours fail to migrate appropriately into skin windows of normal volunteers.[60] Furthermore, the deformability of granulocytes will decrease during storage at 4°C and after approximately 24 hour disintegration starts.[6] Thus, one may conclude that the direct adhesion capacity of granulocytes will decrease[30] and the mechanical entrapment will increase if RCC stored at 4°C will be filtered. Bodensteiner,[61] using polyester flatbed filters, indeed showed that depletion of leukocytes from RCC stored for at least 29 days at 4°C was less efficient compared to pre-storage leukocyte depletion.

Lymphocytes survive well during storage at 4°C. The changes in cell morphology and deformability are less outspoken than those of granulocytes. Storage at 4°C will probably not influence the filtration mechanisms of lymphocytes.

Non-deformable red cells may also influence filter efficiency. Red cell deformability depends on the morphology and temperature. The red cell morphology changes from discocytes to sphero-echinocytes during storage at 4°C.[32] The latter cells have protrusions and may have difficulties passing pores of less than 5 µm.[51] Preliminary experiments in our laboratory showed that storage of RCC at 4°C indeed influenced the red cell retention in the filters. The red cell recovery after filtration, including a rinsing step, dropped from 94% with fresh RCC to 84% with RCC stored for 21 days at 4°C [personal observation]. These captured red cells may compete with leukocytes, causing early saturation of the filters, which may be another explanation of the results found by Bodensteiner.[61] Furthermore, in RCC stored in the presence of leukocytes and platelets, microaggregate formation will occur.[6,62] These microaggregates may form a gel on the filter surface, clog the filter and/or compete with leukocytes.

Platelets will easily adhere to fibers, especially when activated. The activation of platelets may be induced by the preparation method, increases during storage at 22°C and is highly affected by decrease of temperature below 18°C. PC prepared by the platelet-rich plasma (PRP) method showed the first 2 days of storage a higher expression for GP IIb/IIIa complex and a more spheric morphology compared to platelets prepared by the buffy coat method.[63] Moreover, lactate production, LDH leakage and beta-tromboglobuline release were higher in PRP derived PC, indicating activation.[63] During prolonged storage up to 5 days the differences between PRP and buffy coat derived PC disappeared.[63] Based on these findings it could be expected that filtration of fresh PRP will induce a high platelet loss in the filters and a good leukocyte removal, whereas filtration of 5-day-old PRP will have a better platelet yield but is less efficient regarding leukocyte removal.[64]

COMPOSITION OF THE BLOOD COMPONENT

Plasma Proteins

Before blood cells can adhere to the fiber surface adsorption of plasma protein occurs when the filter materials are exposed to blood. Thus, leukocyte adhesion onto fiber surfaces will be largely influenced by preadsorped proteins of the blood components.[20,65-67] During the filtration there will be a gradual displacement of plasma proteins at the surface, known as the Vroman effect.[68] This will occur in the following sequence: albumin, immunoglobin G, fibrinogen, fibronectin, high molecular weight kininogen and factor XII.[68] Albumin is known to reduce the adhesiveness of leukocytes,[20,65] whereas globulins,[66] fibronectin,[67] C1 complex or properdin[35] seem to increase the adhesion of platelets and leukocytes. The rate and amount of protein adsorption is dependent on the physico-chemical properties of the fiber material.[69]

Resuspension of RCC in saline-adenine-glucose-mannitol (SAGM) influenced the trapping pattern of red cells. Steneker et al[37] showed that about 6% of the red cells of RCC resuspended in SAGM were found between the fibers of polyester flat-bed filters as clusters of pseudo-agglutinated cells compared to 3% of captured red cells from RCC suspended in plasma. Loss

of deformability of the red cells or a change in zeta-potential due to the replacement of plasma by a crystalloid solution may be the cause.

Recently, Szuflad and Dzik,[70] using a polyester flat bed filter for PC showed that the retention of granulocytes suspended in PRP differed from granulocytes suspended in a crystalloid solution.

The Effect of Anticoagulants

The effect of anticoagulant is, except for heparin, primarily due to the reduction of the concentration of divalent ions. Divalent ions, Ca^{2+} and Mg^{2+} in particular, are known to promote leukocyte adhesion.[20,35] In the complete absence of divalent ions the adhesion of granulocytes onto glass slides is markedly reduced.[20] The addition of Ca^{2+} alone did not restore basal levels of granulocyte adhesion, whereas addition of Mg^{2+} alone restored almost completely normal adhesiveness. In citrate-anticoagulated blood the concentration of Ca^{2+} and Mg^{2+} is still high enough to permit leukocyte adhesion in vitro, whereas EDTA-anticoagulated blood inhibits leukocyte adhesion.[35]

The Effect of the Cellular Composition of RCC

The significance of leukocyte-platelet interaction on the efficiency of leukocyte depletion from RCC by filtration has as yet had little attention. However, nowadays there is increasing demand for PC, which are prepared from whole blood prior to filtration, thus leaving RCC depleted of platelets. Moreover, the number of leukocytes and platelets in RCC will depend on the preparation method of PC.[37] Steneker et al[37] showed that platelet depletion of RCC prior to filtration did not change the capture of lymphocytes and monocytes in the filters. In contrast, the granulocyte depletion clearly depended on the platelet content in the RCC. Indeed a positive correlation between leukocyte depletion capacity of the filters and the platelet count in the RCC prior to filtration was found.[37] This phenomenon was due to a diminished capacity of the filters for granulocyte depletion. These results were confirmed by Pietersz et al.[71]

Since the above results were found with filters designed for leukocyte depletion from RCC, the influence of red cells must be considered. There is evidence that red cells transport platelets and leukocytes towards a surface (vessel wall) and that this is dependent on the local shear rate.[72] This is the so called margination effect.

The Effect of the Cellular Composition of PC

The composition of PC differs from RCC, i.e., platelets and leukocytes are suspended in either plasma or a crystalloid platelet storage medium. Moreover, the method of preparation, PRP, buffycoat or apheresis, may also influence the composition of PC, i.e., activation of platelets and the leukocyte differentiation. These variables are difficult to standardize in routine processing. Also, the effect of the cellular composition of PC on the leukocyte depletion mechanisms is yet not systematically studied.

Extrapolating the mechanisms found with RCC filtration, it may be postulated that lymphocytes will be captured by cell sieving in the smaller pores of the filter, independent of the composition of the PC. An increased filter length (inlet to outlet) may increase filter efficiency.

In red cell filters, granulocytes were most prominently captured by direct adhesion (Fig. 4.3C) onto the fibers and cell-cell interactions (Fig. 4.3B).[50] Direct adhesion of granulocytes will be increased by the margination effect of red cells and the attraction by the fiber material. Because red cells are absent in PC filtration, only the fiber material will play a role. Direct adhesion will be best when granulocytes are less than 24 hour old and in the presence of plasma.[70] The method of PC preparation will decide the loss of (activated) platelets in the filters.[63] In PC older than 24 hours, granulocytes will also be removed by sieving but detachment and fragmentation may occur. Indirect adhesion of granu-

locytes onto the fibers (Fig. 4.3B) is based on platelet-granulocyte interactions and platelet activation. Both events will variably occur but cause platelet loss in the filter. To prevent platelet loss, platelet activation by the method of preparation and by the fiber material should be avoided.

FILTRATION METHOD

Temperature

Leukocyte depletion from RCC by filtration requires a sufficient deformability of red cells[24] and an optimal adhesive capacity of leukocytes and platelets.[37] Based on the literature, it was expected that a temperature of 20°C would favor both features.

With regard to leukocyte depletion filters for RCC, there are only a few publications concerning the optimal temperature of filtration. Davey et al[39] concluded that the most efficient method of leukocyte removal with an integral in-line filter (cellulose acetate) was a hard spin followed by room temperature filtration. The same results were reported for column filters filled with cotton-wool[17] and cellulose acetate fibers.[48] In contrast, Beaujean et al[38] concluded that leukocyte removal of 2-10-days-old platelet poor RCC by a polyester flat-bed filter was better at 7-10°C compared to 24-28°C. Preliminary results obtained with cellulose acetate filters and polyester filters partly confirmed above results [personal observation]. Cellulose acetate column filters loaded with fresh RCC, either stored at 20°C or at 4°C, showed no difference in leukocyte depletion capacity (the number of leukocytes in the RCC applied to the filter which resulted in a residual leukocyte amount of 5.0 x 10^6).[37] In contrast, the leukocyte depletion capacity of polyester filters was higher for RCC stored at 4°C compared to those stored at 20°C [personal observation].

Filtration of PC will be performed at ambient temperature, i.e., the storage temperature of PC, promoting direct adhesion of granulocytes.

Flow and Contact Time

The adhesion of leukocytes onto fibers is a process which requires sufficient contact time. A flow rate of more than 100 ml per min may prevent adherence and, in addition, may induce disruption of blood cells. Olijslager et al[48] showed that the flow rate was inversely correlated with the hematocrit of the blood component being applied to the filter. A longer filtration time may increase the risk of leakage of cell remnants or intact leukocytes from the filter because the strength of adherence declines over the incubation period.[36] It would be of interest to examine the cell morphology in relation to contact time inside the filter.

To provide optimal leukocyte depletion from blood components by filtration, the flow rate should be sufficiently low to allow contact between leukocytes and fibers. On the other hand, the flow rate should be high enough to prevent detachment of leukocytes and allowing unacceptable duration of the filtration for routine use in blood banks. Rinsing the filters after filtration of RCC at high speed may also induce detachment of leukocytes. Especially for the filtration of PC, the flow rate should be adjusted to the type of filter to allow appropriate removal of leukocytes.

CONCLUSION

1. Routine leukocyte depletion by filtration is the result of several processes, i.e. adhesion, mechanical sieving and cell-cell interactions.
2. The composition of blood components and the physical as well as functional properties of blood cells will affect the filtration process.
3. These properties are highly dependent on changes exerted on the blood cells during collection of the blood and processing and storage of blood components; therefore, optimal leukocyte depletion by filtration can only be obtained after standardization of these conditions and of the filtration procedure itself.
4. Since satisfactorily filtered blood products depend on the use of standardized and controlled techniques, optimal leukocyte depletion by filtration will never be achieved under routine hospital bed-side conditions.

REFERENCES

1. Svedberg T, Rinde H. The determination of the distribution of size of particles in disperse systems. J Am Chem Soc 46:2677, 1923.
2. Meryman HT, Hornblower M. Red cell recovery and leukocyte depletion following washing of frozen-thawed red cells. Transfusion 13:388, 1973.
3. Crowley JP, Wade PH, Wish C, et al. The purification of red cells for transfusion by freeze-preservation and washing. V. Red cell recovery and residual leukocytes after freeze-preservation with high concentrations of glycerol and washing in various systems. Transfusion 17:1, 1977.
4. Goldfinger D, Lowe C. Prevention of adverse reactions to blood transfusion by the administration of saline-washed red blood cells. Transfusion 21:277, 1981.
5. Meryman HT, Bross J, Lebovitz R. The preparation of leukocyte-poor red cells: a comparative study. Transfusion 20:285, 1980.
6. Swank RL. Alteration of blood on storage: measurement of adhesiveness of 'aging' platelets and leukocytes and their removal by filtration. New Engl J Med 265:728, 1961.
7. Perkins PA, Payne R, Ferguson J, et al. Nonhemolytic febrile transfusion reactions. Vox Sang 11:578, 1966.
8. Brand A, Claas FHJ, Voogt PJ, et al. Alloimmunization after leukocyte depleted multiple random platelet transfusions. Vox Sang 54:160, 1988.
9. Fisher M, Chapman JR, Ting A, et al. Alloimmunization to HLA antigens following transfusion with leukocyte-poor and purified platelet suspensions. Vox Sang 49:331, 1985.
10. Gilbert GL, Hayes K, Hudson IL, et al. Prevention of transfusion-acquired cytomegalovirus infection in infants by blood filtration to remove leukocytes. Lancet I:1228, 1989.

11. deGraan-Hentzen YCE, Gratma JW, Mudde GC, et al. Prevention of primary cytomegalovirus infection in patients with hematologic malignancies by intensive leukocyte depletion of blood products. Transfusion 29:757, 1989.

12. Okochi K, Sato H. Transmission of adult T-cell leukemia virus (HTLV-1) through blood transfusion and its prevention. AIDS Research 2:5157, 1986.

13. Rawal BD, Busch MP, Endow R, et al. Reduction of human immunodeficiency virus-infected cells from donor blood by leukocyte filtration. Transfusion 29:460, 1989.

14. Wagner SJ, Friedman LI, Dodd RY. Approaches to the reduction of viral infectivity in cellular blood components and single donor plasma. Transfusion Med Rev 1:18, 1991.

15. Fleming A. A simple method of removing leukocytes from blood. Br J Exp Path 7:281, 1928.

16. Greenwalt TJ, Gajewski M, McKenna JL. A new method for preparing buffy-coat poor blood. Transfusion 2:221, 1962.

17. Diepenhorst P, Sprokholt R, Prins HK. Removal of leukocytes from whole blood and erythrocytes suspensions by filtration through cotton-wool. I. Filtration technique. Vox Sang 23:308, 1972.

18. European patent application. Publication number: 0155003. Application number: 85102975:3, 1985.

19. Fiore JV, Olson WP, Holst SL. Depth filtration, in Methods of Plasma Fractionation, (ED. J.M. Curling), Academic Press, London, 239, 1980.

20. Forrester JV, Lackie JM. Adhesion of leukocytes under conditions of flow. J Cell Sci 70:93, 1984.

21. Absolom DR, Thomson C, Hawthorn, Zingg W, Neumann AW. Kinetics of cell adhesion to polymer surfaces. J Biomed Mater Res 22:215, 1988.

22. van Oss CJ, Gillman CF, Neumann AW. in: Phagocytic engulfment and cell adhesiveness as cellular surface phenomena. Dekker, New York, 1975.

23. Loos JA, Blok-Schut B, Kipp B, et al. Size distribution, electronic recognition and counting of human blood monocytes. Blood

48:473, 1976.

24. Williamson JR, Shanahan MO, Hodimuth RM. The influence of temperature on red cell deformability. Blood 46:611, 1975.

25. Milner GR, Fagence R, Darnborough J. Temperature dependence of leukocyte depletion of blood with an automatic blood cell processor. Transfusion 22:48, 1982.

26. Albelda SM, Buck CA. Integrins and other cell adhesion molecules. FASEB J 4:2868, 1990.

27. Jungi TW, Spycher MO, Nydegger UE. Platelet-leukocyte interactions: selective binding of thrombin stimulated platelets to monocytes, polymorphonuclear leukocytes and related cell lines. Blood 67:629, 1986.

28. Hamburger SA, McEver RP. GMP-140 mediates adhesion of stimulated platelets to neutrophils. Blood 75:550, 1990.

29. Yeo EL, Kennington J, Feurstein I. Role of PADGEM/GMP-140 in leukocyte adherent platelet interaction under flow conditions. Blood 78:278a, 1991.

30. Lederman DM, Cumming RD, Petschek HE, Levine PH, Krinsley NI. The effect of temperature on the interaction of platelets and leukocytes with materials exposed to flowing blood. Trans Am Soc Artif Intern Organs 24:557, 1978.

31. Manara FS, Schneider DL. The activation of the human neutrophil respiratory burst occurs only at temperatures above 17°C: evidence that activation requires membrane fusion. Biochem Biophys Res Comm 132:696, 1985.

32. Truter EJ, Murray PW le R. Morphological classification by scanning electron microscopy of erythrocytes stored at 4°C in citrate-phosphate-dextrose anticoagulant. Med Lab Sci 47:113, 1990.

33. Humbert JR, Fermin CD, Winsor EL. Early damage to granulocytes during storage. Sem Hematol 28:10, 1991.

34. Forrester JV, Lackie JM. Adhesion of neutrophils under conditions of flow. J Cell Sci 70:93, 1984.

35. Lang EY, Lang JH, Lasser EC. Adherence of granulocytes to nylon fibers. Evidence for a plasma granulocyte adherence factor. Tromb Res 50:243, 1988.

36. Unarska M, Robinson GB. Adherence of

human leukocytes to synthetic polymer surfaces. Life Support Systems 5:283, 1978.

37. Steneker I, Prins HK, Florie M, Loos JA, Biewenga J. Mechanisms of white cell reduction in red cell concentrates by filtration: the effect of the cellular composition of the red cell concentrates. Transfusion 33:42, 1993.

38. Beaujean F, Segier JM, le Forestier C, Duedari N. Leukocyte depletion of red cell concentrates by filtration: Influence of Blood product Temperature. Vox Sang 62:242, 1992.

39. Davey RJ, Carmen RA, Simon TL, et al. Preparation of white cell-depleted red cells for 42-day storage using a integral in-line filter. Transfusion 29:496, 1989.

40. Kikugawa K, Minishima K. Filter columns for preparation of leukocyte-poor blood for transfusion. Vox Sang 34:281, 1978.

41. Stuart J, Stone PCW, Bareford D, et al. Effect of pore diameter and cell volume on erythrocyte filterability. Clin. Hemorheol 5:449, 1985.

42. van Kampen CL. Effect of implant surface chemistry upon arterial thrombosis. J Biomed Mater 13:517, 1979.

43. Gingell D, Vince S. Long-range forces and adhesion: an analysis of cell-substratum studies. In Cell adhesion and motility (eds. Curtis ASG, Pitts JD), University Press, Cambridge 1, 1980.

44. Vassar PS, Hards JM, Seaman GVF. Surface properties of human lymphocytes. Biochem Biophys Acta 291:107, 1973.

45. Polliack A, Lampen N, Clarkson BD, et al. Identification of human B and T lymphocytes by scanning electron microscopy. J Exp Med 138:607, 1973.

46. Curtis ASG, Forrester C, McInnes C, Lawrie F. Adhesion of cells to polystyrene surfaces. J Cell Biol 97:1500, 1983.

47. Lim F, Cooper SL. The effect of surface hydrophilicity on biomaterial-leukocyte interactions. Asaio Transactions 37: M146-M147, 1991.

48. Olijslager J, Hennink WE, Prins HK. Leukocyten filter fase II: invloed van vezelmateriaal en vezel diameter. Instituten voor kunstoffen, rubber, verpakking en verf (TNO). 487:41, 1986.

49. Steneker I, Biewenga J. Histological and immunohistochemical studies on the preparation of leukocyte-poor red cell concentrates by filtration. The filtration process on cellulose acetate fibers. Vox Sang 58:192, 1990.

50. Steneker I, Biewenga J. Histological and immunohistochemical studies on the preparation of leukocyte-poor red cell concentrates by filtration. The filtration process using three different polyester filters. Transfusion 31:40, 1991.

51. Steneker I, Luyn MJA van, Wachem PB van, Biewenga J. Electronmicroscopic examination of white cell depletion on four white-cell reduction filters. Transfusion 32:450, 1992.

52. Bruil A, Aken WG van, Beugeling T, Feijen J, Steneker I, Huisman JG, Prins HK. Asymmetric membrane filters for the removal of leukocytes from blood. J Biomed Mat Res 25:1459, 1991.

53. Kora S, Kuroki H, Kido T, Katsurada N, Daso M. Mechanism of leukocyte removal by porous material. In: Clinical application of leukocyte depletion. Ed: Sekiguchi S. Blackwell Sci Pub 119, 1993.

54. Takemoto Y, Matsuda T, Kishimoto T, et al. Molecular understanding of cellular adhesion on artificial surfaces. Trans Am Soc Artif Intern Organs 35:354, 1989.

55. Kuypers TW, Koenderman L, Weening RS, et al. Continous cell activation is necessary for stable interaction of complement receptor 3 with its counter structure in the aggregation response of human neutrophils. Eur J Immunol 20:501, 1990.

56. Adams GA, Feuerstein IA. Kinetics of platelet adhesion and aggregation on protein coated surfaces: morphology and release of dense granules. Asaio J 4:90, 1981.

57. Wester MR, Prins HK, Huisman JG. A new radioimmuno assay for detection of small amounts of white cells and platelets in red cell concentrates: implications for blood transfusion. Transfusion 30:117, 1990.

58. Buesher ES, Gallin JI. Effects of storage and radiation on human neutrophil function in vitro. Inflammation 11:401, 1987.

59. Eastlund T, Charbonneau T, Britten A. Changes in neutrophil aggregation and

chemotaxis response during 18-hour cold storage. Transfusion 24:513, 1984.

60. McCullough J, Weiblen BJ, Fine D. Effects of storage of granulocytes on their fate in vivo. Transfusion 23:20, 1983.

61. Bodensteiner DC. Leukocyte depletion in older units of blood. Transfusion 31:18S, 1991.

62. Prins HK, de Bruijn JCGH, Henrichs HPJ, et al. Prevention of microaggregate formation by removal of "buffycoats". Vox Sang 39:48, 1980.

63. Fijnheer R, Pietersz RNI, de Korte D, Gouwerok CWN, Dekker WJA, Reesink HW, Roos D. Platelet activation during preparation of platelet concentrates: a comparison of the platetelet-rich plasma and the buffy coat methods. Transfusion 30:634, 1990.

64. Elias MK, Smit JW, Weggemans M, et al. In vitro evaluation of a high-efficiency leukocyte adherence filter. Ann Hematol 53, 1991.

65. Curtis ASG, Forrester JV. The competitive effects of serum proteins on cell adhesion. J Cell Sci 71:17, 1984.

66. Katoaka K, Maeda T, Nishimura T, et al. Estimation of cell adhesion on polymer surfaces with the use of the 'column-method'. J Biomed Mater Res 14:817, 1980.

67. Garcia-Pardo A, Ferreira OC. Adhesion of human T-lymphoid cells to fibronectin is mediated by two different fibronectin domains. Immunol 69:121, 1990.

68. Elwing H, Askendal A, Lundstrom I. Competition between adsorbed fibrinogen and high-molecular-weight kininogen on solid surfaces incubated in plasma (the Vroman effect): influence of solid surface wettability. J Biomed Mater Res 21:1023, 1987.

69. Absolom DR, Zingg W, Neumann AW. Protein adsorption to polymer particles: role of surface properties. J Biomed Mater Res 21:161, 1987.

70. Szuflad P, Dzik WH. Do platelet-WBC interactions promote wbc removal during filtration? Transfusion 33:S199, 1993.

71. Pietersz RNI, Steneker I, Reesink HW, et al. Comparison of five different filters for the removal of leukocytes from red cell concentrates. Vox Sang 62:76, 1992.

72. Mellema J, Blom C. Rheology, its basic concept. Tijdschrift NVKC 15:78, 1990.

73. Roos D, de Boer M. Purification and cryopreservation of phagocytes from human blood. Meth Enzymol 132:225, 1986.

CHAPTER 5

ROLE OF CONTAMINATING WHITE BLOOD CELLS IN THE STORAGE LESIONS OF RED CELLS AND PLATELETS

Joseph D. Sweeney, Stein Holme, Andrew Heaton

SUMMARY

Red cell concentrates prepared from whole blood donations without buffy coat removal contain the majority of the original white cells contained in the whole blood donation. These white cells are predominantly granulocytes. Granulocytes may be metabolically active and release oxidant radicals. They certainly degenerate rapidly on storage, releasing proteolytic enzymes. Such substances may damage the red cell membrane, resulting in accelerated glycolysis, possibly to supply ATP for the sodium/potassium pump, followed by in vitro hemolysis and diminished in vivo recovery or survival.

Early studies on buffy coat-depleted additive-suspended red cells showed less hemolysis after storage as compared to nonbuffy coat-depleted concentrates. Furthermore, studies on pre-storage filtration of red cells have consistently shown a favorable effect of early leukocyte removal on in vitro hemolysis and 24-hour recovery in red cell concentrates stored in PVC-DEHP containers, though this improvement was only significant with >4 $\log_{10}$ leukodepletion. Recent studies have also indicated that early removal of leukocytes from red cell concentrates stored in *non-DEHP* containers is also beneficial, though not enough to compensate for the lack of the protective effect of DEHP on red cell membrane integrity.

Platelet concentrates (PC) prepared from whole blood donations or apheresis devices show great variation in white cell content. The predominant cell is the mononuclear cell, except in situations where there

Clinical Benefits of Leukodepleted Blood Products, edited by Joseph Sweeney, M.D. and Andrew Heaton, M.D. © 1995 R.G. Landes Company.

is poor cell separation, in which granulocytes may be present in large numbers. Contaminating leukocytes may potentially damage platelets by competing for available oxygen or metabolic substrates, by releasing enzymes which degrade platelet membrane glycoproteins, or by releasing substances which act on platelets to cause activation or degranulation.

Some studies have implied an adverse indirect or direct effect of leukocytes on platelet properties during storage. Most of these studies have involved high residual leukocyte levels in platelet concentrates platelet stored in first-generation containers where insufficient oxygen for cell respiration may have led to a fall in pH. In addition, some studies involved spiking concentrates with buffy coat leukocytes. However, no convincing data indicates that modest levels of mononuclear white cell contamination ($<1 \times 10^8$) in second-generation containers affect the platelet storage lesion, and no differences in in vivo recovery or survival have been demonstrated.

In a number of plateletpheresis concentrate studies where mononuclear cells were predominant and present in the 10^5-10^8 range, there was no evidence that this was associated with an adverse effect on platelet quality. Manufacturing protocols which result in high residual granulocyte content may affect platelets, but, in practice, this is uncommon.

RED CELL CONCENTRATES

CHANGES IN RED CELLS DURING STORAGE

Red cell concentrates (RCC), prepared from CPD-anticoagulated whole blood units are routinely suspended in a plasma-free additive solution containing saline, adenine, and glucose for storage.[1] In some commercially available solutions, mannitol, sorbitol, guanosine, citrate, and/or phosphate are included for additional membrane stabilization and/or metabolic support. Storage is carried out at 4°C in polyvinyl chloride plastic containers with di-2-ethylhexylphthalate (DEHP) or butyryl-tri-n-hexyl-citrate (BTHC) as plasticizers.[1-3]

During storage at 4°C in CPDA-plasma or in currently manufactured additive solutions, the red cells undergo morphologic/membrane and metabolic alterations (Table 5.1) which lead to progressive loss of viability with increasing storage time.[1,4,5] The metabolic storage lesion includes a rapid loss of 2,3-diphosphoglycerate (DPG) during the first 2 to 3 weeks.[1,4] Furthermore, during storage there is a decreasing rate of glycolysis associated with falling pH levels.[6,7] From pre-storage levels of 6.9, pH levels fall below 6.5 after 5 to 6 weeks. As a result of the decreased rate of glycolysis, metabolic depletion occurs with ATP levels dropping from approximately 4-5 μmoles/g Hb at 2 to 3

Table 5.1. Changes associated with in vitro storage of red cells

Metabolic Depletion	Morphologic Changes
Loss of 2,3 DPG	Discocyte → Echinocyte
Glycolytic Metabolism↓	Echinocyte → Spheroechinocyte
	Membrane Microvesiculation
	Cell Swelling (↑ MCV)
	↑ Cell Rigidity
Reduction in ATP	Hemolysis
	K⁺ Leakage

weeks to levels below 2 μmoles/g Hb at 7 weeks of storage. ATP levels in stored red cells have been shown to predict approximately 50% of the variance post-transfusion viability after infusion (r = -0.7).[5] The metabolic depletion may be retarded by addition of modifiers of energy metabolism such as ammonium chloride and phosphate.[7-11] Phosphate stimulates glycolysis through activation of phosphofructokinase (PFK),[12] as well as the synthesis of ribonucleotides from purines through the salvage pathway.[13] It may also act as a buffer to maintain pH extracellular and intracellular. Greenwalt[10] has suggested that the beneficial effect of ammonium chloride may be through its stimulation of the pentose-phosphate pathway, thereby increasing the formation of phosphoribosylpyrophosphate which is needed for the phosphorylation of adenine by adenyl phosphoribosyltranferase. It may also stimulate glycolysis by relieving the inhibition of ATP on PFK.[8,9]

The morphologic/membrane storage lesions include loss of cellular potassium with swelling[14] and loss of membrane lipid vesicles (microvesicles).[15,16] Approximately 5% membrane phospholipid is lost during 42 days of storage. The latter is probably responsible for the increased levels of extracellular hemoglobin (reaching levels between 0.3-1.0% of total hemoglobin at 42 days of storage) rather than red cell disintegration per se.[16] The microvesicles contain approximately 70% of the extracellular hemoglobin released during storage.

It has been suggested that the microvesicle membrane loss is responsible for the morphological changes with a characteristic discocyte-echinocyte-spheroechinocyte transformation occurring during storage.[17-19] These changes have also been related to loss of cellular deformability as measured by an osmotic fragility test or by aspiration of the red cells through a 1 to 3 μm pipette[15] as well as loss of viability.[19]

It is uncertain whether the membrane lesions are indirectly caused by the metabolic depletion with ATP loss or due to more direct causes. Studies by Wolfe et al[15] have indicated that cell metabolic depletion caused by starvation at 37°C, resulted in a rapid ATP fall and similar membrane/morphological lesions to those observed during storage at 4°C. Furthermore, in studies where the metabolic lesions were retarded by metabolic modifiers, improvements in morphology and reduced hemolysis were also observed.[8,10,20-22]

The plasticizer, DEHP, impairs platelet and granulocyte function either due to adherence to cell membrane surface or to solubility in phospholipids in the membrane resulting in an inhibition of cell motility or recognition.[23] For the red blood cell, the plasticizer's incorporation into the lipoprotein in the membrane and cytosol has been shown to have a protective effect on the red cell membrane resulting in reduced storage hemolysis, erythrocyte fragility, and microvesiculation.[24-27] In order to store refrigerated red cells in plastic containers without leachable plasticizer, an improved preservative which can compensate for the stabilizing effects of the DEHP is, therefore, needed. Inclusion of an osmotic agent such as mannitol (licensed for in vivo use in the United States) or sorbitol (used in Europe) may decrease storage-related hemolysis. Mannitol may prevent hemolysis by prevention of red cell osmotic swelling that occurs in additive solutions.[14,28] It is also possible that its influence on hemolysis is through an antioxidant effect, perhaps by prevention of oxidative damage to spectrin.[29] However, it did not prevent the accelerated membrane damage found with RBC stored in non-DEHP containers such as the CLX® (polyvinylchloride plastic container from Miles, Inc., Berkeley, CA) which incorporates a non-leachable tri-(2-ethylhexyl) trimellitate (TOTM) plasticizer. This study, which used the licensed red cell additive solution AS-3 (Miles, Inc.) and various concentrations of mannitol, showed unacceptable levels of hemolysis of more than 1% after only 5 weeks.[30]

The combination of adenine and guanosine together with sorbitol as membrane solution, PAGGS (phosphate-adenine-glu-cose-guanosine-sorbitol, from Biotrans, Drieich, Germany) used in Europe, has also been shown to support prolonged red cell storage. Post-storage metabolic parameters, maintenance of normal RBC morphology, and decreased echinocyte formation were also observed.[1] An additive solution containing mannitol to reduce hemolysis and guanosine to maintain ATP may, therefore, offset the losses in red cell quality and morphology due to storage in the absence of DEHP. However, in a recent study conducted in our laboratory where red cells stored in a combination of PAGGS additive solution and CLX containers were compared to red cells stored in a standard AS-3/DEHP PVC container, the superior protective effect of DEHP was evident in terms of post-storage erythrocyte viability, osmotic fragility, and hemolysis.[30] Thus, neither the addition of guanosine nor mannitol used in this study appeared to offset the membrane deterioration during storage without DEHP stabilization.

POTENTIAL MECHANISMS OF LEUKOCYTE-MEDIATED RED CELL INJURY

There are indications that contaminant leukocytes in red cell transfusion products are not only associated with adverse transfusion outcomes, but may also affect the quality of the red cells. During centrifugation of whole blood units for processing into various components, most of the leukocytes are sedimented into a layer between the (platelet-rich-) plasma and the red cells, the so-called "buffy coat" layer. Early studies with red cells suspended in additive solutions showed that pre-storage removal of the buffy coat resulted in a substantial reduction in hemolysis.[28,31]

There are good reasons to suspect that the presence of contaminating leukocytes was the cause for the detrimental effect of the buffy coat on the red cell membrane during storage. Studies by Humbert[32] have suggested that both neutrophil stimulation and leukocyte disintegration takes place in the early phases of refrigerated storage: by

two weeks 40% of the leukocytes (90% granulocytes) have disintegrated, by six weeks 75% of the cells have disintegrated. Morphologically, changes can be observed within 1-2 days with marked damage including vacuolization and disintegration of internal structure, and with disruption of membrane observed after one week. At 10 days of storage, there is almost total destruction with dissolution of nucleus and fragmentation. Fragments, granules, and microvesicles from this destruction were observed to pass through infusion filters. It was suggested that in the early stages, within hours after collection, the oxidative enzymatic system may be activated with release of oxidant free radicals, which together with serine proteases, may cause the damage to the leukocyte membrane components.

Leukocytes contain metabolites such as acid hydrolases, histamine, a chymotrypsin-like enzyme, and also two serine proteases, (elastase and cathepsin G), which are considered to be proteolytic enzymes of high potency.[33,34] It has been demonstrated that both enzymes have the ability to change the structure and function of platelets and neutrophil membranes.[35-38] Furthermore, as shown in recent studies, these serine proteases also have the ability to degrade erythrocyte surface components with preferential digestion of glycophorins and band 3 protein.[33,39,40] Plasma contains inhibitors of these serine proteases which may be able to prevent most of the detrimental effect of these enzymes on red cell membrane.[41,42] In fact, this was suggested by the early studies with plasma-free red cell storage media described by Högman.[28,31]

With storage in a saline-adenine-glucose (SAG) additive solution, in the absence of plasma, the additive-suspended red cells exhibited increased hemolysis unless enzyme inhibitors were added[28] or the buffy coat was removed, or plasma returned to the unit.[31] In these studies, red cells were concentrated to a 90% hematocrit and diluted in a 100 mL saline-adenine-glucose (SAG) medium. Hemolysis and potassium leakage were found to be higher in SAG-stored RBC than in CPDA-1 whole blood, suggestive of a protective effect of plasma proteins. This hemolysis was prevented by buffy coat depletion or by storage in the presence of synthetic enzyme inhibitors. Subsequent studies showed that hemolysis in SAG medium with buffy coat removal could be further reduced by the addition of mannitol for stabilization of the red cell membrane, and SAGM is still the most commonly used European red cell additive solution.[19]

Another potential cause of damage to red cells during storage by residual white cells may be activation of the oxidative enzymatic system with the release of oxidant radicals. These agents have been shown to deactivate the natural plasma inhibitors of serine proteases.[41,42] It has been suggested by Weiss et al[39] that the combination of oxidant radicals and serine proteases may be responsible for the shortening of lifespans of red cells in anemias accompanying inflammatory diseases.

In conclusion, during storage at 4°C, residual white cells may potentially release oxidant radicals that, together with released esterases and other serine proteases, may be responsible for accelerated breakdown/activation of leukocytes that then potentiate the effect of serine proteases on red cell membrane. Therefore, there is reason to believe that some improvement in in vitro quality may be achieved by pre-storage reduction of the number of leukocytes in the stored units. It is also possible that some of the beneficial effect of DEHP observed with storage of red cells may be caused by the plasticizer on the membrane integrity of *white cells,* thus preventing the release of esterases and other proteases that may damage the red cell membrane. It will, therefore, be of interest to evaluate if white cell removal prior to storage can prevent increased red cell hemolysis during storage in DEHP-free containers.

STUDIES AIMED AT INVESTIGATING THE ROLE OF CONTAMINATING WBC IN THE RED CELL STORAGE LESION USING FILTRATION FOR WBC REMOVAL

One of the early studies reporting the effect of pre-storage removal of white cells by filtration was described by Lovric et al[43] using in-line filtration as an alternative to buffy coat leukodepletion of red cells. These studies showed that there was an effect on storage-induced potassium leakage and hemolysis preventing damage to the red cell membrane as well as improvement in the oxygen dissociation characteristics of stored red cells. This suggested an effect on the maintenance of 2,3 DPG levels,[43] which was confirmed by subsequent studies by Angue et al.[44] In addition, glucose consumption and lactate production were reduced during storage. It was not clear, however, whether this effect was due to reduced *leukocyte* metabolism (following filtration) or due to slower red cell metabolism through a secondary effect of the absence of leukocyte enzymes on the membrane of the stored red cells. The effects of

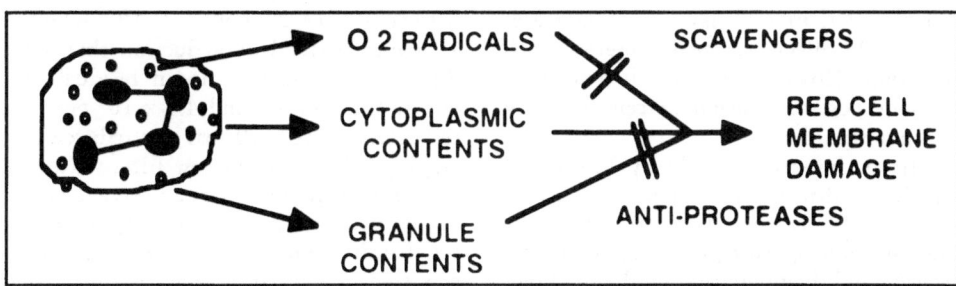

Fig. 5.1. Potential mechanisms of leukocyte-mediated red cell injury during in vitro storage and possible sites of counteraction of such injury.

brane of the stored red cells. The effects of prestorage WBC removal on storage of red cells were later confirmed by others. In a study by Pietersz et al,[45] a "Cellselect" filter composed of cellulose acetate from NPBI (Amstelveen, The Netherlands) was used for filtration. A whole blood unit was separated into plasma, buffy coat, and RBC concentrate. SAG with mannitol added was used as additive for the red cells. The WBC count in the RBC unit before filtration was 6.6×10^8 (due to buffy coat removal) and, after filtration, this was reduced to levels less than 10^6, representing more than 99% removal. RBC loss during filtration was 11%. It was shown that filtered units had lower levels of extracellular hemoglobulin, potassium, and LDH than unfiltered units at day 42 of storage, indicative of an effect of the contaminating WBC on the stability of the red cell membrane. In addition, ATP, glucose, and pH levels were higher and lactate levels lower in the filtered units, which confirmed a metabolic effect of pre-storage leukocyte removal.

Similar findings were reported by Davey et al.[46] In these studies, a "Leukotrap system" with a cellulose acetate filter was used and buffy coat was not removed prior to filtration. WBC counts in the filtered units averaged 1.1×10^8, representing a 97.7% ± 2.7% removal. RBC loss by filtration was 10% ± 1%. Complement 3a was shown to be generated by filtration. Following 42 days of storage, pre-storage filtration was associated with reduced microaggregate formation, and reduced hemolysis (0.41 ± 0.68% for filtered vs. 1.15 ± 1.54% for unfiltered units). An improvement in ATP levels, suggestive of a metabolic effect, was again observed with filtration. However, the improvement in 24-hour post-transfusion percent recovery was not significant.

In an important study by Brecher et al,[47] it was directly demonstrated that pre-storage WBC removal prevented the accumulation during storage of neutrophil activation and disintegration products. Blood was collected into CP2D and the AS-3 red cells were filtered through an integral pro-

totype third-generation polyester filter, "Leukotrap"® (Miles, Inc.). Leukocyte counts in unfiltered units decreased from a mean of 8.6×10^9/L on day 0 to 2.2×10^9/L on day 42, representing a 74% decrease. Filtration resulted in a 3-4 $\log_{10}$ removal. It was shown that leukocyte metabolites such as acid hydrolases, granulocyte elastase, histamine, and a chymotrypsin-like enzyme accumulated during storage in the unfiltered units and that pre-storage leukocyte depletion prevented any significant accumulation of these metabolites. Beneficial effects of filtration were observed after 42 days of storage with mean hemolysis reduced in filtered units from 0.83% to 0.34% for the unfiltered units. In these studies the effect on ATP levels, osmotic fragility, or 24-hour post-transfusion percent recovery of filtration was not significant.

Recently, a large four-center study involving 43 donors in a paired study design was conducted to examine the effect of pre-storage leukocyte removal using a new, high-efficiency filter (RC-300, Pall Corp. Glen Cove, NY) in-line in a blood container system (Leukotrap®RC system, Miles, Inc.).[48] The studies were designed to evaluate the effect of two different processing conditions on 42 day AS-3 red cell storage. Filtration was performed either at 22°C within 8 hours or at 4°C within 24 hours of phlebotomy. The study showed that pre-storage leukocyte depletion with the integral filter consistently achieved leukoreduction in the 4-5 $\log_{10}$ range such that residual red cell leukocyte levels were below < 1×10^6 per product. Surprisingly, filtration after 24 hours at 4°C achieved 10 times better leukoreduction than after 8 hours at 22°C with mean residual leukocyte units of 3.2 and 4.1×10^4 per unit respectively. Red cell loss was reduced (averaging 6%) with the new filter. After 42 days of storage, there was an average of 2% better post-transfusion recovery with filtered units compared to unfiltered, which was statistically significant in this paired study. In vitro parameters associated with in vivo quality such as pH, ATP levels, extracellular K+, osmotic fragility, and hemolysis levels were also significantly improved. Reduced glycolytic activity was observed in the filtered units, and in control units lactate production correlated with the prestorage leukocyte load. In the filtered units, the improved red cell quality post storage was not directly correlated with the degree of residual leukocytes prior to storage, and there was no correlation with red cell energy consumption. Poststorage ATP levels were significantly less in the unfiltered units held for 8 hours at 22°C and it was in these units that the correlation between final ATP levels and posttransfusion recoveries was the most significant ($r = .80$). Consequently, it is possible that the presence of leukocytes in stored red cell units was associated with a red cell membrane lesion resulting in potassium leakage and hemolysis which caused accelerated red cell glycolysis with more rapid pH fall, and that this may lead to a more rapid fall in ATP with loss of viability.

The question whether the benefit of DEHP on red cell storage is due to stabilization of WBC membrane rather than RBC membrane, thereby preventing release of harmful enzymes during storage, was investigated in a recent study reported by Davey et al.[49] In this study, two laboratories examined whether the positive effect of leukodepletion could offset the negative effect of the absence of DEHP. Laboratory 1 studied the effect of 1 $\log_{10}$ leuko-filtration with storage of standard and leukopoor AS-3 red cells in a non-DEHP TEHTM plastic container for 42 days. Hemolysis was elevated in both storage conditions, but was significantly higher in the unfiltered units (1.8 vs. 0.8%, respectively). No difference was found with regard to osmotic fragility, or post-storage supernatant potassium levels, red cell ATP levels, or percent recovery. The studies in Laboratory 2 utilized 3-4 $\log_{10}$ leuko-filtered AS-3 red cells which were stored in TEHTM containers and compared to unfiltered AS-3 suspended red cells in standard DEHP-PVC containers. Higher potassium and osmotic fragility values were found in the

filtered units, confirming a direct stabilizing effect of DEHP on red cell membrane which was not replaced by leuko-filtration. In spite of the leukoreduction, there was substantial decrease in the 24-hour posttransfusion percent recovery as compared to standard control units, 69 ± 7% vs. 77 ± 5%. Glucose consumption was greater in the standard units and ATP preservation similar suggesting that leukoreduction partially ameliorated the metabolic effects of DEHP absence but not enough to avoid the membrane lesion, or the reduction in post transfusion recoveries. This study suggested that the beneficial effect of DEHP plasticizer was of sufficient magnitude that this (or other leachable plasticizers such as BTHC) could not be omitted from the plastic formulation container. The beneficial effects of pre-storage leukodepletion of red cell concentrates on in vitro and in vivo parameters are illustrated in Table 5.2 and Figure 5.2.

PLATELET PREPARATIONS

THE PLATELET STORAGE LESION

The platelet storage lesion refers to a reduced capacity to survive post-infusion in vivo and to respond hemostatically to physiologic stimuli. Attempts to define and quantitate this storage injury by in vitro tests have recently been reviewed.[50-52] In vitro tests which are commonly employed are outlined in Table 5.3. In practice, most investigators have used a battery of tests when evaluating a new storage condition,[53] and for the present, this would appear to be the most satisfactory approach.

The in vivo tests of platelet viability and function are outlined in Table 5.4. The most widely used and accepted test of viability is the in vivo infusion of autologous radio-labeled platelets with subsequent measurement of recovery and survival.[54] This is a valuable test in assessing the platelet storage injury and has become the benchmark against which the in vitro tests are compared. Measurement of corrected count increments in transfused thrombocytopenic recipients has also found acceptance.[55-57] However, recipient-associated variables such as allosensitization, ABO incompatibility, fever, or medications are known to impact on platelet count increments in a manner which is unrelated to the intrinsic quality of stored platelets.[58]

To evaluate platelet function, post-infusion tests have also been used, such as bleeding time estimation in aspirinized volunteers[59] or ex vivo aggregation of radio-labeled platelets.[60] None of these tests, while interesting, has achieved either common place use or general acceptance and, as a result, both in vitro and in vivo tests continue to be used to evaluate the platelet storage injury when potential improvements, such as leukodepletion, are being analyzed.

Table 5.2. Post storage in vivo and in vitro values of prestorage leukocyte depleted red cells

	Ref.	% Leuko-reduction	Number	% Post Transfusion Recovery	Red Cell Filtration Loss %	Hemolysis %	ATP (µM/g Hb)
Test	46	97.7 ± 2.7	17	80 ± 6	10 ± 1	*.41 ± .68[T]	*3.5 ± 0.9[T]
Control		–	17	79 ± 6	–	1.15 ± 1.54	2.9 ± 0.9
Test	48	>99.99	43	*84 ± 5	6.4 ± 0.7	*.18 ± .14	*2.6 ± 0.6
Control		–	43	81 ± 6	–	.54 ± .46	2.4 ± 0.6

* p <.05 to controls   [T]N = 6

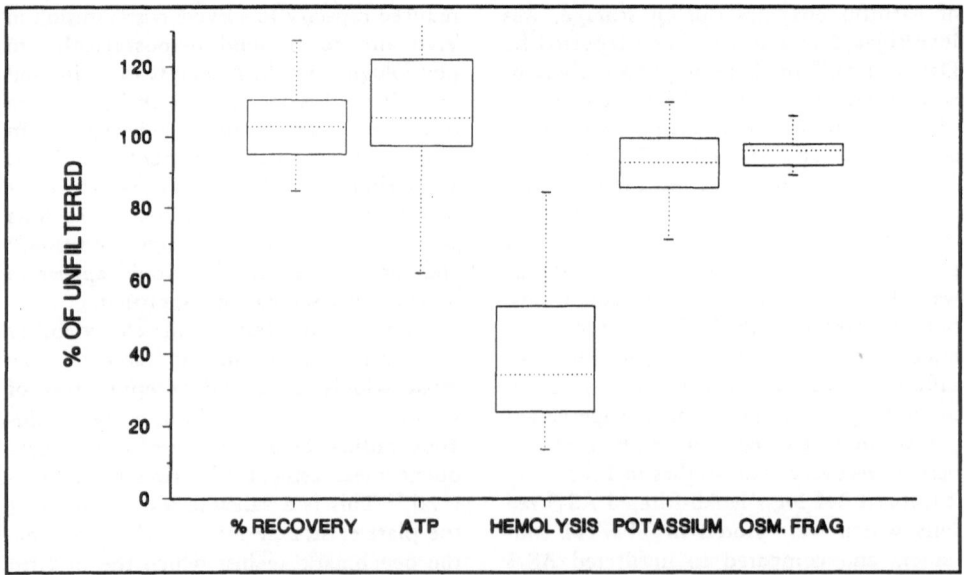

Fig. 5.2. The effect of pre-storage leukodepletion of red cell concentrates. Data is derived from paired sequential studies, in vitro and in vivo, where the abscissa represents the mean value of the unfiltered products expressed as 100%.

POTENTIAL MECHANISMS OF IN VITRO LEUKOCYTE-MEDIATED PLATELET INJURY

Several mechanisms exist whereby the presence of leukocytes in platelet preparation could conceivably accelerate or exacerbate the platelet storage injury. Both leukocytes and platelets have active oxidative phosphorylating mechanisms and thus competition for oxygen could jeopardize the metabolic integrity of the stored platelet. This is especially likely in a storage container in which there is a limited transport of oxygen. Second, granulocytes store poorly in vitro with loss of membrane integrity and release of intracellular proteases such as elastase or cathepsin G. These could proteolytically cleave platelet surface glycoproteins, rendering the platelet hemostatically effete or inert.[35,36,37,61,62] Third, products of leukocyte metabolism, such as substances resembling platelet activating factor, could be secreted and activate platelets resulting in irreversible degranulation.[63] Surface expression of activation epitopes such as P-selectin could also induce leukocyte platelet clumping[64] (Fig. 5.3).

THE MANUFACTURE OF PLATELET PREPARATIONS

Different manufacturing practices exist to produce the platelet preparations currently used in transfusion practice. From whole blood donations, platelet concentrates are derived using either platelet-rich-plasma or buffy coat as an intermediate product. The different manufacturing schemes for whole blood-derived products are outlined in Figure 5.4. Platelet concentrates may also be produced from a single donor using a variety of cell separator devices. In addition, the platelet concentrates may be filtered for WBC removal prior to storage. The yield and volume characteristics of the end products vary greatly depending on the preparation protocols. On account of this, clinical studies will be examined separately for each product type (Table 5.5).

Table 5.3. In vitro tests of the quality of stored platelets

1. Tests of metabolic processes: pH, pO_2, pCO_2, glucose consumed, lactate generated, platelet ATP.

2. Physiologic "stress" tests: In vitro aggregation to platelet agonists; shape change in response to ADP, osmotic challenge test (hypotonic stress ratio).

3. "Leakage" tests: LDH (from cytoplasm); B thromboglobulin and von Willebrand factor (α-granule), lysosomal enzymes, (lysosomes), thrombin induced ATP release (dense bodies), Intracellular calcium (dense tubular system).

4. Surface alteration: Loss (glycoprotein 1b, glycoprotein IIb/IIIa) or gain (P-selectin) of glycoproteins.

5. Alterations in soluble components: Cytokine production, activation of complement, fibrinolytic or coagulation systems.

6. Structural: morphology score (evaluation of relative number of discs to spheres to microscopy), "swirling" of platelets, presence of macroscopic clumps, analysis of platelet proteins using one-dimensional or two-dimensional gels, microvesicle formation, electron microscopy.

Table 5.4. In vivo and ex vivo tests of the quality of stored platelets

1. Infusion of radio isotopically or fluorescence labelled autologous stored platelets with estimation of recovery and survival.

2. Transfusion of allogeneic stored platelets with estimation of platelet count increments (single or serial) in the recipient.

3. Physiologic challenge tests: e.g. bleeding time estimation post-infusion of autologous stored platelets in an aspirin-treated donor, post-infusion ex vivo agonist-induced aggregation of radio-isotopically labelled stored autologous platelets.

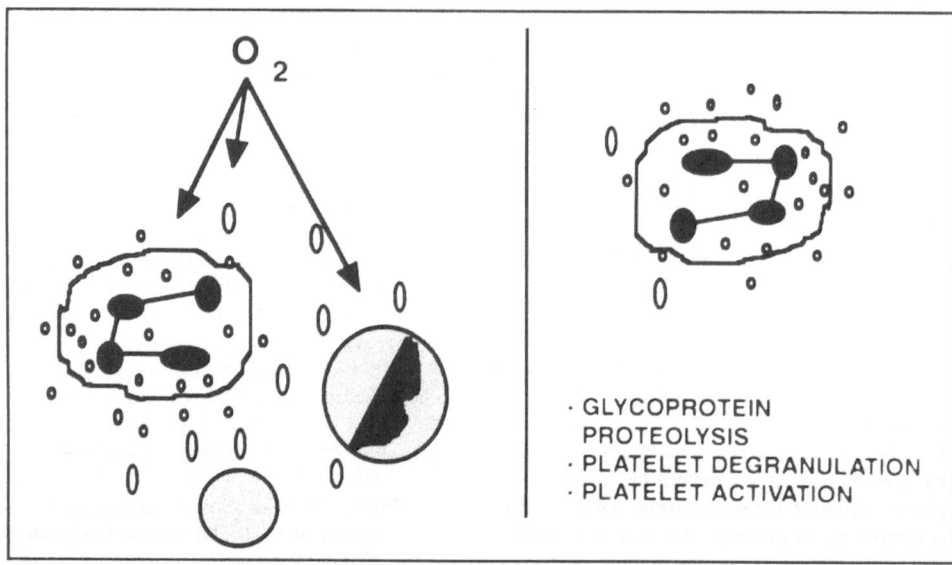

Fig. 5.3. Potential mechanisms of leukocyte-mediated platelet injury during in vitro storage (a) competition for available oxygen (O₂) in solution, (b) release of substances which exert a deleterious effect on platelet integrity.

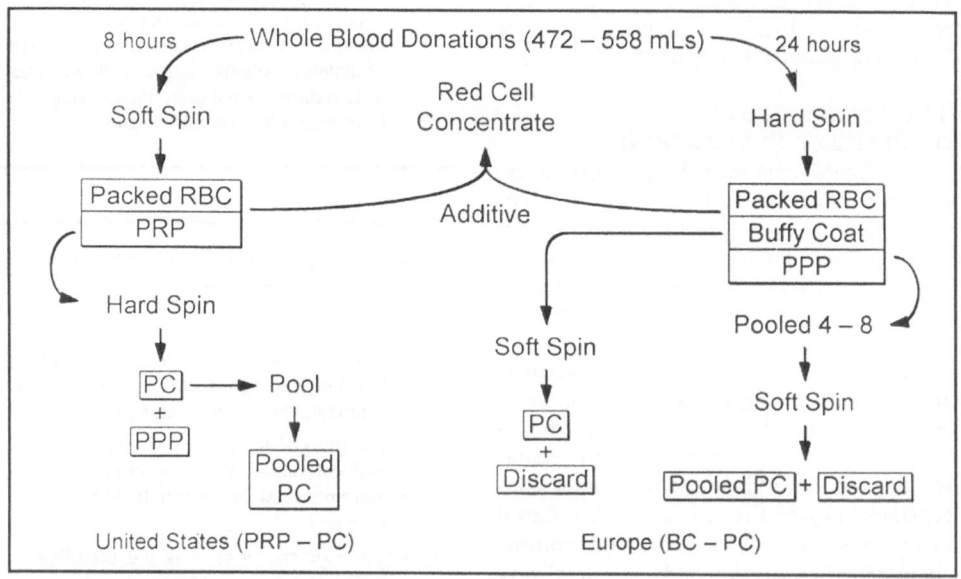

Fig. 5.4. Manufacturing schemes for the production of platelet concentrates from whole blood donations.

CLINICAL STUDIES DESIGNED TO EVALUATE THE EFFECT OF LEUKOCYTE CONTAMINATION ON THE PLATELET STORAGE INJURY

Platelet-Rich-Plasma Derived Platelet Concentrates (PRP-PC)

Early work by Gottschall et al,[65] using platelets stored in first-generation containers, showed that residual white cells increased glucose consumption, lactate production, and lowered pH levels at the end of the storage period (72 hours). The authors suggested that white cell reduction would result in an improved product. This work was, however, performed in polyvinylchloride (PVC) containers plasticized with diethyl-hexylphthalate (DEHP) which are known to have unfavorable gas diffusion characteristics. An alternative explanation could be that white cell competition for limited dissolved oxygen and limited container CO_2 diffusion capacity resulted in anaerobic platelet energy metabolism with accelerated lactate production and inadequate bicarbonate buffering activity. This work therefore, may not be relevant to storage containers in current use. Taylor et al[66] studied paired "split" platelet concentrates stored in non-DEHP containers. These authors showed an adverse effect of the addition of buffy coats to the platelet-rich-plasma prior to platelet concentrate manufacture. An effect of leukocyte concentration on hypotonic stress ratio and glucose consumption was demonstrated, but not on the binding of AN 51, a monoclonal antibody against the von Willebrand binding site of glycoprotein $1b\alpha$. Although this work is interesting, the buffy coat additive to the platelet-rich-plasma contained allogenic, in addition to autologous, leukocytes, and would likely have had a high content of granulocytes. The buffy coats were not characterized prior to addition to the platelet-rich-plasma nor was the final leukocyte content measured. Despite the performance of these studies in second-generation containers, the relevance to current practice is questionable. Studies by Holme et al in which fil-

---

Table 5.5. Different types of platelet products

1. Platelet concentrate manufactured from a whole blood donation using platelet rich plasma as an intermediate product (PRP-PC).
2. Platelet concentrate manufactured from a whole blood donation using the buffy coat as an intermediate product (BC-PC).
3. Platelet concentrate manufactured from a single donor using an automated device or manual apheresis method (platelets, pheresis).

---

tered apheresis platelet concentrates and pooled PRP-PC were compared with unfiltered products showed no difference when in vitro platelet properties were measured during a 5-day storage period.[67]

Studies by Wallvik et al,[68] using a PVC-DEHP container (Terumo XT612), showed an inverse relationship between supernatant LDH, pH, and leukocyte content after 5 to 7 days storage. An increase in elastase also correlated with leukocyte content. However, the leukocyte concentrations in the high leukocyte platelet concentrate were high (13×10^9/L) and unlikely to be encountered with current manufacturing practices. The higher platelet content in the high leukocyte platelet concentrates could also have exacerbated the competition for metabolic oxygen, especially in this type of container with low oxygen transport capacity. Dzik et al[69] used a concurrent design in which three similar platelet suspensions were used to perform in vitro studies in stored platelet concentrates. These suspensions were unfiltered, filtered, or leuko-enriched with autologous leukocytes. Leuko-enriched concentrates had a lower pO_2 and pH, but no difference in glycocalicin or supernatant LDH. In the same publication, a second study was reported in which two unpaired groups, one consisting of leukodepleted platelets, the other standard (non-leukodepleted) platelets, were studied using ^{111}In survival studies. No differences were evident in recovery or survival between the groups. Sweeney et al[70] used a similar filter to produce leukodepleted and non-leukodepleted PRP-PC's from the same donor on the same day. Leukodepleted PRP-PCs showed a wide variation in WBC content, but with 95% less WBC than the non-filtered units. This paired concurrent design used a battery of in vitro studies with subsequent in vivo double labeling using ^{51}Cr and ^{111}In. No effect of pre-storage leukodepletion on in vitro measures or in vivo recovery or survival was measurable.

Buffy Coat Platelets

There has been considerable interest in using buffy coats as an intermediate product in the manufacture of platelet concentrates.[71] Early studies showed variable and slightly lower platelet yields but less white cell contamination[72] than with PRP-PCs. Modification in preparation protocols associated with prolonged (16 to 20 hour) periods of 22°C hold as whole blood or as buffy coats resulted in buffy coat platelet products in which white cell content was reduced by one $\log_{10}$ (90%), but with an associated platelet yield of approximately 20% less than that found in conventional PRP-derived platelet concentrates. Advocates of this production protocol point to the reduced white cell contamination,[73] lesser degrees of platelet activation in the period immediately after platelet concentrate preparation,[74] the possible harvesting of platelet subpopulations which are intrinsically superior to those harvested in the more standard PRP-derived platelets[75] and lastly, the amenability of these preparation protocols to automation. Early work by Pietersz[73] showed an inverse correlation between leukocyte content and both pH and glucose consumption and a direct relation with supernatant LDH and lactic acid production. These platelet products were stored in PVC DEHP containers with risk of hypoxia. The most pronounced changes in pH and LDH release were in BC-PCs with the highest white cell content. This group had a large percentage of granulocytes, many of which disintegrated during storage. Interestingly, morphology score was not related to leukocyte content after five days of storage. The authors concluded that a detrimental effect of leukocytes on platelet quality was likely. No in vivo studies were performed. An alternative explanation is that the presence of leukocytes, particularly granulocytes, in a container with limited gas exchange characteristics, results in oxygen deprivation of both granulocytes and platelets; the former disintegrate and damage platelets; the latter are also affected by the limited oxygen available. These data may not be relevant to second-generation container storage. In a subsequent study[76] in which a variety of containers were used, no such container effect could be demonstrated. However, in this study the white cell content was much lower (1×10^7) than the groups studied in the previous publication (8×10^6 - 8×10^8), and the mean platelet yield was approximately 10% less. Thus, the interpretation of the absence of a container effect may only be relevant to products with lower platelet yields ($< 5.6 \times 10^{10}$) and lower white cell content ($\leq 1 \times 10^7$). Keegan et al,[77] using a paired sequential design in which autologous donors gave on two separate occasions, showed no difference between platelet concentrates prepared from buffy coat and PRP as measured by in vivo recovery and survival. Buffy coat platelet concentrates had approximately 20% lower platelet yield, and 1 $\log_{10}$ less white cell content. Some differences were observed in in vitro tests with lower pO_2 in the PRP-PC. Morphology score and osmotic challenge were not different. Tandy et al[78] surveyed automated processing devices currently in use in Europe. Superior in vitro characteristics of buffy coat platelet concentrates were presented relative to historical PRP-PC controls. BC-PCs showed higher pH, lower lactate, and less supernatant von Willebrand factor and glycocalicin. The clinical relevance is in question however, as concurrent PRP-PCs were not studied and, especially as no in vivo data was available. It is noteworthy that the hypotonic stress test did not show a difference of any significant degree between the historically PRP-PC and the BC-PCs.

Pheresis Products

There have been fewer studies on the role of leukodepletion on the quality of pheresis platelets. Early work by Snyder et al[79] showed that storage of platelets in the presence of autologous granulocytes as a combined platelets-granulocyte pheresis product was unfavorable to the stored platelet when compared to whole blood-derived platelets. Again, these studies were performed with preparations stored in PVC-DEHP (PL146 containers). Release of lysosome was evident, especially with agitation. Sloand and Klein[80] showed that the addition of ficoll-separated autologous granulocytes to platelet concentrates exerted an adverse effect on in vitro measures of platelet integrity. No effect of autologous mononuclear cells was evident. The authors concluded that autologous granulocytes, but not mononuclear cells, would adversely affect stored platelets, and speculated that the release of granulocyte enzymes may be a possible mechanism of injury. However, platelet pheresis concentrates tend to be largely contaminated with mononuclear cells,[81] and thus, this study would likely suggest that, in practice, there would be no effect of leukocytes on platelet integrity. Garcia et al,[82] using a concurrent paired design and centrifugational reduction of leukocytes, failed to demonstrate an effect of pre-storage leukodepletion on glycoprotein 1B surface expression as measured by flow cytometry, ristocetin-induced platelet aggregation, or von Willebrand factor in the supernatant or platelet granules. White cell content was high (>10[9]) in the non-white cell- reduced suspensions. Sweeney et al,[83] using products produced in both the Haemonetics MCS and Cobe Spectra, studied the effect of pre-storage leukocyte depletion by filtration. Each product was divided into two suspensions, one of which was filtered. A large range of white cell content was present (10^4 - 10^8). Using a variety of in vitro measures, flow cytometry for GP1b and P-selectin, concurrent in vivo survival using ^{51}Cr and ^{111}In labeling, and post-infusion ex vivo aggregation to ADP, no differences were present between the leukodepleted and nonleukodepleted suspensions. Bock et al,[84] studying apheresis products from a Fenwal CS3000 stored in second-generation containers (PL-732), demonstrated increased levels of products of leukocyte disintegration in stored platelets but no evidence of an effect of such on platelet integrity. Furthermore, studies by Holme et al where the WBC contamination in the CS3000 PC in PL-732 containers ranged from 10^5 to 10^9 cells per container showed no significant correlations between WBC counts and platelet post-transfusion viability or any morphologic, functional, or metabolic in vitro variables, including lactate and pH after five days of storage. An exception was the oxygen consumption rate which correlated positively (r = 0.54) with the WBC count.[85] Recently Wallvik et al[86] failed to show any effect of mononuclear cells (76 - 96% of total leukocytes) on pH, pCO_2, lactate production, or glucose consumption of apheresis platelets produced using an IBM 2997 device.

Data from the studies do not indicate an adverse effect of contaminating leukocytes on the intrinsic quality of pheresis platelets. The absence of leukocyte effect is illustrated in Figure 5.5.

CONCLUSIONS

1. Pre-storage leukodepletion of red cell concentrates may exert a slight effect in ameliorating the red cell storage injury, but is of questionable clinical significance.
2. Storage of the currently available platelet concentrates in a leukodepleted milieu in second-generation containers does not appear to exert a beneficial influence on the platelet storage lesion.

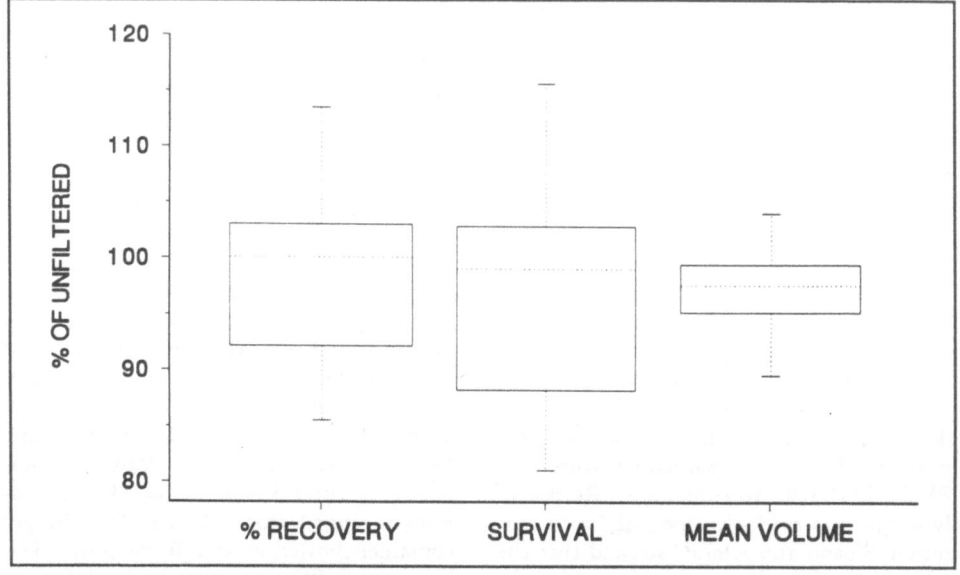

Fig. 5.5. In vivo effects and change in mean platelet volume associated with pre-storage leukodepletion of platelet concentrates. Data is derived from paired concurrent studies (n = 21), where the mean of the unfiltered products is expressed as 100%.

REFERENCES

1. Heaton W. Enhancement of cellular elements. In: Wallas, CH and McCarthy, LJ (eds). New Frontiers in Blood Banking. Arlington VA, AABB,p 89, 1986.

2. Carmen R. The selection of plastic materials for blood bags. Trans Med Rev 7:1, 1993.

3. Hogman C, Eriksson L, Erickson A, et al. Storage of saline-adenine-glucose-mannitol suspended red cells in a new plastic container: polyvinylchloride plasticized with butyryl-n-trihexyl-citrate. Transfusion 31:26, 1991.

4. Moore G. Red blood cell preservation: A survey of recent research. In Sohmer PR, Schiffer CA (eds): Blood storage and preservation. A technical workshop. Arlington VA, AABB, p 9, 1982.

5. Heaton W. Evaluation of posttranfusion recovery and survival of transfused red cells. Trans Med Rev 6:153, 1992.

6. Moroff G, Holme S, Heaton A, et al. Storage of ADSOL-preserved red cells at 2.5-5.5° C. Comparable in vitro properties. Vox Sang 59:136, 1990.

7. Meryman H, Hornblower M. Manipulating red cell intra- and extracellular pH by washing. Vox Sang 60:99, 1991.

8. Kay A, Beutler E. The effect of ammonium, phosphate, potassium, and hypotonicity on stored red cells. Transfusion 32:37, 1992.

9. Greenwalt T, McGuiness C, Dumswala U, et al. Studies on red cell preservation 3. A phosphate-ammonium-adenine-additive solution. Vox Sang 58:94, 1990.

10. Greenwalt T, Dumaswala U, Dhingra N, et al. Studies in red cell preservation. Vox Sang 65:87, 1993.

11. Mazor D, Dvilansky A, Meyerstein N. Prolonged storage of red cells with ammonium chloride and mannitol. Transfusion 30:150, 1990.

12. Jacobach G, Minakami S, Rapoport S. Glycolysis of the erythrocyte; in Yoshikawa H, Rapoport SM (eds): cellular and molecular biology of erythrocytes. Baltimore, University Park Press, p 55, 1974.

13. Hershko A, Razin A, Mager J. Regulation of the synthesis of 5-phosphoribosyl-1-pyrophosphate in intact red blood cell and in cell-free preparations. Biochem Biophys Acta 184:64, 1969.

14. Olivieri O, de Franceschi L, de Gironcoli M, et al. Potassium loss and cellular dehydration of stored erythrocytes following incubation in autologous plasma: Role of the KCL cotransport system. Vox Sang 65:95, 1993.

15. Wolfe L. The membrane and the lesions of storage in preserved red cells. Transfusion 25:185, 1985.

16. Greenwalt T, Bryan D, Dumaswala U. Erythrocyte membrane vesiculation and changes in membrane composition during storage in citrate-phosphate-dextrose-adenine-1. Vox Sang 47:261, 1984.

17. Rumsby M, Trotter J, Allan D, et al. Recovery of membrane microvesicles from human erythrocytes stored for transfusion. A mechanism for the erythrocyte discocyte-to-spherocyte shape transformation. Biochem Soc Trans 5:126, 1977.

18. Trotter J, Rumsby M. Lipids of the erythrocyte membrane during storage for transfusion. Correlation of lipid changes with the discocyte to spherocyte shape transformation. J Appl Biochem 3:19, 1981.

19. Hogman C, de Verdier C, Borgstrom L. Studies on the mechanism of human red cell loss of viability during storage at +4_C. II. Relation between cellular morphology and viability. Vox Sang 52:20, 1987.

20. Meryman H, Hornblower M, Keegan T, et al. Refrigerated storage of red cells. Vox Sang 60:88, 1991.

21. Hogman C, Eriksson L, Gong J, et al. Half-strength citrate CPD and new additive solutions for improved blood preservation. I. Studies of six experimental solutions. Transfusion Med 3:43, 1993.

22. Sasakawa S, Mitomi Y. Di-2-ethylhexyl phthalate (DEHP) content of blood or blood components stored in plastic bags. Vox Sang 34:81, 1978.

23. Miyamoto M, Sasakawa S. Effects of plasticizers and plastic bags on granulocyte function during storage. Vox Sang 53:19, 1987.

24. Horowitz B, Stryker M, Waldman A, et al. Stabilization of red blood cells by the plasticizer, diethylhexylphthalate. Vox Sang 48:150, 1985.

25. Estep T, Pedersen R, Miller T, et al. Characterization of erythrocyte quality during the refrigerated storage of whole blood containing di-(2-ethylhexyl) phthalate. Blood 64:1270, 1988.

26. AuBuchon J, Estep T, Davey R. The effect of the plasticizer di-2-ethylhexyl phthalate on the survival of stored red cells. Blood 71:448, 1988.

27. Waldman A. Effects of plasticizers on red blood cells and platelets during storage. Plasma Ther Transfus Technol 9:317, 1988.

28. Högman C, Hedlund K, Akerblom O, Venge P. Red blood cell preservation in protein-poor media: I. Leukocyte enzymes as a cause of hemolysis. Transfusion 18(2):233, 1978.

29. England M, Cavarocchi N, O'Brien J. Influence of antioxidants (mannitol and allopurinol) on oxygen free radical generation during and after cardiopulmonary bypass. Circulation (Suppl. III):134, 1986.

30. Whitley P, McNeil D, Holme S. The evaluation of red cell viability with and without leukodepletion, stored in DEHP and non-DEHP containers. In: Proc. of Mid-Atlantic Association of Blood Banks Annual Meeting, Fredericksburg, VA, May, 1992.

31. Högman CF, Hedlund K, Sahlestrom Y. Red cell preservation in protein-poor media: III. Protection against in vitro hemolysis. Vox Sang 41:274, 1981.

32. Humbert J, Fermin C, Winsor E. Early damage to granulocytes during storage. Sem in Hematol 28:10, 1991.

33. Weiss D, Murtaugh M. Activated neutrophils induce erythrocyte immunoglobulin binding and membrane protein degradation. J Leukocyte Biol 48:438, 1990.

34. Janoff A. Elastase in tissue injury. Ann Rev Med 36:207, 1985.

35. Bykowska K;, Kaczanowska J, Karpowicz M, Stachuiska Z, Kopec M. Effect of neutral proteases from blood leukocytes on human platelets. Thromb Haemostas 50:768, 1983.

36. Bykowska K, Kaczanowska J, Karpowicz M, et al. Alterations of blood platelet function induced by neutral proteases from human leukocytes. Thromb Res 38:535, 1985.

37. Brower M, Levin R, Garry K. Human neutrophil elastase modulates platelet function by limited proteolysis of membrane glyco-

proteins. J Clin Invest 75:657, 1985.

38. Selak M, Chignard M, Smith J. Cathepsin G is a strong platelet agonist released by neutrophils. Biol J 251:293, 1988.

39. Weiss D, Aird B, Murtaugh M. Neutrophil-induced immunoglobulin binding to erythrocytes involves proteolytic and oxidative injury. J Leukocyte Biol 51:19, 1992.

40. Bykowska K, Duk M, Kusnierz-Alejska G, et al. Degradation of human erythrocyte surface components by human neutrophil elastase and cathepsin G: preferential digestion of glycophorins. Brit J Haematol 84:736, 1993.

41. Travis J. Structure, function and control of neutrophil proteinases. Am J Med 84:37 (Suppl.6A), 1988.

42. Weiss S. Tissue destruction by neutrophils. New Eng J Med 320:365, 1989.

43. Lovric V, Schuller M, Raftos J, et al. Filtered microaggregate-free erythrocyte concentrates with 35-day shelflife. Vox Sang 41:6, 1981.

44. Angue M, Chatelain P, Fiabane S, et al. Viabilite des globules rouges humains conserves pendant 35 jours apres depletion en leucocytes (etude in vitro). Rev Fr Transfus Hemobio 32:27, 1989.

45. Pietersz R, Reesink H, deKorte D, et al. Storage of leukocyte-poor red cell concentrates: filtration in a closed system using a sterile connection device. Vox Sang 57:29, 1989.

46. Davey R, Carmen R, Simon T, et al. Preparation of white cell-depleted red cells for 42-day storage using an integral inline filter. Transfusion 29:496, 1989.

47. Brecher M, Pineda A, Torloni A, et al. Prestorage leukocyte depletion: effect on leukocyte and platelet metabolites, erythrocyte lysis, metabolism, and in vivo survival. Sem Hematol 28:3, 1991.

48. Heaton WAL, Holme S, Smith K, Brecher ME, Pineda A, Aubuchon JP, Nelson E. Effects of 3-5 log_{10} pre-storage leucocyte depletion on red cell storage and metabolism. Brit J of Haem 87:363, 1994.

49. Davey R, Heaton W, Sweat L, et al. Characteristics of leukocyte-reduced red cells stored in tri(2-ethylhexyl) trimellitate plastic. Transfusion 34:895-898, 1994.

50. Murphy S. Platelet storage for transfusion.

Semin Haematol 22:65, 1985.

51. Holme S. Platelet storage in a liquid environment. Transfusion Science 15(2):7, 1994.

52. Murphy S, Rebulla P, Bertolini F, Holme S, Moroff G, Snyder E, and Stromberg R. In vitro assessment of the quality of stored platelet concentrates. Trans Med Rev 8:29, 1994.

53. Slichter SJ. In vitro measurements of platelet concentrates stored at 4°C and 22°C: Correlation with post transfusion platelet viability and function. Vox Sang 40:72, 1981.

54. Murphy S. Use of an arithmetic model for evaluation of in vivo platelet survival. Transfusion 26:26, 1986.

55. Leach MF, Aubuchon JP. Effect of storage time on clinical efficacy of single donor platelet units. Transfusion 33:661, 1993.

56. Peter-Saloren K, Bucher U, Nydegger UE: Comparison of post transfusion recoveries achieved with either fresh or stored platelet concentrates. Blut 54:207, 1987.

57. Shanwell A, Wikman A, Ringden O. Pretransfusion incubation of apheresis platelets at 37°C improves post transfusion recovery. Transfusion 32:71S, 1992.

58. Bishop JF, McGrath K, Wolf MM. Clinical factors influencing the efficacy of pooled platelet transfusion. Blood 71:383, 1988.

59. Button LN, DeWolf WL, Newburger PE. The effects of irradiation on blood components. Transfusion 21:419, 1981.

60. Owens M, Holme S, Heaton A, Sawyer S, Cardinali S. Post transfusion recovery of function of 5 day stored platelet concentrates. Brit J Haematol 80:539, 1992.

61. Taki M, Miura T, Inagaki M, et al. Influence of granulocyte elastase-like proteinase (ELP) on platelet function. Thromb Res 41:837, 1986.

62. Bykowska K, Pawlowska Z, Cierniewki E, Lopaciuk S, Kopec M. Different effects of human neutrophil elastase on platelet glycoproteins IIb and IIIa of resting and stimulated platelets. Thromb Haemostas 64:69, 1990.

63. Silliman CC, Thurman GW, Ambruso DR. Stored blood components contain agents that prime the neutrophil NADPH oxidase through the platelet activating factor receptors. Vox Sang 63:133, 1992.

64. Palabrica T, Lobb R, Furie B. et al. Leukocyte accumulation promoting fibrin deposition is mediated in vivo by P-selectin on adherent platelets. Nature 359:848, 1992.

65. Gottschall JL, Johnston VL, Rzad L, Anderson AJ, Aster RH. Importance of white blood cells in platelet storage. Vox Sang 47:101, 1984.

66. Taylor MA, Tandy NP, Fraser ID. Effect of new plastics and leukocyte contamination on in vitro storage of platelet concentrates. J Clin Pathol 36:1382, 1983.

67. Holme S, Dunn S, Sawyer S, Gambill P, Heaton A. Storage of filtered apheresis and filtered pooled platelet concentrates. American Association of Blood Banks/International Society of Blood Transfusion Joint Congress; Los Angeles, CA (abstract), 1990.

68. Wallvik J, Suonkaka AM, Blomback M. Proteolytic activity during storage of platelets in plasma. Transfus Med 2:135, 1992.

69. Dzik WH, Cusack WF, Sherburne B, Vickler T. The effect of pre-storage white cell reduction on the function and viability of stored platelet concentrates. Transfusion 32:334, 1992.

70. Sweeney JD, Holme S, Heaton WAL, Nelson E. Leukodepleted platelet concentrates prepared by in-line filtration of platelet rich plasma. Transfusion (in press).

71. Prins HK, deBruijn H, Henrichs HPJ, Loos JA. Prevention of microaggregate formation by removal of buffy coats. Vox Sang 39:48, 1980.

72. Racz Z, Thek M. Buffy coat or platelet-rich plasma. Vox Sang 47:108, 1984.

73. Pietersz RNI, deKorte D, Reesink HW, van der End A, Dekker WJA, Roos D. Preparation of leukocyte poor platelet concentrates from buffy coats. Vox Sang 55:14, 1988.

74. Fijnheer R, Pietersz RNI, de Korte D, Gouwerak CWN, Dekker WJA, Reesink HW, Roos D. Platelet activation during preparation of platelet concentrates a comparison of the platelet-rich plasma and the buffy coat methods. Transfusion 30:634, 1990.

75. Mohr R, Goor DA, Yellin A, Moshkovitz Y, Shinfield A, Martinowitz U. Fresh blood units contain large potent platelets that improve hemostasis after open heart surgery.

Ann Thorac Surg 53:650, 1992.

76. Pietersz RNI, Reesink HW, Dekker WJA. Preparation of leukocyte-poor platelet concentrates from buffy coats. II. Lack of effect on storage of different plastics. Vox Sang 53:208, 1987.

77. Keegan T, Heaton A, Holme S, Owens M, Nelson E, Carmen R. Paired comparison of platelet concentrates prepared from platelet-rich plasma and buffy coats using a new technique with ^{111}In and [51]Cr. Transfusion 32:113, 1991.

78. Tandy NP, Seghatchian MJ, Bessus H. Automated processing of leukocyte-poor platelet concentrates. Blood Coag Fibrin 3:625, 1992.

79. Snyder EL, Ezekowitz MD, Malech HL, et al. In vitro characteristics and in vivo viability of platelets contained in granulocyte-platelet apheresis concentrate. Transfusion 27:10, 1987.

80. Sloand EM, Klein HG. Effect of white cells on platelets during storage. Transfusion 30:333, 1990.

81. Skinnider L, Wrobel H, McSheffrey B. The nature of the leukocyte "contamination" in platelet concentrates. Vox Sang 49:309, 1985.

82. Garcia GI, Fitzpatrick JE, Hoernig LA, Stewart CC, Sweeney JD. Effects of prestorage white cell reduction of apheresis platelets on platelet glycoprotein Ib and von Willebrand factor. Transfusion 32:148, 1992.

83. Sweeney JD, Holme S, Heaton WAL, Stromberg RR. In vitro and in vivo effects of prestorage filtration of apheresis platelets. Transfusion (in press).

84. Bock M, Glaser A, Pfosser A, Schleuning M, Heim MV, Mempel W. Storage of single donor platelet concentrates: metabolic and functional changes. Transfusion 33:311, 1993.

85. Holme S, Heaton A, Smith K, Buchholz DH. Evaluation of apheresis platelet concentrates collected with a reduced (30 mL) collection chamber with resuspension and storage in a synthetic medium. Vox Sanguinis 67:149, 1994.

86. Wallvik J, Soontaka AM. Limited metabolic effect of mononuclear cells in platelet storage. Throm Res 70:255, 1993.

CHAPTER 6

LEUKODEPLETION TO PREVENT TRANSFUSION REACTIONS:
EFFECTS ON CYTOKINES AND OTHER BIOLOGIC RESPONSE MODIFIERS

Gary Stack, Edward L. Snyder

SUMMARY

The role of allogeneic leukocytes in causing febrile nonhemolytic transfusion (FNHTR) reactions has been known since the mid-1950s. Recent data suggests plausible mechanisms in which pro-inflammatory cytokines (IL-1α, IL-1β, IL-6 and TNF-α) mediate the symptom complex of this reaction to blood transfusion. Furthermore, the source of these cytokines may be host leukocytes reacting to allogeneic leukocytes or donor leukocytes producing these cytokines in vitro during storage or in vivo post transfusion. Leukodepletion post-storage, reduces the occurrence of FNHTRs by the former mechanism and pre-storage leukodepletion should be effective to prevent these reactions by either mechanism. Formal comparisons of pre-storage leukodepleted cellular products versus post-storage leukodepleted cellular products have not yet been performed.

The clinical features of hemolytic transfusion reactions may also be due to cytokines, but allogeneic leukocytes are not known to be implicated in the pathophysiology of these reactions. In transfusion related acute lung injury, a small percentage (6%) of occurrences may be caused by these cells. Allergic reactions are usually attributed to allogeneic soluble proteins, but particulate matter derived from leukocytes disintegrating in vitro or substances produced by stored allogeneic leukocytes, such as IL-8 or histamine, may be important promoters. The role of leukodepletion in amelioration of the above reactions is unknown. Transfusion-associated graft-versus-host disease is a rare but catastrophic adverse effect of blood transfusion due to donor T lymphocytes. Leukodepletion

Clinical Benefits of Leukodepleted Blood Products, edited by Joseph Sweeney, M.D., and Andrew Heaton, M.D. © 1995 R.G. Landes Company.

should theoretically prevent this reaction, but it is considered that the level of residual leukocytes currently obtainable is not low enough to prevent this effect.

INTRODUCTION

Leukocytes are responsible for many, if not most, of the transfusion reactions that result from immunologic incompatibilities between the blood donor and the transfusion recipient. In some cases passenger leukocytes, i.e., residual leukocytes in cellular blood components, are directly responsible for inciting an immunologic rejection reaction in the transfusion recipient. These donor leukocytes may be the target of attack by the host immune system (e.g. febrile, non-hemolytic transfusion reactions; FNHTR) or may themselves attack host tissue (i.e. transfusion-associated graft-versus-host disease; TA-GVHD). In other cases the transfusion recipient's leukocytes may be targeted for immunologic attack by infused anti-leukocyte antibodies (e.g. transfusion-related acute lung injury, TRALI). Recipient leukocytes also may be recruited into a cascade of events by an incompatibility involving other cell types (e.g. hemolytic transfusion reactions), by contaminating bacteria in the blood component (i.e. septic transfusion reactions), or by antigen-antibody complex formation with soluble antigens (e.g. allergic/anaphylactoid reactions). Passenger leukocytes that remain metabolically active during blood component storage may synthesize and/or secrete soluble cytokines and other biologic response modifiers into the plasma/supernatant portion of the blood component in vitro. It is possible that infusion of these storage-related biologic response modifiers during transfusion also may provoke immunologic reactions (e.g. FNHTR, septic reactions, allergic/anaphylactic reactions).

Cytokines are polypeptides that serve as intercellular signaling molecules for a wide range of local and systemic responses.[1-4] Cytokines can act in an autocrine, paracrine and/or endocrine fashion. Cytokines may be subdivided into several families defined largely by structural simi-larities of their receptors.[1,2] The cytokine families include the hematopoietins, interferons, tumor necrosis factor-related molecules, the chemokines, and the immunoglobulin superfamily members. Despite these groupings, one cytokine can have multiple and divergent effects and multiple cytokines may mediate similar responses. Cytokines may also be grouped according to biological activities rather than by structural similarities. For example, the pro-inflammatory subset of cytokines, which may be of potential relevance in the transfusion setting, consists of members from several different cytokine families. The pro-inflammatory group includes cytokines such as tumor necrosis factor-α (TNF-α), interleukin-1 (IL-1), interleukin-6 (IL-6), interleukin-8 (IL-8), monocyte chemoattractant protein-1α (MCP-1α) and macrophage inflammatory protein-1 (MIP-1).[5-11] IL-1β, IL-6, TNF-α and MIP-1 are pyrogenic.[5-8] IL-8 is a neutrophil chemotactic and activating factor, while MCP-1 is chemotactic for monocytes.[9-11] It is clear from studies on septic shock in animals and humans that these pro-inflammatory cytokines are important mediators of the acute phase response and the systemic inflammatory response syndrome (SIRS).[3,7,12-14] The acute phase response is the multi-system response that the body makes to changes in homeostasis, such as tissue injury or immunologic disturbances.[7] The acute phase response often includes, but is not limited to, fever, leukocytosis, activation of complement and coagulation cascades, and secretion of acute phase proteins. SIRS is a specifically defined subset of the acute phase response that describes changes in vital signs and white blood cell count and is manifested by two or more of the following: fever or hypothermia, tachycardia, tachypnea, and either leukocytosis, leukocytopenia or an increased band count.[14] Ironically, these responses can be excessive and lead to greater morbidity and mortality in some cases than the initiating insult itself. The infusion of allogeneic blood cells during transfusion can constitute a significant immunologic insult to the recipient despite the therapeutic intent of the ordering physician. During the transfusion reactions that sometimes ensue, such as with FNHTR, hemolytic, and septic transfusion reactions, the transfusion recipient may develop symptoms that approach or in some cases fulfill the criteria of SIRS or the acute phase response. Accordingly, it may be reasonable to predict that pro-inflammatory cytokines mediate some of the symptom complex of these acute transfusion reactions.

The prevention of many transfusion reactions is likely to require the prevention of generation of cytokines and other biologic response modifiers. Leukocytes, particularly monocytes/macrophages, are a major source of cytokines. The two possible sources of leukocytes in the transfusion setting are the donor, i.e., the transfused blood component, and the recipient. Thus, a means to prevent cytokine generation is to remove one possible source and/or stimulus of cytokine generation by removing leukocytes from the donor unit. In succeeding sections we will consider the role of leukocytes, pro-inflammatory cytokines, as well as other cytokines and biological response modifiers in the pathogenesis of a variety of transfusion reactions. We will discuss the theoretical and/or actual advantage of leukodepletion in preventing those reactions and where relevant we will discuss the possible advantages of prestorage versus bedside leukodepletion.

FEBRILE NON-HEMOLYTIC
TRANSFUSION REACTIONS (FNHTR)

A FNHTR is often defined as a 1°C rise in body temperature and/or chills occurring within several hours of transfusion. The fever must be unrelated to hemolysis or infection and often lasts a few hours, but rarely as long as 24 hours. A chill sensation and in more severe reactions, shaking chills, can precede the onset of fever. In mild reactions there may be a chill without a detectable febrile response. In recent years the pathogenesis of fever in general has become increasingly well-understood.[15] Some disturbance of homeosta-

sis, such as an immunologic reaction or infection, stimulates monocytes, macrophages, endothelial cells, fibroblasts and other cells to synthesize and secrete pro-inflammatory cytokines (Fig. 6.1). According to current models the pyrogenic cytokines (e.g. IL-1, IL-6, TNF-α) reach the thermoregulatory center of the anterior hypothalamus via the systemic circulation.[5,15] They initiate fever by inducing the synthesis of arachidonic acid and prostaglandins, including prostaglandin E_2 (PGE$_2$). PGE$_2$ acts on the anterior hypothalamus to raise the thermostatic set point by altering the firing rate of thermoregulatory neurons. This in turn sets in motion a series of responses intended to elevate the body temperature to the new set point. These include muscle contraction and shivering to increase heat generation and peripheral vasoconstriction to conserve heat. During the period that the body temperature is below the new set point an individual may subjectively feel a chill. The chill is probably a manifestation of the heat-conserving cutaneous vasoconstriction and usually is a prelude to a fever. As noted above, a chill may occur in the apparent absence of a documented fever, particularly when body temperature is not monitored at frequent intervals. Nevertheless, chills in the setting of transfusion should be considered a mild FNHTR since the mechanism is presumably the same that underlies an actual fever.

FNHTRs have been associated with and attributed to recipient antibodies to transfused leukocytes or platelets. Frequently the implicated antibodies have specificity for human leukocyte antigens (HLA) antigens, but may also be granulocyte- or platelet-specific.[16-19] Those at greatest risk for making such antibodies, such as previously transfused or pregnant recipients, are most likely to suffer FNHTRs. The role of donor leukocytes in the pathogenesis of FNHTR is supported by the finding that the infusion of the leukocyte-rich portion of whole blood is capable of inducing fever in transfusion recipients.[20] A minimum of approximately

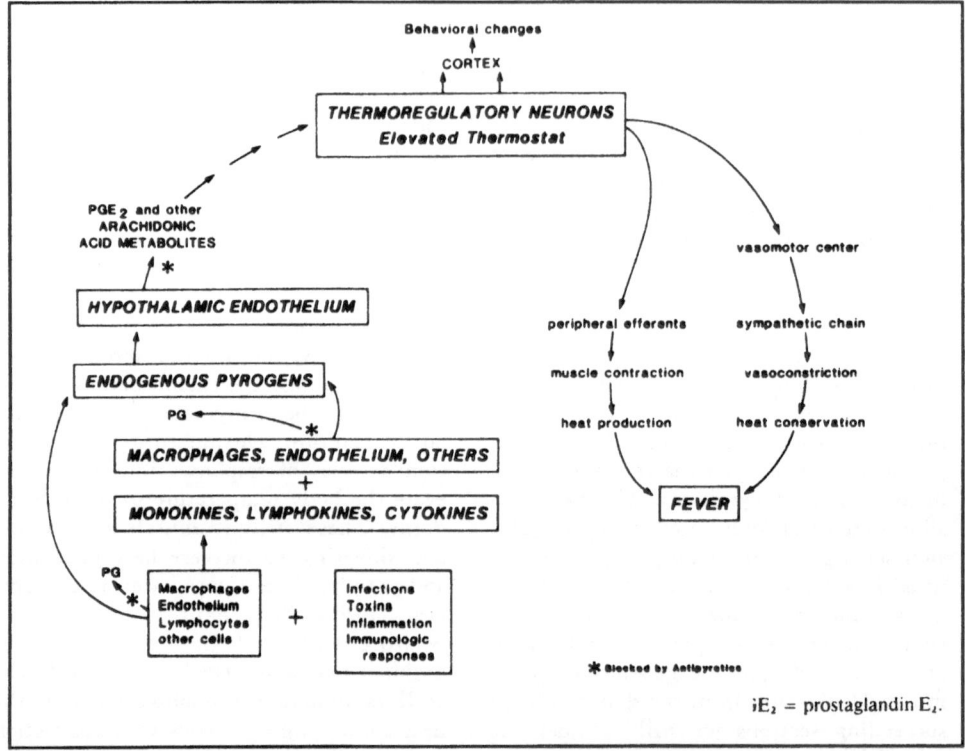

Fig. 6.1. Proposed mechanism for the development of fever. (Reprinted with permission from Dinarello CA, Cannon JC, Wolff SM. Rev Infect Dis 1988; 10:168. © University of Chicago Press)

5×10^8 leukocytes per unit appears necessary to cause a FNHTR, although this number varies somewhat for different patients.[21-24] A variety of techniques that produce about a 90% or one-log reduction of the leukocyte content of cellular blood components, such as saline washing, freezing and deglycerolization, and microaggregate filtration, reduce the leukocyte content below that threshold and reduce the incidence of FNHTR.[22-24] (See chapter 2) Newer leukodepletion filters, which provide the most efficient leukodepletion technique yet, are capable of a 3 log leukocyte depletion or more. However, published and anecdotal reports indicate that febrile reactions are still reported with these bedside filters at a rate greater than expected from the degree of leukodepletion.[25] In some cases this may be due to the failure of filtration to remove as many leukocytes

as expected due to problems in technique or filter variability. However, this also raises several questions regarding the pathogenesis and prevention of FNHTR: (1) Is leukocyte removal alone sufficient to prevent all FNHTR? (2) Is an element in the filtrate remaining after leukodepletion responsible for mediating some FNHTRs? The recent discovery of cytokines in the plasma/supernatant portion of cellular blood components, several of which are capable of inducing fever and various other acute reactions, may provide an explanation for the apparent filter failures, as well as for FNHTR occurring in recipients that have no leukocyte or platelet antibodies or in those who receive autologous blood.[26-33]

Based on our understanding of the pathogenesis of fever, FNHTRs are expected to be the result of elevated levels of pyrogenic cytokines in the transfusion recipient.[15] This may occur by one or more of several different mechanisms. First, recipient cells (leukocytes, endothelial cells, etc.) may be stimulated directly or indirectly by infused foreign cells or plasma to produce pyrogenic cytokines. Secondly, donor leukocytes may be stimulated in vivo to produce cytokines upon infusion into the recipient. For example, this may occur when anti-leukocyte antibodies in the recipients in vitro bind to the infused donor leukocytes. Third, donor leukocytes in the component bag may be stimulated to produce pyrogenic cytokines during storage. If sufficient quantities of pyrogenic cytokines accumulate during blood component storage, they might induce a febrile response upon passive infusion into a recipient during the transfusion. While it is possible that all three potential cytokine sources play a role, only the latter has been well-documented in the transfusion setting. That is, cytokine accumulation occurs in vitro in the plasma/supernatant portion of some blood components presumably due to synthesis and secretion by passenger leukocytes during blood bank storage. IL-8 was the first reported cytokine to be detected in the plasma portion of stored platelet concentrates (PC) prepared for blood bank use.[26] Stack and Snyder showed that the percentage of PC with detectable IL-8 ranged from 30% of 2-day-old units up to 83% of 5-day-old units.[27] These PC were stored as single, unpooled units. As such, no immunologic humoral or cellular incompatibility could have existed as a stimulus. In a given unit of PC the IL-8 concentration in the plasma portion increased with both storage time and total white blood cell count (Fig. 6.2).

Subsequently, several groups have shown that other pro-inflammatory cytokines, including IL-1β, IL-6, TNF-α, and MIP-1α are generated and accumulate in stored PC.[27-33] Since these cytokines have pyrogenic activity, they could be expected, if present in high enough concentration, to induce febrile responses in transfusion recipients. In fact, Muylle et al found an association between high levels of IL-6 and

TNF-α in the plasma portion of PC with the occurrence of FNHTR in transfusion recipients.[28] A report by Heddle et al, also supports a role of cytokines in the plasma portion of PC in mediating FNHTR.[31] In their study PCs were divided into a cellular portion and a plasma/supernatant portion. Patients requiring platelet transfusion received the two portions in two infusions separated by a 2 hour interval. Febrile reactions were noted to be significantly higher following the plasma/supernatant portion of the PC than following the cellular portion. Moreover, the plasma/supernatant portions that caused FNHTR contained higher levels of IL-1β and IL-6 than those that did not cause a febrile response. These data support the role of the plasma/supernatant portion of PC as a source of pro-inflammatory cytokines and a possible important stimulus of FNHTR.[31]

To examine the potential role of cytokines in mediating FNHTR to RBC transfusion, pro-inflammatory cytokines have also been measured in the supernatant portion of stored RBC. Since RBC are stored in the cold (1-6°C), the capacity for passenger leukocytes in RBC units to synthesize and secrete cytokines should be reduced compared to PC due to the inhibitory effect of cold on cellular metabolism. Despite cold storage, however, Stack et al and Smith et al measured IL-8 and IL-1β in stored RBC.[32,33] IL-8 reached levels in some units of RBC in the range at 200 to 2000 pg/mL by 42-days of storage.[32] The levels of IL-1β generated during RBC storage would appear to be too low (≤20 pg/mL) to mediate significant physiologic reactions, particularly after dilution in the systemic circulation. However, low levels of cytokines are known to have additive or synergistic effects with other cytokines.[34-36]

IL-8 appears to be present in higher concentrations in stored blood components than other leukocyte-derived pro-inflammatory cytokines measured to date. Levels as high as 200 ng/mL have been detected in 5-day-old platelet concentrates.[27] Since

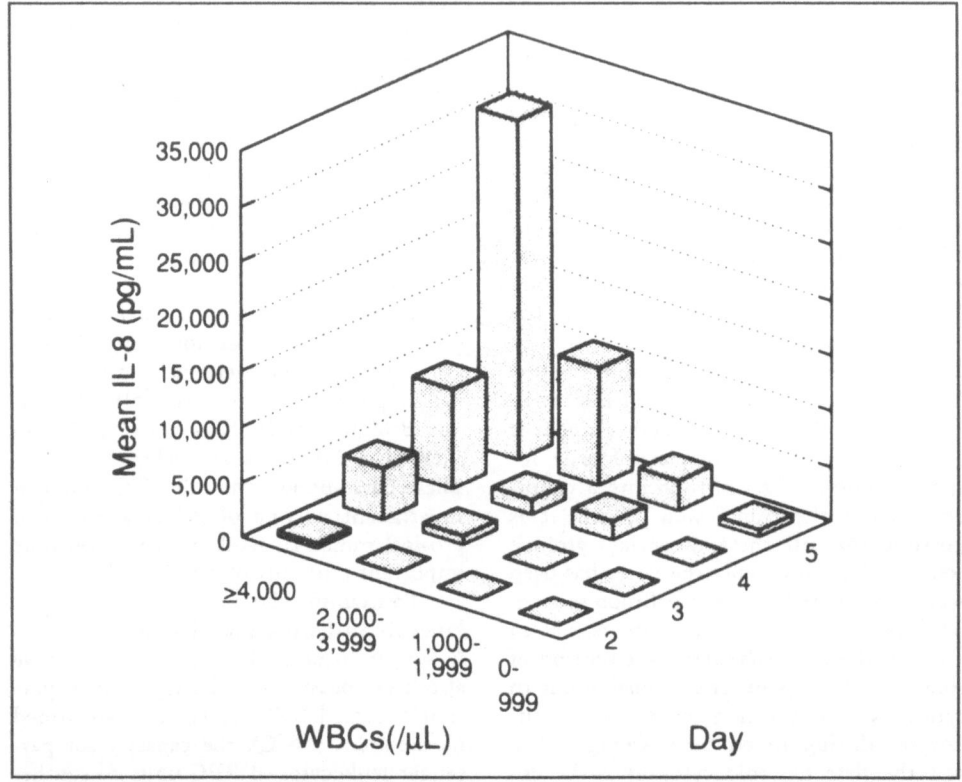

Fig. 6.2. Relationship of IL-8 levels in platelet concentrates to storage time and white blood cell count. (Reprinted with permission from Transfusion 1993;34:20, published by the American Association of Blood Banks.)

IL-8, unlike IL-1β, IL-6, and TNF-α, is not known to have pyrogenic activity in humans, it is not clear at this time whether it mediates acute reactions or other adverse consequences to RBC or platelet transfusions. IL-8 is a member of the chemokine family of pro-inflammatory cytokines.[2,10,11] IL-8 stimulates the migration of leukocytes to sites of inflammation, neutrophil activation and degranulation, and basophil release of histamine.[10,11,37,38] Levels of plasma IL-8 are increased in sepsis and correlate with the severity of the sepsis syndrome.[39,40] The intravenous infusion of human recombinant IL-8 in non-human primates induces a transient granulocytopenia followed by a prolonged rebound granulocytosis.[41] In addition, intravenous IL-8 administration inhibits neutrophil migration to sites of acute inflammation.[42] Repeated intravenous IL-8 administration has been reported to cause lung injury in rats with features similar to the human adult respiratory distress syndrome.[43] IL-8 has a priming effect on leukocytes that renders them more sensitive to the effects of other pro-inflammatory cytokines, such as TNF-α.[36] Thus, in theory IL-8 may mediate or exacerbate a variety of reactions, including allergic reactions and transfusion-related acute lung injury (TRALI). Through its priming effect, IL-8 may augment the pyrogenic activities of other cytokines, both endogenous and exogenous. However, none of these reactions to IL-8 has been documented to date in the transfusion setting and they remain theoretical possibilities that require further investigation.

The clinical significance of infused IL-8 and several other chemokines may be decreased by the presence of an erythrocyte chemokine receptor on RBC membranes.[44-46] Recent evidence indicates that the Duffy blood group antigen is a promiscuous and high affinity receptor for at least several chemokines, including IL-8, melanoma growth stimulatory activity (MGSA), MCP-1 and RANTES, but not MIP-1α.[44,46] The receptor may serve in vivo as a sink to pull these chemokines effectively out of circulation. This raises the intriguing possibility that the biological effect of intravenously infused IL-8 and other chemokines generated in stored blood components may be greater in Duffy-negative than in Duffy (Fy^a or Fy^b)-positive individuals. However, no data has been reported that demonstrates the actual function of the erythrocyte chemokine receptor, nor has a similar erythrocyte receptor been reported for other pro-inflammatory cytokines such as IL-1β, IL-6, and TNF-α.

While the cell source of the storage-generated cytokines has not yet been directly demonstrated, it is evident that cytokine production particularly in platelet concentrates, is proportional to the leukocyte content of the unit.[27,28] In addition, pre-storage or early storage (within one to two days of duration) leukodepletion by third generation filtration prevents their generation in stored PC and RBC.[27,30,32,33,47] Therefore, whether or not leukocytes produce the cytokines themselves, their participation in storage-related cytokine production is nevertheless essential. The stimulus for cytokine generation during blood component storage remains to be determined. There are at least several possibilities. First, leukocytes may be subject to contact activation upon interaction with the plastic blood component bag wall. Adherence to plastic is a known stimulus of cytokine production by monocytes.[48-51] Also, bacterial products such as endotoxin or certain exotoxins are known inducers of cytokine secretion by leukocytes.[5,40] The presence of bacteria in stored blood components has been shown to increase the levels of some storage-related cytokines, particularly in platelet concentrates (see below).[32,52] While this mechanism could account for storage-related cytokines in some blood component bags, it seems unlikely that enough units are sufficiently contaminated to account for all of the published observations. One can also speculate that other potential stimuli, such as shear stress during the manipulations carried out for blood component preparation or continuous agitation of platelet concentrates during storage, may also stimulate storage-related cytokine generation.

Estimates have been made regarding the number of passenger leukocytes in platelet concentrates necessary for storage-related cytokine generation. Stack and Snyder observed that 97 percent of units with IL-8 levels $\geq$1000 pg/mL had either $\geq$2000 WBC per L or storage time $\geq$4 days.[27] Cytokine levels (IL-8, IL-1β, IL-6, TNF-α) were not detected in units with <1000 passenger leukocytes per L and that had been stored 4 days or less. Muylle et al observed TNF-α, IL-6, or IL-1 generation only in platelet concentrates with $\geq$3000 passenger leukocytes per L.[28] Prestorage or early storage leukoreduction by third-generation filters appears to prevent storage-related cytokine generation because it reduces passenger leukocytes to well below these apparent threshold levels. If cytokine infusion proves to be a cause of a significant number of nonhemolytic transfusion reactions, then this may represent an important justification for pre- or early-storage leukoreduction by filtration. Bedside leukoreduction filtration would not offer this advantage since the leukocytes would still be present and would generate cytokines during storage. In all there appears to be reasonable evidence to suspect that cytokines in transfused PC contribute to the FNHTRs that occur despite the use of third-generation filters at the bedside. However, definitive clinical studies have yet to be published demonstrating that storage-related cytokines actually cause FNHTR or other adverse effects.

Table 6.1. Some probable mediators of systemic inflammatory response syndrome accompanying hemolytic transfusion reactions

Complement-derived anaphylatoxins (C3a, C5a)

Kinins

Cytokines: Including TNF-α, IL-1, IL-6, IL-8, MCP-1

Mast cell/platelet products: Serotonin, histamine

HEMOLYTIC TRANSFUSION REACTIONS

A hemolytic transfusion reaction occurs when allogeneic red blood cells are infused intravenously into a recipient who has antibodies to membrane antigens on the infused RBC. The formation of the RBC antigen:antibody complex sets in motion a complex series of humoral and cellular events, the nature of which depends often, but not exclusively, on the molecular characteristics (e.g. isotype) of the antibody. In some cases, as with IgM antibodies directed against ABO system antigens, the outcome is intravascular hemolysis. The signs and symptoms that accompany intravascular hemolysis include fever, chest pain, hypotension, nausea, flushing, and dyspnea.[53] Severe reactions progress to shock, disseminated intravascular coagulation, renal failure, and sometimes death. In other cases, for example with IgG antibodies directed against blood group antigens of the Rh system, the outcome is a generally less clinically severe extravascular hemolysis. The transfusion reaction signs and symptoms of extravascular hemolytic reactions commonly include fever and jaundice. Detailed descriptions of which blood group systems are implicated in which kind of reactions as well as detailed descriptions of the clinical reactions can be found elsewhere.[54,55]

The symptom complex of intravascular hemolytic reactions often includes SIRS and is part of an acute phase response. SIRS accompanying hemolytic reactions is prob- ably mediated by a network of several classes of biologic response modifiers (Table 6.1).[56] Models of the pathogenesis of these reactions attribute many of these responses to the initial activation of complement and the generation of anaphylatoxins C3a and C5a.[54,56] In addition, activation of factor XII (Hageman factor) by immune complexes may set in motion a cascade leading to the generation of bradykinin. Activation of factor XII also is the first step in the intrinsic coagulation pathway, which, along with procoagulant effect of RBC stroma generated by hemolysis, may contribute to the onset of disseminated intravascular coagulation. Anaphylatoxin- activated mast cells and immune complex- activated platelets are probable sources of histamine and serotonin.

More recent data indicate that cytokines also play a key role in mediating hemolysis-associated SIRS. IL-8, TNF-α, MCP-1 (monocyte chemoattractant protein-1) are generated in a test tube model of intravascular hemolysis.[57-59] Hemolysis results when ABO-incompatible, washed RBC are added to heparinized whole blood at 37 in vitro. During the ensuing 6 hours cytokines are synthesized and secreted by leukocytes present in the whole blood specimen. Peak TNF-α levels have been detected at 2-4 hours after addition of incompatible RBC.[58] IL-8 is detected by 4 hours and MCP-1 between 6 and 24 hours.[57,59] While levels of IL-8 and MCP-1 continue to increase, TNF-α levels return to baseline by 24 hours. Analogous studies of cytokine generation during incompatible transfusions in vivo have not be done in humans. However, a case report indicates that TNF-α was generated and detected in the bloodstream of a type O patient who by error received 100 ml of type A RBC.[60] The direct biochemical stimulus of cytokine production in the setting of RBC incompatibility and hemolysis has not been determined. However, preliminary data indicates that complement may be required in some cases.[57]

Extravascular hemolytic reactions, where IgG-coated RBC are taken up by phagocytic cells of the reticuloendothelial system, also result in fever and in some cases a milder version of the acute inflammatory response. An in vitro model system of extravascular hemolytic transfusion reactions has also been developed. In this model IgG-sensitized RBC were added to monocyte cell cultures. IL-1, IL-6, and TNF-α were synthesized and secreted by the monocytes beginning 2-6 hours after exposure to IgG-coated RBCs.[61,62] Thus, pro-inflammatory cytokines may be one of the classes of biologic response modifiers that play an important role in the symptom complex of extravascular hemolytic transfusion reactions.

The generation of the pro-inflammatory cytokines could help explain many of the symptoms and signs of intravascular and extravascular hemolytic transfusion reactions, in particular the late or delayed symptoms. For example, IL-1β is known to induce fever, somnolence, and at high doses hypotension and shock.[6] TNF-α has similar effects and can stimulate the production of and act synergistically with other pro-inflammatory cytokines.[5,14,63] IL-6 also induces fever and the acute phase response.[7] During the in vitro studies of hemolysis the generation of cytokines was delayed several hours presumably due to the need for new synthesis as demonstrated by increased cytokine RNA levels.[57,59] This lag phase would argue against these cytokines mediating the immediate signs and symptoms of intravascular hemolysis. More immediate reactions, such as flushing, tachypnea, tachycardia and hypotension seen in intravascular hemolysis would more likely be attributable to other mediators, such as histamine and bradykinin, which can be generated more rapidly by secretion from pre-existent intracellular pools or by generation via enzymatic cascade. Later reactions such as fever, on the other hand, occur on a time course consistent with the generation and activity of pyrogenic inflammatory cytokines.

Leukodepletion of RBC is unlikely to have any impact on the majority of hemolytic transfusion reactions. The underlying immune incompatibility exists in virtually all cases with RBC, not WBC antigens. Rarely, hemolytic reactions have been reported which have been attributed to antibodies to Bg antigens, which are actually human leukocyte antigens (HLA).[64,65] It is possible that leukodepletion of RBC units either at the bedside or pre-storage could decrease or delay the development of Bg antibodies in transfusion recipients, as has been demonstrated for HLA antibodies in general, and prevent such reactions. However, Bg antibody-mediated hemolysis appears to be a rare event and clinically mild when it occurs. Of greater significance, leukodepletion should reduce the number of hemolytic reaction investigations. The major reason for investigating any febrile response to transfusion is to rule out immune hemolysis, since fever is the most common manifestation of a hemolytic transfusion reaction.[53] Because leukodepletion should decrease FNHTR (see above), such transfusion reaction investigations also should be reduced, resulting in savings in laboratory and clinical staff time and expense. In addition, transfusion delays and patient discomfort should be decreased.

ALLERGIC TRANSFUSION REACTIONS

Allergic transfusion reactions are most commonly attributed to the infusion of plasma proteins. Allergic manifestations vary from mild urticaria to severe anaphylactoid reactions. These allergic reactions result from antigen-antibody interactions that stimulate the release of histamine from mast cells and basophils and in all likelihood the generation of other vasoactive biological response modifiers such as kinins and complement-derived anaphylatoxins. Elevated plasma levels of histamine, in fact, have been measured in patients undergoing anaphylactoid transfusion reactions.[66] Based on our understanding of allergic reactions in other clinical and experimental settings, allergic transfusion reactions likely have at least two pathogenetic mechanisms: (1) immediate-type hypersensitivity reactions mediated by IgE, and (2) anaphylactoid reactions resulting from the interaction of transfused IgA (or other soluble donor plasma molecules) with recipient anti-IgA (or antibodies directed against some other soluble molecule in the donor plasma).

Donor leukocytes, in particular basophils, may also play a role in allergic reactions due to the release of histamine during blood component storage. Evidence from in vitro studies indicates that the level of histamine in the plasma or supernatant portion of stored platelets concentrates and red blood cells increases with increasing blood bank storage time. Frewin et al measured a progressive increase in plasma histamine levels in unfiltered additive solution red blood cells that reached a peak mean value of 67 ± 17 ng/mL after 42 days of storage.[67] Units of red blood cells that were leukodepletion post-storage by buffy coat removal had lower levels of histamine at 18 ± 10 ng/mL. However, pre-storage leukodepletion by filtration gave units with even lower histamine levels, ranging from 0.4 to 7 ng/mL depending on the filter. These results are in agreement with other reports showing that plasma histamine levels increase progressively during both platelet and red blood cell storage and that removal of leukocytes from units of blood before storage reduces the increase in histamine.[66,68-70] The extent of leukocyte removal parallels the reduction in plasma histamine. By reducing the amount of infused histamine, leukodepletion could decrease the degree or frequency of allergic transfusion reactions that are attributable to storage-generated histamine. However, leukodepletion, whether pre-storage, post-storage, or bedside, cannot prevent allergic reactions that result from biological response modifiers that are generated in vivo. The relative extent to which storage-generated as opposed to in vivo generated histamine contributes to allergic transfusion reactions is unknown. Since microgram quantities of histamine may need to be infused to give a clinically significant level in transfusion recipients,[70] storage-generated histamine would seem to be less significant. However, clinical correlations have shown that older units of red blood cells are more likely to be associated with anaphylactoid transfusion reactions, which suggests that a storage-related change, such as in vitro histamine generation, could be contributing to these reactions.[66]

Based on their biologic activities, the complement-derived anaphylatoxins, C3a and C5a, are expected to be generated and to play a role in transfusion recipients undergoing anaphylactoid transfusion reactions. While C3a and C5a appear not to be generated in vitro during red blood cell storage, Holme et al have reported the generation of the complement fragment C3a, but not C5a, during platelet storage.[71,72] Furthermore, passage of platelet concentrates through some leukocyte depletion filters made of cotton wool as well as one polyester filter also results in the generation of C3 activation products.[72-74] The transfusion of C3a generated in vitro in stored platelets has been shown to be associated with an increase in the post-transfusion levels of C3a in transfusion recipients.[72] The C3a complement component is believed to be generated due to an internal thioester bond rearrangement which occurs spontaneously and upon contact with plastic surfaces.[75] C5 is not as easily or readily activated. Two reports have shown that not all leukocyte depletion filters (LDF) are associated with the generation of the C3a complement component.[73,74] Indeed, the Pall PL50 and PL100 filters were reported to decrease levels of C3a post-filtration on the order of 90-95%.[74,76] A recent submitted abstract by Snyder et al reported similar findings for a new generation of bedside filter (Pall PXL-8) as well.[77] The mechanism of this removal is unclear and may relate to the adherence of the C3a to the filter media or to the polymer coating of the polyester filter fiber.[75] However, there have been no reports of clinically symptomatic allergic transfusion reactions clearly attributable to infusion of preformed C3a. Thus, the clinical relevance of this phenomenon is uncertain. Regardless, it is generally considered prudent to avoid infusion of any biological response modifier. Bedside filtration would seem to offer a possible advantage over pre-storage filtration for the removal of storage-generated C3a in platelet concentrates. However, not all leukodepletion filters have the same effect and some may even increase C3a levels.

TRALI

Transfusion-related acute lung injury (TRALI) is characterized by acute respiratory distress resulting from noncardiogenic pulmonary edema usually occurring within several hours of transfusion.[78,79] Other associated signs and symptoms include fever, hypoxemia, and hypotension. TRALI is associated in the majority of reported cases with passive transfer of donor HLA- or granulocyte-specific antibodies or anti-5b antibodies to the transfusion recipient.[78-81] For an as yet unexplained reason the interaction of donor antibodies with recipient cells initiates a response in which the lung is targeted for injury. In an animal model complement appears to be essential for the induction of TRALI.[82] Therefore, in one conceptual model the donor anti-body-recipient leukocyte interaction would lead to the activation of complement as the initial event leading to TRALI. The concomitant generation of C5a, a granulocyte chemotaxin, would result in granulocyte migration to the lungs. The reason for the apparent pulmonary specificity is unclear, but lung inflammation has been reproduced in rabbits following the injection of C5a.[83] Activation of the recruited granulocytes presumably results in the activation of CD11a/CD18 and CD11b/CD18 complexes on the cell surface.[84] This would promote adherence of the granulocytes to the vascular endothelial wall and permit diapedesis whereby they would enter the alveolar interstitial space (Fig. 6.3). Subsequent degranulation would result in the release of destructive lysosomal enzymes and the development of a capillary leak syndrome and non-cardiogenic pulmonary edema. Activated granulocytes also may produce oxygen radicals which could damage pulmonary endothelial cells, resulting in an increase in pulmonary vascular permeability and the further passage of fluid into alveolar spaces.

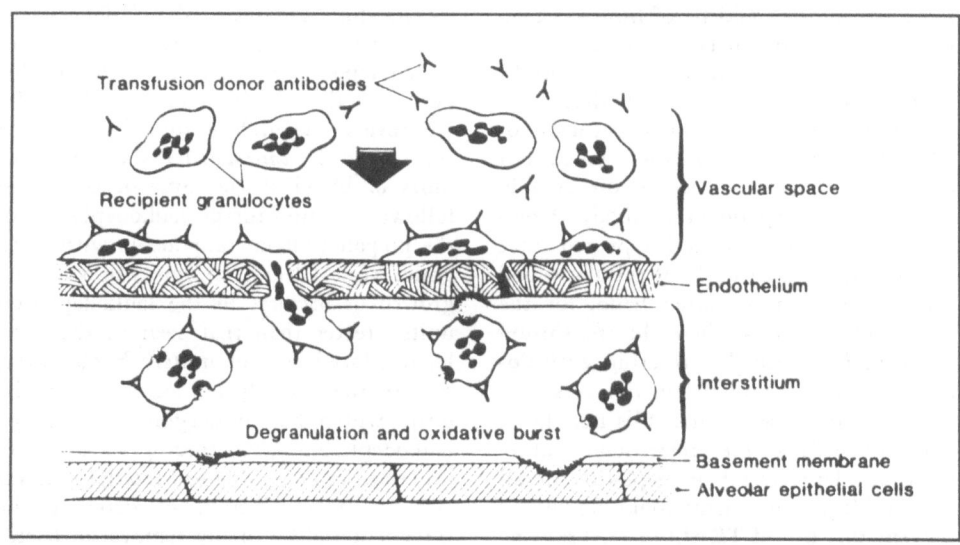

Fig. 6.3. Proposed mechanism of transfusion-related acute lung injury. (Reproduced with permission from Swank DW, Moore SB. Roles of the neutrophil and other mediators in adult respiratory distress syndrome. Mayo Clin Proc 1989; 64:1118-1132.)

IL-8, which is produced in stored units of platelet concentrate and red blood cells, is known to produce acute lung injury upon repeated intravenous administration in laboratory animals.[43] In addition, IL-8 is chemotactic for granulocytes and is emerging as an important mediator involved in recruiting neutrophils to the lung in human acute lung injury in general.[38] In the lungs alveolar macrophages appear to be a major source of IL-8, although type II pneumocytes, lung fibroblasts, and pulmonary endothelial cells also can produce IL-8.[38] Thus, based on known biological activity, it is feasible that IL-8, in addition to C5a, could play a role in TRALI, Although it is mere speculation at this time, the infusion of IL-8 generated in vitro during blood component storage could also plausibly play a role in inducing TRALI. Pre-storage leukodepletion would offer a potential benefit should that be the case since it would decrease the in vitro generation and subsequent infusion of IL-8 during transfusion.

Since Popovsky et al[78] reported that 89% of TRALI in their series of 36 cases was caused by donor antibody reacting with recipient leukocytes, leukodepletion of the donor unit should be of limited or no value for the majority of cases. Donor screening and rejection of units with high-titer leukocyte or HLA antibodies is of theoretical benefit in the prevention of TRALI. In addition, saline-washed red blood cells or platelets would presumably help by removing donor antibody. However, this is not a practical approach since it is not feasible to wash all cellular blood components. On the other hand, for the 6% of TRALI cases where the transfusion recipient has antibodies reacting with donor leukocytes,[78] rather than vice versa, removal of transfused neutrophils may be of clinical benefit for the prevention of future reactions. Universal leukodepletion of all cellular blood components could potentially prevent this 6% of TRALI cases. Pre-storage or bedside leukodepletion would seem to offer equal benefit for this purpose. However, since the number of donor leu-

kocytes necessary to cause TRALI is unknown in these cases, leukodepletion for the prevention of TRALI is a theoretical concept only.

SEPSIS

Despite strict arm cleansing protocols, it is impossible to completely sterilize the donor arm prior to venipuncture. This is because bacteria reside in the outer layer of squamous epithelium over the antecubital fossa. Accordingly, when a needle is inserted into the arm, some bacteria may enter the blood bag along with the first few drops of blood collected. Rarely, the bacteria can proliferate to produce an infected blood component unit.[85,86] Numerous studies have been published evaluating whether use of prestorage leukodepletion filters would result in a higher or lower incidence of bacterially-contaminated blood products.[87-91] Some researchers posed the hypothesis that pre-storage leukodepletion would increase the risk of bacterial growth since the granulocytes present in units of blood or blood component may serve the important function of phagocytosis of bacteria present in the unit.[92-94] Concerns were raised that pre-storage leukodepletion would allow an increased proliferation of any contaminating bacteria. Published research reports, however, have shown this not to be the case in actual practice.[87-91]

Several research groups have shown that when *Y. enterocolitica* was added to units of blood at the time of collection followed by pre-storage leukodepletion of the prepared blood components with third generation filters, in no case was the growth of bacteria in the leukodepletion units greater than that seen in the non-leukoreduced control units.[87-90] Moreover, growth was actually less or absent in the units which had undergone pre-storage leukodepletion. This finding is generally explained as being due to bacterial removal either by direct adherence of bacteria to the filter material.[87,95] or by removal of bacteria because they are associated with leukocytes by adherence or phagocytosis.[89,92] Högman et al demonstrated that bacteria proliferated to a greater extent when added to already leukodepleted units as compared with the nonleukodepleted control units.[92] Their study supports the role of passenger leukocytes in limiting bacterial growth in stored blood, but is not a good model for what actually occurs during blood donation. In reality bacteria will be present in the donated blood prior to leukodepletion. Nevertheless, bacterial adherence to leukocytes or phagocytosis of bacteria by leukocytes in blood during the first few hours after collection appears to play a significant role in reducing bacterial contamination and growth in blood components. Overall, the data indicate that in actual practice pre-storage leukodepletion will not result in a higher incidence of *Y. enterocoliticia* contamination of red blood cells. On the contrary, *Y. enterocolitica* contamination appears to be significantly reduced by prestorage, leukocyte filtration. Similar findings have been obtained for some other bacteria and for platelet concentrates.[91,96] However, it is unlikely that the filter manufacturers will attempt, or that the FDA will permit, leukodepletion filters to be labeled as being acceptable for bacterial removal. The presence of so many species and serotypes of bacteria and the likely influence of many donor-specific factors preclude such labeling.

Based on our understanding of the role of cytokines in the response syndrome that accompanies sepsis,[7,12,13] cytokines are likely to play a major role in the symptom complex of septic transfusion reactions. Cytokines may be generated from several potential sources in the setting of septic transfusion reactions: (1) recipient leukocytes, endothelial cells, and other cell types in response to infusion of bacteria, (2) donor leukocytes after infusion into recipients, or (3) donor leukocytes in vitro during storage in the presence of bacteria or bacterial products. While the recipient leukocytes and other cells would seem to be the major potential source of cytokines in septic transfusion reactions, a recent preliminary report by Stack et al has also documented that bacteria in stored PC may

stimulate a large increase in plasma cytokines in the component bag.[52] For example, *E. coli* contamination of PC resulted in up to 10- to 20-fold higher plasma/supernatant concentrations of the cytokines IL-8 and IL-1β in the platelet storage bag after 5 days of storage than in sterile control PC. In addition, *Y. enterocolitia* stimulated IL-8 and IL-1β generation in stored RBC.[32] The magnitude of the effect of bacterial contamination on cytokine generation in RBC units is substantially less than that observed in PC. This could be due to several factors, including the nature and growth characteristics of the organism, the temperature of storage, degree of WBC contamination, and metabolic activity of the leukocytes and bacteria. Because of the more modest effect of bacteria on cytokine generation in stored RBC, as opposed to stored PC, the most severe septic transfusion reactions to contaminated RBC are less likely to be mediated by storage-related cytokines alone than by the in vivo generation of cytokines and other biologic response modifiers. These findings indicate that pro-inflammatory cytokines produced in vitro during the storage of bacterially-contaminated blood components, especially PC, are another source of biologic response mediators that may mediate the symptoms of septic transfusion reactions. Storage-generated cytokines have the potential to stimulate immediate responses in the transfusion recipient following infusion of a bacterially-contaminated unit. By contrast cytokines generated in vivo in the transfusion recipient are more likely to stimulate responses with a longer lag time following transfusion due to the apparent need for new synthesis of many of these cytokines.

Leukocyte depletion by third generation filters early in platelet or red blood cell storage prevented or significantly decreased the generation of cytokines during storage even in units heavily contaminated with bacteria.[32,52] Thus, through a combination of removing some bacteria prior to storage as well as preventing cytokine generation during storage, pre-storage leukodepletion offers several theoretical advantages over bedside leukodepletion in reducing septic transfusion reactions. Bedside leukodepletion after several days of storage is not likely to be effective in removing the large numbers of bacteria that may have proliferated by that time nor is there any reason to expect that bedside filtration will remove bacterial products such as endotoxin or exotoxins.

TA-GVHD

Transfusion-associated graft-versus-host disease (TA-GVHD) results from the infusion of viable T lymphocytes into immunosuppressed recipients.[97,98] However, even immunocompetent transfusion recipients may at times be at risk for TA-GVHD when the donor is homozygous and the recipient is heterozygous for the same HLA haplotype.[99] In both cases the transfused T cells are insufficiently opposed by the recipient's immune system and are free to attack host tissue. Effects on skin, liver, gastrointestinal tract and bone marrow are clinically most evident.[97] TA-GVHD is over 90% fatal due to the involvement of the bone marrow, resulting in aplasia and pancytopenia. This is in contrast to GVHD following bone marrow transplantation, where the bone marrow is spared.[100] The major cytokines responsible for GVHD in animal models, are believed to be IL-2, γ-interferon, and TNF.[97] Some preliminary evidence suggests that IL-8 may also play a role.[101] Host tissue damage appears to be mediated principally by the secretion of TNF-α and lymphotoxin (TNF-β) by donor cytotoxic T and NK cells.[97] While there is little data to indicate the minimum number of donor lymphocytes required to mediate TA-GVHD, 10^7 lymphocytes per kg is a frequently quoted estimate largely based on animal studies.[96-98,102,103] However, the number of leukocytes reported to cause TA-GVHD in a child with severe combined immunodeficiency syndrome who received fresh plasma (not FFP) was only 10^4 leukocytes per kilogram body weight.[104]

Gamma irradiation of donor blood, not leukodepletion, is the recommended treatment for inactivating the immunocompetent donor leukocytes in order to prevent TA-GVHD in susceptible transfusion recipients.[105,106] The FDA has recently ruled that the minimum acceptable dose of radiation to prevent TA-GVHD is 2500 cGy to the center of the blood bag with at least 1500 cGy to the edge of the bag.[106] Since TA-GVHD is caused by infused passenger lymphocytes, it is theoretically possible that leukodepletion of blood components, if efficient enough, could decrease or prevent this complication.[107] At the present time, however, there is no actual clinical data to support the use of leukodepletion for prevention of TA-GVHD. As such, any reliance on leukodepletion to prevent TA-GVHD, an almost always fatal disease, would be ill-advised. In fact, Akahoshi et al reported a death due to failure of a third generation filter to prevent TA-GVHD in a recipient who received non-irradiated blood.[108] The role of leukodepletion in the prevention of GVHD should remain on issue for research only and not employed in clinical practice at the present time. Until the minimum number of donor leukocytes needed to produced GVHD is determined and leukodepletion becomes more efficient, it is mandatory that gamma radiation be used to prevent GVHD.

CONCLUSIONS

1. Leukocytes, whether from the transfusion donor or recipient, are responsible for most immune-mediated transfusion reactions.

2. Cytokines and other biologic response modifiers secreted or induced by donor or recipient leukocytes presumably are responsible for the symptom complex of many transfusion reactions. (Table 6.2)

3. Leukodepletion of donor blood components decreases the incidence of FNHTR. In addition, leukodepletion by filtration theoretically can decrease several other classes of transfusion reactions by the mechanisms summarized in Table. 6.3.

4. Biological response modifiers, such as the cytokines IL-1β, IL-6, IL-8, MIP-1α, as well as histamine, are gen-

erated during platelet storage. IL-8, IL-1β, and histamine also have been detected in the plasma/supernatant portion of stored RBCs.

5. The passive infusion of storage-generated cytokines and histamine during transfusion of stored blood components correlates with the onset of FNHTR and allergic reactions, respectively. A causal relationship between passive administration of storage-generated biologic response modifiers and transfusion reactions is strongly suggested.[31]

6. Pre-storage or early storage leukodepletion eliminates or significantly decreases storage-related cytokine and histamine-generation presumably by removing passenger leukocytes. This would be an advantage for preventing febrile, allergic, or septic reactions that might be induced by storage-related cytokines. (Table 6.3)

Table 6.2. Biologic response modifiers implicated in acute transfusion reactions

Sign/Symptom	Putative Mediator	Predominant Reaction Type
Fever Chills	IL-1β, IL-6, TNF-α, MIP-1α	FNHTR; hemolytic; septic
Hypotension Shock	C3a, C5a, bradykinin	Hemolytic; anaphylactoid; septic
Flushing	Histamine; serotonin	Allergic; anaphylactoid
Urticaria	Histamine	Allergic; anaphylactoid
Renal Failure Lower Back Pain	Catecholamine-mediated renal vasoconstriction; hypotension; DIC	Hemolytic
Dyspnea	C5a	Hemolytic; anaphylactoid; septic
Pulmonary Edema	C5a; IL-8	TRALI

Table 6.3. Leukoreduction by filtration: theoretical mechanisms for decreasing transfusion reactions

| Reaction Type | Time of Leukodepletion | |
	Prestorage	Bedside
Febrile	↓WBC ↓Storage-generated cytokines	↓WBC
Hemolytic	None	None
Allergic[1,2]	↓Donor Basophils ↓Storage-generated histamine	↓Donor Basophils ↓C3a
TRALI[3]	↓Granulocytes	↓Granulocytes
TA-GVHD[4]	↓T lymphocytes	↓T lymphocytes
Septic[5]	↓Inoculum size of some bacteria ↓Storage-generated cytokines and bacterial products	↓Bacterial load

[1] It is unclear to what extent, if any, donor cells contribute to in vivo histamine generation in transfusion recipients.
[2] Some polyester leukodepletion filters absorb and remove C3a from the plasma/supernatant portion of platelet concentrates (see text).
[3] Leukodepletion is predicted to decrease TRALI only in the small percentage (6%) of cases where the transfusion recipients have antibodies to donor leukocytes.
[4] The effectiveness of present leukodepletion techniques in decreasing TA-GVHD is unproven and not recommended.
[5] "Third generation" filters are variably effective in removing bacteria prestorage. The effectiveness of bedside filtration in removing bacteria from blood components post-storage is unclear and presumably limited to units with low bacterial colony counts.

7. Pre-storage leukoreduction by filtration removes some species of contaminating bacteria such as *Yersinia enterocolitica*, which may help prevent some septic transfusion reactions. (Table 6.3)

8. Leukodepletion theoretically could decrease TRALI in the small percentage (estimated 6%) of cases due to recipient rather than donor anti-HLA or anti-granulocyte specific antibodies. (Table 6.3)

9. While leukodepletion could theoretically decrease the risk of TA-GVHD, its actual effectiveness at the present time for that purpose is unproven. Moreover, a failure of leukodepletion by filtration to prevent TA-GVHD has been reported. Thus, leukodepletion should not be used at the present time to prevent GVHD.

10. Further research is needed to determine whether or to what extent pre-storage and bedside leukodepletion filters prevent transfusion reactions.

REFERENCES

1. Paul WE, Seder RA. Lymphocyte responses and cytokines. Cell 76:241, 1994.
2. Kelvin DJ, Michiel DF, Johnston JA, Lloyd AR, Sprenger H, Oppenheim JJ, Wang J-M. Chemokines and serpentines: the molecular biology of chemokine receptors. J. Leukocyte Biol 54:604, 1993.
3. Kishimoto T, Taga T, Akira S. Cytokine signal transduction. Cell.76:253, 1994.
4. Rees RC. Cytokines a biological response modifiers. J Clin Path 45:93, 1992.
5. Dinarello, CA. The endogenous pyrogens in host-defense interactions. Hosp Prac (Off Ed) 24:111, 1989.
6. Dinarello, CA. Interleukin-1 and interleukin-1 antagonism. Blood 77:1627, 1991.
7. Heinrich PC, Castell JV, Andus T. Interleukin-6 and the acute phase response. Biochem J 265:621, 1990.
8. Wolpe SD, Cerami A. Macrophage inflammatory proteins 1 and 2: members of a novel superfamily of cytokines. FASEB J 3:2565, 1989.
9. Matsushima K, Oppenheim JJ. Interleukin 8 and MCAF: novel inflammatory cytokines inducible by IL-1 and TNF. Cytokine 1:2, 1989.
10. Baggiolini M, Clark-Lewis I. Interleukin-8, a chemotactic and inflammatory cytokine. FEBS Letters 307:97, 1992.
11. Strieter RM, Kasahara K, Allen RM, Standiford TJ, Rolfe MW, Becker FS, Chensue SW, Kunkel SL. Cytokine-induced neutrophil-derived interleukin-8. Am J Pathol 141:397, 1992.
12. Calandra T, Glauser MP. Cytokines and septic shock. Diagn Microbiol Infect Dis 13:377, 1990.
13. Casey LC, Balk RA, Bone RC. Plasma cytokine and endotoxin levels correlate with survival in patients with the sepsis syndrome. Ann Intern Med 119:771, 1993.
14. Strieter RM, Kunkel SL, Bone RC. Role of tumor necrosis factor-α in disease states and inflammation. Crit Care Med 21:S447, 1993.
15. Dinarello CA, Cannon JG, Wolff SM. New concepts on the pathogenesis of fever. Rev Infect Dis 10:168, 1988.
16. Décary F et al. An investigation of nonhemolytic transfusion rections. Vox Sang 46:277, 1984.
17. De Rie MA, van der Plas-van Dalen CM, Engelfriet CP, von dem Borne AE. The serology of febrile transfusion reactions. Vox Sang 49:126, 1985.
18. Heinrich D, Mueller-Eckhardt C, Stier W. The specificity of leukocyte and platelet alloantibodies in sera of patients with nonhemolytic transfusion reactions. Von Sang 25:442, 1973.
19. Brubaker DB. Clinical significance of white cell antibodies in febrile nonhemolytic transfusion reactions. Transfusion 30:733, 1990.
20. Brittingham TE, Chaplin H Jr. Febrile transfusion reactions caused by sensitivity to donor leukocytes and platelets. JAMA 165:819, 1957.
21. Perkins HA, Payne R, Ferguson J, Wood M. Nonhemolytic febrile transfusion reactions. Quantitative effects of blood components with emphasis on isoantigenic incompatibility of leukocytes. Vox Sang 11:578, 1966.
22. Goldfinger D, Lowe C. Prevention of adverse reactions to blood transfusion by the

administration of saline-washed red blood cells. Transfusion 21:277, 1981.

23. Wenz B. Microaggregate blood filtration and the febrile transfusion reaction. A comparative study. Transfusion 23:95, 1983.

24. Lane TA, Anderson KC, Goodnough LT, Kurtz S, Moroff G, Pisciotto PT, Sayers M, Silberstein LE. Leukocyte reduction in blood component therapy. Ann Int Med 117:151, 1992.

25. Mangano MM, Chamber LA, Kruskall MS. Limited efficacy of leukopoor platelets for prevention of febrile transfusion reactions. Am J Clin Path 95:733, 1991.

26. Stack G, Snyder EL. Interleukin-8 generation in platelet concentrates during storage. Blood 78:388a, 1991.

27. Stack G, Snyder EL. Cytokine generation in stored platelet concentrates. Transfusion 34:20, 1994.

28. Muylle L, Joos M. Wouters E, De Bock R, Peetermans ME. Increased tumor necrosis factorα (TNFα), interleukin 1, and interleukin 6 (IL-6) levels in the plasma of stored platelet concentrates: relationship between TNFα) and IL-6 levels and febrile transfusion reactions. Transfusion 33:195, 1993.

29. Cole S, Stack G. Macrophage inflammatory protein-1α generation in stored platelets. Blood 82:398a, 1993.

30. Aye MT, Palmer DS, Giuliva A, Hashemi S. Effect of filtration of platelet concentrates on the production of cytokines and platelet release factors during storage. Blood82:336a, 1993.

31. Heddle NM, Klama L, Singer J, et al. The role of plasma from platelet concentrates in transfusion reactions. New Eng J Med 331:625, 1994.

32. Stack G, Baril L, Napychank P, Snyder E. Cytokine generation in stored units of red blood cells. Blood 82:394a, 1993.

33. Smith KJ, Sierra EF, Nelson EJ. Histamine, Il-1β and IL-8 increase in packed RBCs stored for 42 days but not in RBC leukodepleted pre-storage. Transfusion 33:53S, 1993.

34. Elias JA, Gustilo K, Baeder W, Freundlich B. Synergistic stimulation of fibroblast prostaglandin by recombinant interleukin 1 and tumor necrosis factor. J Immunol 138:3812, 1987.

35. Okusawa S, Gelfond JA, Ikejima T, et al. Interleukin 1 induces a shock-like state in rabbits. Synergism with tumor necrosis factor and the effect of cyclo oxygenase inhibition. J Clin Invest 8:1162, 1988.

36. Yuo A, Kitagawa S, Kasahara T, Matshushima K, Saito M, Takaku F. Stimulation and priming of human neutrophils by interleukin-8: cooperation with tumor necrosis factor and colony stimulating factors. Blood 78:2708-2714, 1991.

37. Dahinden CA, Kurimoto Y, De Wech AL, Lindley I, Dewald B, Baggiolini M. The neutrophil-activating peptide NAF/NAP-1 induces histamine and leukotriene release by interleukin 3-primed basophils. J Exp Med 170:1787, 1989.

38. Kunkel SL, Standiford T, Kasahara K, Strieter RM. Interleukin-8 (IL-8): the major neutrophil chemotactic factor in the lung. Experimental Lung Research 17:17, 1991.

39. Hack CE, Hart M, Van Schijndel RJ, Eerenberg AJ, Nuijens JH, Thijs LG, Aarden LA. Interleukin-8 in sepsis: relation to shock and inflammatory mediators. Infect Immun 60:2835, 1992.

40. van Zee KS, DeForge LE, Fischer E, Marano MA, Kenney JS, Remick DG, Lowry SF, Moldawer LL. IL-8 in septic shock, endotoxemia, and after IL-1 administration. J Immunol 146:3478, 1991.

41. Van Zee KJ, Fischer E, Hawes AS, et al. Affects of intravenous IL-8 administration in nonhuman primates. J Immunol 148:1746, 1992.

42. Hechtman DH, Cybulsky MI, Fuchs HJ, Baker JB, Gimbrone MA Jr. Intravascular IL-8, inhibitor of polymorphonuclear leukocyte accumulation at sites of acute inflammation. J Immunol 147:883, 1991.

43. Rost A. Some aspects of NAP-1 pathophysiology: lung damage caused by a blood-borne cytokine. Adv Exp Med Biol 305:127, 1991.

44. Darbonne WC, Rice GC, Mohler MA, Apple T, Hebert CA, Valente AJ, Baker JB. Red blood cells are a sink for interleukin 8, leukocyte chemotaxin. J Clin Invest 88:1362, 1991.

45. Horuk R, Chintis CE, Darbonne WC, Colby TJ, Rybicki A, Hadley TJ, Miller LH. A receptor for the malarial parasite Plasmodium vivax: the erythrocyte chemokine receptor. Science 261:1182, 1993.

46. Noete K, Darbonne W, Ogez J, Horuk R, Schall TJ. Identification of a promiscuous inflammatory peptide receptor on the surface of red blood cells. J Bio Chem 268:12247, 1993.

47. Muylle L, Peetermans ME. Effect of prestorage leukocyte removal on them cytokine levels in stored platelet concentrates. Vox Sang 66:14, 1994.

48. Eierman DF, Johnson CE, Haskill JS. Human monocyte inflammatory mediator gene expression is selectively regulated by adherence substrates. J Immunol 142:1970, 1989.

49. Haskill S, Johnson C, Eierman D, Becker S, Warren K. Adherence induces selective in RNA expression of monocyte mediators and proto-oncogenes. J Immunol 140:1690, 1988.

50. Kasahara K, Strieter RM, Chensue SW, Standiford TJ, Kunkel SL. Mononuclear cell adherence induces neutrophil chemotactic factor/interleukin-8 gene-expression. J Leuk Biol 50:287, 1991.

51. Sporn SA, Eierman DF, Johnson CE, Morris J, Martin G, Ladner M, Haskill S. Monocyte adherence results selective induction of novel genes sharing homology with mediators of inflammation and tissue repair. J Immunol 144:4434, 1990.

52. Stack G, Cole S, Campbell S, Snyder E, Edberg S. Interleukin-8 generation in bacterially-contaminated platelet concentrates. Transfusion 33:50S, 1993.

53. Pineda AA, Brzica SM Jr, Taswell HF. Hemolytic transfusion reaction. Recent experience in a large blood bank. Mayo Clin Proc 53:378, 1978.

54. Mollison PL, Engelfriet CP, Contreras M. Blood Transfusion in Clinical Medicine, ninth edition, Blackswell Scientific Publications, Boston, 1993.

55. Walker RH, ed, Technical Manual, 11th ed, AABB, Bethesda, 1993.

56. Goldfinger D. Acute hemolytic transfsuion reactions - a fresh look at pathogenesis and considerations regarding therapy. Transfu-

sion 17:85, 1977.

57. Davenport RD, Strieter RM, Standiford TJ, Kunkel SL. Interleukin-8 production in red blood cell incompatibility. Blood 76:2439, 1990.

58. Davenport RD, Strieter RM, Kunkel SL. Red cell ABO incompatibility and production of tumor necrosis factor-alpha. Br J Haematol 178:540, 1991.

59. Davenport RD, Burdick M, Strieter RM, Kunkel SL. Monocyte chemoattractant protein production in red cell incompatibility. Transfusion 34:16,1994.

60. Butler J, Parker D, Pillai R, Shole DJ, Rocker GM. Systemic release of neutrophil elastase and tumor necrosis factor alpha following ABO incompatible blood transfusion. Br J Haemotol 79:525, 1991.

61. Davenport RD, Burdick M, Moore SA, Kumkel SL. Cytokine production in IgG-mediated red cell incompatibility. Transfusion 33:19, 1993.

62 Hoffman M. Antibody-coated erythrocytes induce secretion of tumor necrosis factor by human monocytes: a mechanism for the production of fever by incompatible transfusions. Vox Sang 60:184, 1991.

63. White CW, Ghezzi P, Dinarello CA. Recombinant tumor necrosis factor/cachectin and interleukin 1 pretreatment decreases lung oxidized glutathione accumulation, lung injury, and mortality in rats exposed to hyperoxia. J Clin Invest 79:868, 1987.

64. Nordhagen R, Aas M. Association between HLA and red cell antigens. VII. Survival studies of incompatible red blood cells in a patient with HLA-associated haemagglutinins. Vox Sang 35:319, 1978.

65. Panzer S, Mayr WR, Graninger W, et al: Haemolytic transfusion reactions due to HLA antibodies: a proospective study combining red-cell serology with investigations of Chromium-51-labelled red-cell kinetics. Lancet 1:474, 1987.

66. Frewin DB, Jonsson JR, Frewin CR, et al. Influence on blood storage time and plasma histamine levels of the pattern of transfusion reactions. Vox Sang 56:243, 1989.

67. Frewin CB, Dyer SM, Haylock DN, Bates IR, Davis KG, Beal RW. A comparative study of the effect of three methods of leu-

kocyte removal on plasma histamine levels in stored human blood. Sem Hematol 28 (Suppl)5:18, 1991.

68. Frewin DB, Jonsson JR, Head RJ, Russell WJ, Beal RW. Histamine levels in stored human blood. Transfusion 24:502, 1984.

69. Frewin DB, Jonsson JR, Davis KG, et al. Effect of microfiltration on the histamine levels in stored human blood. Vox Sang 52:191, 1987.

70. Muylle L, Laekeman G, Hermon AG, Peetermans ME. Histamine levels in stored platelet concentrates. Transfusion 28:226, 1988.

71. Holme S, Ross D, Heaton WA. In vitro and in vivo evaluation of platelet concentrates after cotton wool filtration. Vox Sang 57:112, 1989.

72. Holme S, Snyder S, Heaton A, et al. In vitro and in vivo evaluation of cotton wool filtration of platelet concentrates obtained by automated and manual apheresis. Transfusion 32:328, 1992.

73. Hetland G, Mollnes TE, Larsen J, Garred P. Biocompatibility of white cell filters as evaluated by complement activation. Transfusion 32:557, 1992.

74. Shimizu T, Uchigiri C, Mizuno S, Kamiya T, Kokubo Y. Adsorption of anaphylatoxins and platelet-specific proteins by filtration of platelet concentrates with a polyester leukocyte reduction filter. Vox Sang 66:161, 1994.

75. Janatova J, Cheung AK, Parker CJ. Biomedical polymers differ in their capacity to activate complement. Complement and Inflammation 8:61, 1992.

76. Wenz B. Leukodepletion filters should be used with apheresis platelets. J Clin Apheresis 7:149, 1992.

77. Snyder E, Napychank P, Baril L. Removal of complement component C3a and interleukin-8 from platelet concentrate by a bedside leukodepletion filter. Transfusion 1994 (Submitted).

78. Popovsky MA, Moore SB. Diagnostic and pathogenetic considerations in transfusion-related acute lung injury. Transfusion 25:573, 1985.

79. Swank DW, Moore SB. Roles of the neutrophil and other mediators in adult respiratory distress syndrome. Mayo Clinic Proc 64:1118, 1989.

80. van Buren NL, Stroncek DR, Clay ME, McCullough J, Dalmasso AP. Transfusion-related acute lung injury caused by an NB2 granulocyte-specific antibody in a patient with thrombotic thrombocytopenic purpura. Transfusion 30:42, 1990.

81. Nordhagen R, Conradi M, Dromtorp SM. Pulmonary reaction associated with transfusion of plasma containing anti-5b. Vox Sang 51:102, 1986.

82. Seeger W, Schneider U, Kreusler B, von Witzleben E, Walmrath D, Grimminger F, Neppert J. Reproduction of transfusion-related acute lung injury in an ex vivo lung model. Blood 76:1438, 1990.

83. Larsen GL, McCarthy K, Webster RV, Henson J, Henson PM. A differential effect of C5a and C5b des Arg in induction of pulmonary inflammation. Am J Path 100:179, 1980.

84. Arnaout MA. Structure and function of the leukocyte adhesion molecules CD11/CD18. Blood 75:1037, 1990.

85. Goldman M, Blajchman M. Blood product associated bacterial sepsis. Transfus Med Reviews 5:73, 1991.

86. Anderson KC, Lew MA, Gorgone BC, Martel J, Leamy C, Sullivan B. Transfusion-related sepsis after prolonged platelet storage. American J Med 81:405, 1986.

87. Buchholz DH, AuBuchon JP, Snyder EL, Kandler R, Edberg S, Piscitelli V, Pickard C , and Napychank P. Removal of *Yersinia enterocolitica* from AS-1 red cells. Transfusion 32:667, 1992.

88. Wenz B, Burns ER, Freundlich LF. Prevention of growth of *Yersinia enterocolitica* in blood by polyester fiber filtration. Transfusion 32:663, 1992.

89. Hogman CF, Gong J, Hambraeus A, Johansson CS, Eriksson L. The role of white cells in the transmission of *Yersinia enterocoliticia* in blood components. Transfusion 32:654, 1992.

90. Kim DM, Brecher ME, Bland LA, Estes TJ, McAllister SK, Aguero SM, Carmen RA, Nelson EJ. Prestorage removal of *Yersinia enterocolitica* from red cells with white cell-reduction filters. Transfusion 32:658, 1992.

91. Wenz B, Ciavarella D, Freundlick. Effect of prestorage white cell reduction on bacterial growth in platelet concentrates. Transfusion 33:520, 1993.

92. Högman CF, Gong J, Eriksson L, Hambracus A, Johansson CS. White cells protect donor blood against bacterial contamination. Transfusion 31:620, 1991.

93. Heal JM, Cohen HJ. Do white cells in stored blood components reduce the likelihood of posttransfusion bacterial sepsis? Transfusion 31:581, 1991.

94. Nusbacher J. *Yersinia enterocolitica* and white cell filtration. Transfusion 32:597, 1992.

95. Rawal BD, Vyas GN. Complement-mediated bactericidal action and the removal of *Yersinia enterocolitica* by white cell filters. Transfusion 33:536, 1993.

96. Gong J, Hogman CF, Hambraeus A, Johansson CS, Eriksson L. Transfusion-associated *Serratia marcescens* infection: studies of the mechanism of action. Transfusion 33:802, 1993.

97. Brubaker DB. Transfusion-associated graft-versus-host disease. In:Scientific Basis of Transfusion Medicine, Anderson KC, Ness PM, eds, W.B. Saunders Company, Philadelphia, pp. 544-579.

98. Anderson KC, Weinstein HJ. Transfusion-associated graft-versus-host disease. N Engl J Med 323:315, 1990.

99. McMilin KD, Johnson RL. HLA homozygosity and the risk of related-donor transfusion-associated graft-versus-host disease. Trans Med Rev 7:37, 1993.

100. Ferraro JLM, Deeg HS. Graft-versus-host disease. N Engl J Med 324:667, 1991.

101. Gasbarrini G, Facchini A. Elevated interleukin-8 serum concentrations in beta-thalassemia and graft-versus-host disease. Blood 81:2252, 1993.

102. von Fliedner V, Higby DJ, Kim U. Graft versus host disease following blood product transfusion. Am J Med 72:951, 1982.

103. Van Bekkum DW. Transfusion or transplantation? Isr J Med Sci 1:879, 1965.

104. Rubinstein A, Radl J, Cothier H, Rossi E, Gugler E. Unusual combined immunodeficiency syndrome exhibiting kappa-IgD paraproteinemia, residual gut immunity and graft-versus-host reaction after plasma infusion. Acta Paediatr Scand 62:365, 1973.

105. Moroff G, Luban NLC. Prevention of transfusion-associated graft-versus-host disease. Transfusion 32:102, 1992.

106. FDA Memorandum. Recommendations regarding license amendments and gamma irradiation of blood products. FDA Regulations, 22 July, 1993, Rockville, MD, pp 1-19.

107. Dzik WH, Jones KS. The effects of gamma irradiation versus white cell reduction on the mixed lymphocyte reaction. Transfusion 33: 4493, 1993.

108. Akahoshi M, Takanashi M, Masuda M, et al. A case of transfusion-associated graft-versus-host disease not prevented by white cell reduction filters. Transfusion 32:169, 1991.

CHAPTER 7

LEUKODEPLETION
AND ALLOIMMUNIZATION

Irena Sniecinski

SUMMARY

Platelet alloimmunization remains a dilemma in the management of hematology patients since so little can be done to provide the necessary platelet transfusion support. A number of recent studies have provided information about the role of the passenger leukocytes that remain in blood products and how these initiate antibody development by participating in the immunization process. Small numbers of leukocytes, 10^6-10^7, may induce antibody development. As leukodepletion methods have developed from buffy coat depletion and platelet centrifugation to the use of third generation filters, it is now possible to routinely supply blood products with less than 1×10^6 residual leukocyte content for a small (5-10%) loss of the component. Most clinical studies have suggested that the relative risk of refractoriness to platelet transfusions is reduced by blood component leukodepletion. Although the relative risk of refractoriness is reduced by 70-90% in some studies, in others the reduction was not significant. Clearly further studies are needed to better define the immunizing dose of leukocytes, the effects of concurrent chemotherapy and to better relate improvements in clinical outcomes, such as bleeding or number of transfusion episodes, to the levels of leukodepletion. Lastly, the use of ultraviolet irradiation remains an intriguing option in that immunization may be avoided by inhibiting the function of the passenger leukocytes. Further trials are clearly necessary to better define the immunizing dose of leukocytes, the place of UVB irradiation and the role of leukocyte fragments or soluble antigens in order to allow the development of logical strategies to prevent immunization.

INTRODUCTION

Platelet transfusions have permitted advances in the treatment of hematologic and oncologic malignancies by reducing the risk of

Clinical Benefits of Leukodepleted Blood Products, edited by Joseph Sweeney, M.D. and Andrew Heaton, M.D. © 1995 R.G. Landes Company.

thrombocytopenic hemorrhage that occurs with intensive and potentially curative levels of chemotherapy. Hematopoietic stem cell transplantation for a variety of conditions would be impossible without the widespread availability of platelet transfusions. However, in spite of improvements in transfusion support of thrombocytopenic patients, refractoriness to platelet transfusions due to HLA-alloimmunization presents a substantial logistic and financial problem, thereby limiting the efficacy of novel therapies. Since alloimmunization and refractoriness to platelets are principally provoked by leukocytes present in routinely prepared platelet and red cell concentrates, the risk of alloimmunization is influenced by both the number of contaminating leukocytes and the type of leukocytes present. Effective methods have now been developed to reduce the level of contaminating leukocytes in blood products and are currently available for clinical use. This review will focus on the preventive measures of leukodepletion to reduce or prevent alloimmunization.

HLA alloimmunization is the formation of antibodies to foreign class I human leukocyte antigens that are found on all nucleated cells and platelets. Alloimmunization to leukocyte antigens may occur after transfusion of cellular blood components, pregnancy or organ transplantation. Although the mechanism of alloimmunization by blood transfusions is not proven, it is evident that donor leukocytes are the dominant cells, responsible for provocation of primary immune response to foreign antigens.[1,2]

MECHANISMS OF ALLOIMMUNIZATION

The recognition of foreign antigen by the recipient T cell is generally preceded by processing of antigen by the antigen presenting cells (APC).[3,4] These are bone marrow derived dendritic cells with class I and class II major histocompatibility complex (MHC) molecules on the surface, capable of presenting antigens in a form recognizable by T lymphocytes. The APC processes foreign antigens and expresses a modified peptide derived from them on its surface in conjunction with the class II MHC. The class II MHC-peptide complex is recognized by the CD4 or helper T cell, which contacts the MHC-peptide complex through its receptor. Recognition of foreign peptide on the APC by the CD4 cell, results in expression of interleukin-2 (IL-2) receptor on the T-cell surface and in a clustering of other surface molecules around the MHC-T cell attachment.[5] It is believed that this cluster consists of many molecules, including ICAM-1, ICAM-2, CD2, LFA-3, IL-1 and IL-6, which together form a costimulatory (accessory) signal.[6] The costimulatory signal causes the secretion of IL-2 by the CD4 cells which not only leads to proliferation of CD4 cell itself, but also provides the stimulus for proliferation of CD8 (cytotoxic) T cells and B cells.

The class I MHC-peptide complex can also be recognized by the CD8 cytotoxic T cell and by the B cell when presented on the donor APC. This recognition, however, must include CD4 activation and secretion of IL-2 to support CD8 and B cell function. Recently, much emphasis has been placed on the role of the B7-CD28 complex as the costimulatory molecule, necessary for the class I MHC to provoke the response to foreign antigens.

Alloimmunization against the foreign MHC could occur by one of two pathways. First, recipient T cells may recognize the MHC-peptide complex on the surface of viable donor APC.[7] Alternatively, recipient APCs may process and present to recipient T cells a soluble MHC shed from donor cells.[8] The first pathway is primarily the major route of alloimmune response. Alloimmunization by cell-free blood components appears to be relatively uncommon.

APC, B lymphocytes and T lymphocytes express both class I and class II antigens, but the platelets express only class I antigens. Multiple injections of purified platelets failed to stimulate antibodies to major histocompatibility complex class I antigens in rats (equivalent to HLA complex in humans), but injection of leukocytes from the same donor resulted in alloimmunization.[9,10] Dausset and Rappaport reported that intradermal injection of 130- 288 x 10[9] leukocyte-reduced platelets was infrequently accompanied by shortened skin graft survival in humans.[11] In contrast, administration of only 0.15 x 10[9] leukocytes consistently resulted in early graft rejection.[12] The enhanced capacity of leukocytes to induce the development of antibodies to MHC class I antigens is probably not attributable to the fact that they contain approximately 15-fold more MHC class I antigen molecule per cell than do platelets, since platelets greatly outnumber leukocytes in blood components.[10] In fact, the injection of a quantity of platelets sufficient to provide 1000-fold more MHC class I antigen molecules than are present in a sensitizing dose of leukocytes still did not result in immunization in rats.[10] Similar findings were obtained in mice which required approximately 10[3] leukocytes for immunization to MHC class I antigens.[9] Animal studies indicate that platelets alone are poorly immunogenic with respect to HLA transplantation antigens and that the alloimmunization to HLA antigens that accompany platelet and red blood cell transfusion depends mainly on the presence of foreign leukocytes expressing both MHC class I and II antigens in cellular blood components.

CLINICAL CONSEQUENCES OF ALLOIMMUNIZATION

Alloimmunization is a common complication of transfusion therapy which results in two separate difficulties in patient management: (1) clinical intolerance characterized by recurrent febrile reactions and (2) refractoriness to platelet transfusions. Febrile reactions may accompany 0.5 to 4% of transfusions.[13,14] This type of reaction is the most common adverse effect of blood transfusion and of leukocyte alloimmunization and is discussed in chapter 6.

Refractoriness to platelet transfusion occurs in 30-70% of multiply transfused patients.[15-19] Criteria for immune platelet refractoriness are based on a combination of post-transfusion platelet increments and antibody testing results. The management of the alloimmunized patient who is refractory to platelet transfusion represents one of the most difficult challenges in transfusion medicine. As outlined in Table 7.1, several management strategies have been used in alloimmunized patients. None of the available strategies, however, appears to be satisfactory because of their marginal effectiveness, impracticality and expense.

Although the use of HLA matched donors may result in compatible transfusion responses in refractory patients, the complexity of the HLA system makes it difficult to find HLA matched donors. Partially

---

Table 7.1. Approaches to management of alloimmunized patient

Strategy	Limitations
HLA-matched donor platelet transfusions	Expensive, not always effective
Platelet crossmatching	May be impractical for routine use
IV gamma globulin	Expensive, marginal effectiveness
Plasma exchange	Expensive, marginal effectiveness
Immunoadsorption of antibody	Effectiveness not yet established
Splenectomy	Ineffective
Vinblastine-loaded platelets	Limited experience, side effects
Massive platelet transfusions	Expensive, marginal effectiveness

matched single donor platelets are effective when the mismatch of one or two antigens involves cross reactive groups.[20-22] However, approximately 30% of even the best matched donors do not provide good post-transfusion platelet increments.[23] It is difficult to interpret results achieved in different laboratories, since platelet crossmatch testing is currently not standardized. In addition, platelet crossmatch testing does not appear to be cost-effective in cases of highly immunized patients, where screening of the large number of donors is necessary to find the required match for the refractory patient.[24-26]

The effectiveness of intravenous gamma-globulin (IVIgG) in managing patients with alloimmune platelet destruction is unclear. Some studies have shown improved platelet responses in some treated patients whereas other studies shave shown no response (Table 7.2).[27-31] One study suggested that high doses of IVIgG and use of HLA compatible platelets after IVIgG may improve results.[30] In the only randomized placebo-controlled trial in which platelets from the same donor were given before and after treatment, a significant increase of platelet counts in the treated group compared with the untreated group one hour after transfusion was documented.[28] Although platelet increments were improved, platelet survival was increased in only one of the treated patients. Considering the high dose of IVIgG and very transient improvement, this therapy does not appear to be cost-effective.

The removal of platelet alloantibodies by plasma exchange is extremely difficult because most of the alloantibodies are IgG which is distributed within both the intravascular and extravascular spaces. As with IVIgG therapy, this approach is expensive and may at best be only transiently successful unless concurrent immunosuppressive therapy is used.[32]

Recently, two independent pilot studies in the alloimmunized patients indicated that treatment with a Protein A column can diminish the degree of HLA sensitization and improve the responses to platelet transfusions.[33,34] Randomized, controlled trials for this treatment modality of refractoriness are in the early stages of implementation.

PREVENTION OF ALLOIMMUNIZATION

Since it is so difficult to manage the alloimmunized patient who is refractory to platelet transfusion, the prevention of platelet refractoriness is an important goal. Based upon the experimental and clinical data supporting the concept that immunological platelet refractoriness in most patients is mediated by alloantibodies directed against class I antigens and that alloimmunization of this type is dependent on the transfusion of donor antigen presenting cells, three basic approaches to preventing platelet refractoriness have been proposed: (1) immunosuppression of the transfused recipient, (2) limiting exposure to incompatible donor antigens and (3) reduction of immunogenicity of the transfused blood products. Animal platelet transfusion studies have shown that several different types of immunosuppressive therapy may prevent platelet alloimmunization. Slichter and colleagues found that in dogs, administration of cyclosporine dur-

Table 7.2. Trials with intravenous gamma globulin for treatment of platelet refractoriness

Investigator	Type of Study	Improvement in Transfusion Response	
		Study	Control
Schiffer	Unrandomized	0/18 (0%)	N/A
Kickler	Randomized	5/7 (71%)	0/5 (0%)
Zeigler	Unrandomized	13/19 (68%)	N/A

ing platelet transfusion from a random donor prevented alloimmunization even after eight weekly transfusions.[35] Furthermore, 6 of 9 recipients (67%) remained responsive to an additional eight weekly transfusions even after cyclosporine was discontinued. In 6 of 7 (86%) baboons given either prednisone, anti-thymocyte globulin or a combination of these two agents, platelet refractoriness did not occur after repeated weekly platelet transfusions from a single random donor baboon.[36] However, it is unlikely that specific immunosuppressive therapy to prevent platelet alloimmunization will be acceptable because of the side effects and risks of such therapy.

There are three approaches to limiting exposure to incompatible donor antigens: (1) reduction of transfusion frequency, (2) administration of single donor apheresis platelets instead of pooled random donor platelets and (3) administration of antigen compatible donor platelets. The practicality of a more restrictive platelet transfusion policy has been prospectively evaluated in 102 patients being treated for acute leukemia.[37] The results indicate that prophylactic platelet transfusions of afebrile, non-bleeding patient should be carried out only when the platelet decreases to 5,000/μl. This approach, however, may not be useful in the alloimmunized patient who also have prolonged periods of thrombocytopenia requiring multiple platelet transfusions.

Single donor platelet transfusions have been evaluated in one animal study and in three prospective randomized clinical trials. In a canine model, transfusion of a single donor platelets delayed, but did not prevent, platelet refractoriness.[38] In two human studies, the incidence of alloimmunization in recipients of single donor platelet transfusions was reduced compared with patients receiving transfusions from pooled random donors.[39,40] In contrast to these studies, the observations by another group of investigators showed that the alloimmunization rate of single donor platelet recipients did not differ from recipients of random donor platelet concentrates.[41] Thus it is currently unclear whether it is worthwhile to provide all chronic thrombocytopenic patients with the more expensive single donor platelet transfusions when at best alloimmunization is likely to be delayed, rather than prevented.

The role of ABO antigens in platelet transfusion remains controversial, although, two recent studies suggest that ABO identical platelets are a superior transfusion component for patients requiring chronic platelet support.[42,43] ABO unmatched transfusions were associated with reduced platelet increments and higher incidence of lymphocytotoxic antibody formation. The development of HLA antibodies suggested that the recognition of antigens other than ABO occurred during ABO mismatched transfusions.

The benefit of matching single donor platelet for HLA antigens compared to transfusion of unmatched single donor platelets has been evaluated in two transfusion trials.[44,45] In neither of these studies was there evidence that the provision of HLA matched apheresis platelets provided an additional benefit over that achieved with single random donor apheresis transfusions.

LEUKODEPLETION STUDIES

Efforts to modify blood products to render them less immunogenic have focused on two areas, (1) leukocyte removal from the blood products and (2) inactivation of the APC, thus preventing the APCs from sensitizing or releasing immunoregulatory substances that activate T-helper cells. Although the undesirable side effects associated with transfusion of leukocyte-contaminated blood components have long been recognized, attempts to prevent these by leukocyte removal had only minimal success. More recently significant improvements in leukodepletion of blood components have been developed. New generations of filters can reduce the residual leukocyte content of cellular components to 10^7-10^4 cells (a 2-5 log_{10} reduction). These filters remove donor leukocytes by a combination of both barrier retention and leukocyte absorption. In addition, recent enhancements of apheresis equipment have reduced the leukocyte content of platelet products prepared by apheresis. The development of an effective method for high efficiency leukocyte depletion set the stage for studies on the utility of the leukocyte reduction for prevention of platelet refractoriness.

The effect of leukodepletion for prevention of alloimmunization development has been investigated in animal studies. Claas and others reported that intravenous injections of platelet concentrate containing a total of less than 1,000 leukocytes were effective in preventing the development of lymphocytotoxic antibodies in recipient mice.[9] Studies by Kao and others showed that transfusions of 100-300 leukocytes in platelet concentrates each time were sufficient to alloimmunize recipient mice.[46] More recently, Blajchman and others used a rabbit model to study the effect of leukodepletion of blood products on re-

fractoriness to allogeneic donor platelets.[47] Their data provided evidence that the leukodepletion of fresh whole blood significantly reduced the frequency of allogeneic donor platelet refractoriness and increased post transfusion in vivo survival. Furthermore, they concluded that the pre-storage leukodepletion of allogeneic donor blood was associated with a reduced frequency of allogeneic platelet refractoriness and higher in vivo survival when compared to post-storage leukodepletion. Finally, they also observed that refractoriness to allogeneic platelets may be induced by plasma containing non-intact leukocytes or soluble HLA antigens.

The efficacy of leukocyte reduction in delaying or preventing alloimmunization in patients who received intensive platelet and red cell transfusion therapy was evaluated in 5 unrandomized and 6 randomized prospective clinical trials (Table 7.3 and 7.4, respec-

Table 7.3. *Unrandomized studies to evaluate effect of leukocyte reduction on alloimmunization and refractoriness to platelet transfusions*

Investigator (Year)	Residual WBC x10⁶		Refractoriness (%)		Alloimmunization (%)	
	PLTS	**RBCS**	**Study**	**Control**	**Study**	**Control**
Eernisse (1981)	5	<100	24	93	28	71
Fisher (1985)	<5	NR	NR	NR	0	42
Murphy (1986)	20	8	3	23	10	48
Brand (1989)	<20	0.5	9	NR	21	NR
Saarinen (1990)	0.2	<1	0	52	NR	NR

Table 7.4. *Randomized trials to evaluate effect of leukocyte reduction on alloimmunization and refractoriness to platelet transfusions*

Investigator (Year)	Residual WBC x10⁶		Refractoriness (%)		Alloimmunization (%)	
	PLTS	**RBCS**	**WBC Red.**	**Control**	**WBC Red.**	**Control**
Schiffer (1983)	70	100	16	19	20	42
Sniecinski (1988)	6	50	15	50	15	50
Andreu (1988)	151	61	21	47	12	31
van Marwijk Kooy (1991)	<5	<5	11	46	7	42
Oksanen (1991)	<3	<6	13	20	6	13
Handa (1993)	4	<3	3	29	6	38

tively). A synopsis of these studies and the investigator's conclusions is provided below.

UNRANDOMIZED CLINICAL TRIALS

Four of the five unrandomized studies involved prospective follow up of a group of patients receiving leukodepleted blood products and comparison of the level of alloimmunization and/or refractoriness to a retrospective control group.[48-50,52] One study was not controlled.[51] Eernisse and Brand studied 68 patients with aplastic anemia and acute leukemia who received red cell concentrates and platelet concentrates.[48] Red cell transfusions for the historical control patients were partially leukocyte reduced either by "buffy-coat" removal or by granulocyte removal using an adhesion filter. This study showed reductions in both alloimmunization and platelet refractoriness in the study group.

Fisher et al studied 12 patients with renal failure who received three biweekly transfusions of filtered platelet concentrates.[49] None of the 12 patients in the study group who received less than 5×10^6 leukocytes during each transfusion became allosensitized. Five of 12 control patients who received 1.5×10^7 leukocyte per transfusion became alloimmunized. Platelet refractoriness was not evaluated in this study.

In the study report by Murphy et al, patients with acute nonlymphocytic leukemia received leukodepleted platelet concentrates prepared by centrifugation and leukodepleted red cells by filtration.[50] Statistically significant decrease in the incidence of alloimmunization, but not in the development of refractoriness to platelets, was observed in the study group.

Brand et al reported an uncontrolled study of 335 patients who were transfused with filtered red cell concentrates and centrifuged pooled platelet concentrates containing less than 1×10^7 leukocytes.[51] Twenty-one (21%) percent of patients developed lymphocytotoxic antibodies and 9% clinical refractoriness associated with the presence of strong multispecific HLA antibodies.

Saarinen and coworkers investigated a group of 47 pediatric patients with aplastic anemia, acute leukemia or solid tumors with more than half of the patients receiving autologous or allogeneic marrow transplants.[52] The study group received red blood cells and pools of platelets highly leukodepleted by filtration, with each of these products containing less than 1×10^6 leukocytes per transfusion. The historical control group received red blood cells partially leukocyte-reduced by buffy coat depletion. Platelet refractoriness was not observed in the study group, but did occur in 52% of the historical controls. The incidence of alloimmunization was not evaluated in this study.

In each of these unrandomized studies, the results supported the hypothesis that leukodepletion might delay or possibly prevent alloimmunization and decrease the incidence of refractoriness. However, several limitations of these studies were apparent, specifically the incomplete nature of retrospective records and the lack of control over confounding factors. These limit the validity of results generated from such unrandomized studies.

PROSPECTIVE RANDOMIZED LEUKODEPLETION TRIALS

Six randomized trials were designed to determine whether transfusion with leukodepleted blood products resulted in a lower frequency of alloimmunization to HLA antigens and platelet refractoriness.[53-58] In addition, one study compared two methods of leukodepletion, centrifugation and filtration both for effect on leukocyte removal and the prevention of alloimmunization.[56]

Schiffer and colleagues performed a randomized study of patients with acute nonlymphocytic leukemia, excluding those with previous exposure to leukocytes by transfusion or pregnancy.[53] Patients were excluded if they received prior chemotherapy or immunosuppressive therapy for another cancer. Eligible patients were randomized to receive platelet concentrates that were leukodepleted using a centrifugation technique or standard technique. All red cell concentrates transfused to study patients were frozen or washed. Red cells transfused to control patients were prepared by standard technique. Alloimmunization was defined as ≥20% reactivity of cells on a panel of 80-100 lymphocytes. Refractoriness was defined as a corrected count increment (CCI) <7.5 x 10^9/L one hour after platelet transfusion. The study group had a lower rate of alloimmunization than the control group, but the difference was not statistically significant. The failure of this study to demonstrate a significant difference in alloimmunization rates between the study and control groups could be explained by the limited effectiveness of the method of leukodepletion used in the study, leaving more than 10^8 leukocytes in transfused red cell and platelet products.

In our study, the effect of leukodepletion was evaluated in 40 patients with hematological malignancies and aplastic anemia.[54] Patients randomized to the leukodepleted group received filtered pooled platelet concentrates and filtered red blood cell concentrates. The control group received standard red blood cell and platelet concentrates. Alloimmunization was defined by the presence of lymphocytotoxic antibody on a panel of 60 lymphocytes, reactive with ≥10% of cells. Refractoriness was defined as <20% 1 hour post-transfusion platelet recovery on two consecutive transfusions. The follow-up time ranged from 13 to 1,068 days. Patients who received leukocyte-reduced blood components had a significantly lower incidence of alloimmunization and platelet refractoriness than the control group. In addition, a delay in the development of refractoriness was observed in those who developed this complication. Alloimmunization was prevented in the leukocyte reduction group regardless of history of previous pregnancies and transfusions.

In the study by Andreu et al, 69 patients with diagnosis of primary acute leukemia were eligible for the study if they had a high probability of receiving multiple blood transfusions from at least 10 different donors within a 6 month period.[55] Study patients received either pooled random donor platelets or single donor platelets that were filtered and red cell concentrates that were leukodepleted using the same filter. The control group received nonleukodepleted blood products prepared by standard techniques. The rate of previous exposure to leukocytes by transfusion and pregnancy were high in both groups of patients. Alloimmunization was defined by the presence of lymphocytotoxic antibody reactive with ≥10% of cells on a panel of 30 lymphocytes. Refractoriness was defined by two consecutive platelet transfusions with <20% recovery on a 12 to 18 hour post-transfusion specimen. The maximum of patient follow-up was 180 days. The study group had significantly lower rates of alloimmunization and refractoriness despite higher number of platelet transfusions than the control group.

In the study of 53 patients with acute leukemia, van Marwijk Kooy et al excluded patients with previous exposure to leukocytes through pregnancy and transfusions within the 6 week period prior to study.[56] Both control and study group received leukodepleted red cell concentrates that were filtered after removal of buffy coat. Study patients received platelet pools that were leukodepleted using filtration and prostacyclin to prevent platelet aggregation. Control patients received platelet concentrates that were leukodepleted by centrifugation. Alloimmunization was defined by the presence of lymphocytotoxic antibody, reactive ≥10% of cells on a panel of 30 lymphocytes. Refractoriness was defined as ≤20% platelet recovery 1 hour post-transfusion on two consecutive platelet transfusions. Patients were followed for 14-217 days. The study patients which differed from the controls only in the much higher number of the platelet concentrates transfused to them, had a significantly lower rate of alloimmunization and platelet refractoriness than the controls.

Oksanen et al studied 33 patients with newly diagnosed acute lymphocytic and nonlymphocytic leukemia receiving induction chemotherapy.[57] Patients with a history of blood transfusions during the previous 2 years and previous immunosuppressive and cytotoxic therapies were excluded. Study patients received red cell and platelet concentrates leukodepleted by filtration. The control group received standard blood products. Alloimmunization was not defined by the investigators. The refractory state was defined as a corrected count increment of <2.5 x 10⁹/L, 1 hour post-transfusion on two platelet transfusions. The inadequate responses were not required to be on consecutive transfusions. Patient follow-up ranged from 35 to 355 days. Although the study patients showed a decreased rate of alloimmunization and refractoriness, the power of this study was too low to demonstrate a significant difference.

Handa et al conducted a multicenter randomized trial evaluating the benefit of leukodepletion in preventing HLA alloimmunization in 53 patients with hematological malignancies.[58] The study group received leukocyte-depleted 10 unit pools or a single donor apheresis product. The control group received standard platelet products from single or random donors. Patients in both groups received leukocyte-depleted red blood cell products prepared from 200 ml of whole blood by centrifugation and filtration. Alloimmunization was determined by the presence of anti-HLA antibody reactive with >20% of the 10 paneled cells. Refractoriness was determined by the <20% platelet recovery 12 to 18 hours after every transfusion on two successive transfusions. Both alloimmunization and refractoriness to platelet transfusions were found to be significantly less frequent in patients in the filtered group than those in the ocntrol group.

The analysis of the results of the six studies indicate that leukodepletion can result in a significantly lower frequency of alloimmunization and refractoriness. Meta-analysis performed by Heddle showed a common odds ratio for alloimmunization of 0.27 (95% CI, O.13 to 0.55) and a common odds ratio for refractoriness of 0.28 (95% CI, 0.13 to 0.54) in the recipients of leukoreduced products.[59] Three randomized studies showed a significant risk reduction for both alloimmunization and refractoriness (Table 7.5). Handa et al found that the relative risk reduction for alloimmunization was 84% and for refractoriness was 90% for patients who received leukodepleted blood products. In a study performed by van Marwijk Kooy et al, the relative risk reduction for alloimmunization and refractoriness were 82% and 76%, respectively. Finally, our study demonstrated the same significant risk reduction of 70% for both alloimmunization and refractoriness. In three other randomized studies, no significant risk reduction for either alloimmunization or refractoriness could be found due to the smaller difference in the frequency of alloimmunization and refractoriness between the control and study group.

The critical appraisal of the randomized studies leads to the following conclusions: (1) leukodepletion of red blood cell

---

Table 7.5. Relative risks reduction for alloimmunization and refractoriness

Investigator	Relative Risk Reduction for Alloimmunization (%)	Relative Risk Reduction for Refractoriness (%)
Schiffer	20	17
Sniecinski	70	70
Andreu	63	54
van Marwijk Kooy	82	76
Oksanen	38	69
Handa	84	90

and platelet concentrates to levels below 5×10^6 leukocytes per transfusion will prevent and/or delay alloimmunization; and (2) prevention of alloimmunization seems to improve the post-transfusion platelet increment when the clinical factors known to affect the post-transfusion platelet response were absent. The major limitations of the randomized studies to assess the clinical relevance of leukodepleted blood transfusions were: (1) small population of patients in the study and control groups, (2) differences in transfusion and chemotherapy regimens, (3) failure to include a more clinically relevant outcome measures such as days at risk of bleeding or number of platelet transfusions per day in addition to the measures of alloimmunization and refractoriness. Because of the limitations of these clinical trials, a multicenter, randomized trial of leukocyte reduction in patients with acute leukemia has been initiated.

LEUKOCYTE DOSE AND ALLOIMMUNIZATION

It is still a matter of debate as to what extent leukocytes should be removed from platelet and red cell concentrates to prevent primary HLA alloimmunization. The minimum number of leukocytes sufficient to consistently stimulate alloimmunization is unknown and may differ considerably among individuals. In a recent study of patients with acute leukemia, the investigators attempted to address the question of an "immunization threshold" by a reanalysis of their data with respect to the number of leukocytes received per platelet transfusion.[56] They found a significantly higher incidence of alloimmunization in patients who received more than 50×10^6 leukocytes per transfusion compared with patients who received less than 50×10^6 leukocytes per transfusion or 59% versus 8%, respectively. In another study, 24 patients with renal failure who were awaiting transplantation were given three transfusions each of either unmodified random-donor platelets containing 15×10^6 leukocytes per transfusion (control) or leukocyte-reduced platelet concentrates con-

taining fewer than 5×10^6 leukocytes.[49] Five of 12 control patients, but none of the patients in the study group, became alloimmunized. This study suggested that the development of alloimmunization is dose-dependent, with a threshold of between 10^6 and 10^7 leukocytes per transfusion. Although no systemic study of an immunization threshold has been done, it appears from the existing studies that the incidence of alloimmunization can be diminished or delayed in many patients who receive frequent transfusions through the use of modern technologies that are capable of consistently reducing the leukocyte content of blood components to less than 10^7 leukocytes per transfusion.

PREVENTION OF ALLOIMMUNIZATION BY UV-B IRRADIATION

Instead of removing white cells from the transfused blood products, with the inherent problems of complete and effective removal, another method would be to alter the transfused product in order to eliminate immunogenicity. In that regard, a very important observation was made by Lindahl-Kiessling and Safwenberg in 1971.[60] These investigators first demonstrated that UV irradiation (UVR) renders lymphocytes unable to either stimulate or respond in mixed lymphocyte culture, even though HLA antigens were still detected on the surface of the UV irradiated lymphocytes. Exposure of blood transfusion products to UV-C (200-280 nm) or UV-B (280-320 nm) reduces or abrogates their immunogenicity and thereby prevents allosensitization and transfusion refractoriness in several models.[61-65] Although the exact mechanism of action of UV light is unknown, in vitro studies suggest that UV exposure results in a loss of class II histocompatibility antigens from the cell surface, alteration of calcium homeostasis and a lack of interaction between antigen preventing and responding cells (Table 7.6).

Whole body UVR leads to the induction of suppressor cells whereas antigen coupled to UVR-treated cells in vitro leads to antigen-specific suppressor cell formation after in vivo injection.[66-70] In one study, UV-irradiated macrophages did take up antigen, but could not present it normally.[71] With the defective antigen presentation, autologous APCs of the transfusion recipient are unable to process antigen. Dendritic cells are extremely susceptible to UV exposure with resultant cell death after several hours in culture.[72] This may suggest that, if UV-treated blood products were stored prior to injection, they might become even less immunogenic.

T cells that secrete IL-2 can lead B cells to produce both IgG and IgM antibodies in an in vitro culture system.[73] Accessory cells stimulated by UVR express IL-2 receptors, but do not secrete normal amounts of IL-2.[74,75] Furthermore, UVR also impairs IL-1 production by APC.[71] UV-treated macrophages are unable to stimulate T-cell response to alloantigen or to soluble protein antigens.

Finally, UVR reduces or eliminates expression of several cell surface antigens while retaining a normal amount of HLA-A, B and C antigens.[60,76,77] HLA-D region products show reduced expression particularly after in vitro culture.[78] Cell adhesion molecules, such as LFA-1 and ICAM-1 are markedly depressed on the surface of UVR-treated T cells and monocytes, respectively. This interferes with cell-cell interaction and prevents cluster formation from occurring between APCs and T cells that impairs T-cell blastogenesis.[79] In addition, UV-B irradiation of booster cells completely inhibits secondary response in vitro.[80]

Studies have now demonstrated that UV-B irradiation can be used beneficially in several clinical situations, including prevention of alloimmunization. The application of UV-B irradiation in transfusion practice is limited to platelet concentrates. In a dog platelet transfusion model, 11 of 12 recipients (92%) of UV-irradiated platelets did not become refractory to platelets after eight weekly single donor transfusions, compared with 3 of 21 recipients (14%) who were given platelets not exposed to UV.[35] Furthermore, when, after 8 weeks, transfusions of UV-irradiated platelets were stopped and unirradiated transfusions were resumed, two thirds of dogs remained transfusion responsive. This data suggested that the transfusion of UV-irradiated platelets had prevented alloimmunization and induced a state of "tolerance" allowing for subsequent normal platelet survival.

Three pilot clinical trials of UV-B irradiation to prevent HLA alloimmunization have been reported (Table 7.7). Menitove studied 32 patients with newly diagnosed malignancies and anticipated long term platelet transfusion needs.[81] Patients were randomized to receive either UV-irradiated

---

Table 7.6. Ultraviolet B irradiation of blood products

Unique Features:

- Induces abolition of the ability to stimulate and to respond to allogeneic mononuclear cells in MLR.

- Impairs allogeneic antigen presentation to both naive and primed T-cells (effective inhibition of secondary response).

- More effective in the prevention of primary HLA alloimmunization than a 3-log leukocyte removal.

- Induces immunologic anergy.

Table 7.7. Ultraviolet-B studies to prevent alloimmunization

Investigator	Alloimmunization (%)		Refractoriness (%)	
	Study	Control	Study	Control
Menitove	17	36	11	36
Pamphillon	0	9	NR	NR
Andreu	9	62	NR	NR

or unirradiated random donor platelet concentrates. Patients in both groups received red cell concentrates leukodepleted using the Sepacell filter. The study group had a significantly lower rate of alloimmunization and refractoriness. Pamphillon conducted a similar study with UV-B irradiated single donor platelet concentrates.[82] Andreu and others initiated a multi-institutional trial comparing the incidence of alloimmunization and refractoriness between three arms: control, leukodepleted and UV-B irradiated.[83] Preliminary results indicate that the patients in UV-B arm experienced the lowest rate of alloimmunization. It seems likely that these trials, along with the ongoing multi-institutional trial sponsored by the National Heart, Lung and Blood Institute, will demonstrate the merit of UV-B irradiation in the prevention of alloimmunization.

CONCLUSION

1. Immunization to HLA antigens and the development of a refractory state is a complex process that is facilitated by transfusion of donor antigen presenting cells. Once the recipient is immunized there is little that can be done to ameliorate the problem and provision of platelet transfusion support becomes more complex. Residual leukocyte levels of 10^7 or greater are associated with immunization and current standards require less than 5 x 10^6 residual WBC if leukodepletion is indicated for avoidance of HLA immunization.

2. A number of trials have suggested that leukodepletion to levels < 5 x 10^6 may delay immunization, but neither the specific level of leukodepletion nor the specific benefit of blood component processing are adequately defined.

3. In vitro studies indicate that UV-B irradiation can inhibit secondary response by impairing foreign antigen presentation to the primed T cells. Multi-institutional randomized trials will determine the merits of leukocyte depletion and UV-B irradiation in the prevention of platelet alloimmunization.

REFERENCES

1. Dausset J. Leukoagglutinins IV. Leukoagglutinins and blood transfusion. Vox Sang 4:190, 1954.
2. Hogge DE, Dutcher JP, Aisner J, Schiffer CA. Lymphocytotoxic antibody is a predictor of response to random donor platelet transfusion. Am J Hematol 14:363, 1983.
3. Roitt I. Essential Immunology, ed S. Oxford Blackwell Scientific, 1984.
4. Mincheff M, Meryman HT. Stimulation by allo-Ia requires a product of lysosomal processing. XII Int Cong Transplantation Soc., Sydney, p. 177, 1988.
5. Mueller DL, Jenkins MK, Schwartz RH. An accessory cell-derived costimulatory signal acts independently of protein kinase C activation to allow T-cell proliferation and prevent the induction of unresponsiveness. J Immunol 142:2617, 1989.
6. Mincheff MS, Meryman HT. Costimulatory signals necessary for induction of T cell proliferation. Transplantation 49:768, 1990.
7. Mincheff MS, Meryman HT. Induction of primary mixed leukocyte reactions with

ultraviolet B or chemically modified stimulator cells. Transplantation 48:1052, 1989.

8. Takahashi T, Inada S, O'Shea JJ, Brown EJ. Osmotic stress and the freeze-thaw cycle cause shedding of Fc and C3b receptors by human polymorphonuclear leukocytes. J Immunol 134:4062, 1985.

9. Claas FHJ, Smeenk RJT, Schmidt R, van Steenbrugge GH, Eernisse JG. Alloimmunization against the MHC antigens after platelet transfusions is due to contaminating leukocytes in the platelet suspension. Exp Hematol 9:84, 1981.

10. Welsh KI, Burgos H, Batchelor JR. The immune response to allogeneic rat platelets: Ag-B antigen in matrix form lacking Ia. Eur J Immunol 7:267, 1977.

11. Dausset J, Rapaport FT. Transplantation antigen activity of human blood platelets. Transplantation 4:182, 1966.

12. Rapaport FT, Dausset J, Converse JM, Lawrence HS. Biological and ultrastructural studies of leukocyte fractions as transplantation antigens in man. Transplantation 4:490, 1965.

13. Walker RH. Special report: Transfusion risks. Am J Clin Pathol 88:374, 1987.

14. Menitove JE, McElligott MC, Aster RH. Febrile transfusion reaction: What component should be given next? Vox Sang 42:318, 1982.

15. Slichter SJ. Platelet transfusion therapy. Hematol Oncol Clin North Am 4:291, 1990.

16. Howard JE, Perkins HA. The natural history of alloimmunization to platelets. Transfusion 18:496, 1978.

17. Klingemann HG, Self S, Banaji, et al. Refractoriness to random donor platelet transfusions in patients with aplastic anemia: A multvariate analysis of data from 264 cases. Br J Haematol 66:115, 1987.

18. Schiffer CA, Lichtenfield JL, Wiernik PH, Mardiney MR, Joseph JM. Antibody response in patients with acute non-lymphocytic leukemia. Cancer 37:2177, 1976.

19. Klein CA, Blajchman MA. Alloantibodies and platelet destruction. Sem Thromb Hemostas 8:105, 1982.

20. Murphy MF, Metcalfe P, Thomas H, Eve J, Ord J, Lister TA, Waters AH. Use of leukocyte-poor blood components and HLA matched platelet donors to prevent HLA alloimmunization. Br J Haematol 62:529, 1986.

21. Duquesnoy RJ. Donor selection in platelet transfusion therapy of alloimmunized thrombocytopenic patients. In: The Blood Platelet in Transfusion Therapy. Alan R. Liss, New York p.229, 1978.

22. Menitove JE, Aster RH. Transfusion of platelets and plasma products. Clin Haematol 12:239, 1983.

23. Duquesnoy RJ, Filip DJ, Rodey GE, Rimm AA, Aster RH. Successful transfusion of platelets "mismatched" for HLA antigens to alloimmunized thrombocytopenic patients. Am J Hematol 2:219, 1977.

24. Freedman J, Hooi C, Garvey MB. Prospective platelet crossmatching for selection of compatible random donors. Br J Haematol 56:9, 1984.

25. Freedman J, Garvey MB, Salomon de Friedberg Z, et al. Random donor platelet crossmatching: Comparison of four platelet antibody detection methods. Am J Hematol 28:1, 1988.

26. O'Connell BA, Schiffer CA. Donor selection for alloimmunized patients by platelet crossmatching of random-donor platelet concentrates. Transfusion 30:314, 1990.

27. Kekomaki R, Elfenbein G, Gardner R, Graham-Pole J, Mehta P, Gross S. Improved response of patients refractory to random-donor platelet transfusions by intravenous gamma globulin. Am J Med 76:199, 1984.

28. Kickler T, Braine HG, Piantadosi S, et al. A randomized, placebo-controlled trial of intravenous gammaglobulin in alloimmunized thrombocytopenic patients. Blood 75:313, 1990.

29. Zeigler ZR, Shadduck RK, Rosenfeld CS, et al. High-dose intravenous gamma globulin improves responses to single-donor platelets in patients refractory to platelet transfusion. Blood 70:1433, 1987.

30. Zeigler ZR, Shadduck RK, Rosenfeld CS, et al. Intravenous gammaglobulin decreases platelet-associated IgG and improves transfusion responses in platelet refractory states. Am J Hematol 38:15, 1991.

31. Schiffer CA, Hogge DE, Aisner J, et al.

High-dose intravenous gamma globulin in alloimmunized platelet transfusion recipients. Blood 64:937, 1984.

32. Bensinger WI, Buckner CD, Clift RA, et al. Plasma exchange for platelet alloimmunization. Transplantation 41:602, 1986.

33. Christie DJ, Howe RB, Lennon SS, Souro SC. Treatment of refractoriness to platelet transfusion by protein A column therapy. Transfusion 33:234, 1993.

34. Sniecinski I, Delaney G. Response to therapy with Protein-A column in alloimmunized patients (Abstract). Proceedings of International Society of Hematology, Blackwell Scientific Publications, p.17, 1992.

35. Slichter SJ, Deeg HJ, Kennedy MS. Prevention of platelet alloimmunization in dogs with systemic cyclosporine and UV irradiation of cyclosporine loading of donor platelets. Blood 69:414, 1987.

36. Slichter SJ, Weiden PL, Kane PJ, Storb RF. Approaches to preventing or reversing platelet alloimmunization using animal models. Transfusion 28:103, 1988.

37. Gmur J, Burger J, Schanz U, Fehr J, Schaffner A. Safety of stringent prophylactic platelet transfusion policy for patients with acute leukemia. Lancet 338:1223, 1991.

38. Slichter SJ, O'Donnell MR, Weiden PL, Storb R, Schroeder ML. Canine platelet alloimmunization: The role of donor selection. Br J Haematol 63:713, 1986.

39. Sintnicolaas K, Vriesendorp HM, Sizoo W, et al. Delayed alloimmunization by random single donor platelet transfusions. Lancet 1:750, 1981.

40. Gmur J, von Felten A, Osterwalder B, Scali G, Sauter Chr, Frick P. Delayed alloimmunization using random single donor platelet transfusions: A prospective study in thrombocytopenic patients with acute leukemia. Blood 61:473, 1983.

41. Kakaiya RM, Hezzey AJ, Bove JR, et al. Alloimmunization following apheresis platelets vs pooled platelet concentrate transfusion - a prospective randomized study (abstract). Transfusion 21:600, 1981.

42. Lee EJ, Schiffer CA. ABO compatibility can influence the results of platelet transfusion.

Results of randomized trial. Transfusion 29:384, 1989.

43. Carr R, Hutton JL, Jenkins JA, Lucas GF, Amphlett NW. Transfusion of ABO mismatched platelets leads to early platelet refractoriness. Br J Haematol 75:408, 1990.

44. Messerschmidt G, Makuch R, Appelbaum F, et al. A prospective randomized trial of HLA-matched versus mismatched single-donor platelet transfusions in cancer patients. Cancer 62:795, 1988.

45. Murphy MF, Metcalfe P, Thomas H, et al. Use of leukocyte-poor blood components and HLA-matched-platelet donors to prevent HLA alloimmunization. Br J Haematol 62:529, 1986.

46. Kao KJ. Effects of leukocyte depletion and UVB irradiation on alloantigenicity of major histocompatibility complex antigens in platelet concentrate: A comparative study. Blood 80:2931, 1992.

47. Blajchman MA, Bardossy L, Carmen RA, Goldman M, Heddle NM, Singal DP. An animal model of allogeneic donor platelet refractoriness: The effect of pre-storage leukodepletion. Blood 79:1371, 1992.

48. Eernisse JG, Brand A. Prevention of platelet refractoriness due to HLA antibodies by administration of leukocyte-poor blood components. Exp Hematol 9:77, 1981.

49. Fisher M, Chapman JR, Ting A, Morris PJ. Alloimmunization to HLA antigens following transfusion with leukocyte-poor and purified platelet suspensions. Vox Sang 49:331, 1985.

50. Murphy MF, Metcalfe P, Thomas H, et al. Use of leukocyte-poor blood components and HLA-matched-platelet donors to prevent HLA alloimmunization. Br J Haematol 62:529, 1985.

51. Brand A, Claas FH, Voogt PJ, Wasser MN, Eernisse JG. Alloimmunization after leukocyte-depleted multiple random donor platelet transfusions. Vox Sang 54:160, 1988.

52. Saarinen UM, Kekomaki R, Silimes M, Myllyla G. Effective prophylaxis against platelet refractoriness in multitransfused patients by use of leukocyte-free blood components. Blood 75:512, 1990.

53. Schiffer CA. Management of patients refractory to platelet transfusion-an evaluation of

methods of donor selection. Prog Hematol p.91, 1987.

54. Sniecinski I, O'Donnell MR, Nowicki B, Hill LR. Prevention of refractoriness and HLA-alloimmunization using filtered blood products. Blood 71:1402, 1988.

55. Andreu G, Dewailly J, Leberre C, et al. Prevention of HLA immunization with leukocyte-poor packed red cells and platelet concentrates obtained by filtration. Blood 72:964, 1988.

56. van Marwijk Kooy M, van Prooijen HC, Moes M, Bosma-Stants I, Akkerman JW. Use of leukocyte-depleted platelet concentrates for the prevention of refractoriness and primary HLA alloimmunization: A prospective, randomized trial. Blood 77:201, 1991.

57. Oksanen K, Kekomaki R, Ruutu T, et al. Prevention of alloimmunization in patients with acute leukemia by use of white cell-reduced blood components: A randomized trial. Transfusion 31:588, 1991.

58. Handa M, et al. Role of leukocyte depletion from platelet concentrates in reducing HLA alloimmunization and platelet refractoriness in polytransfused patients: A prospective multicenter randomized study in Japan. In: Clinical Application of Leukocyte Depletion. Sekiguchi S [ed], Blackwell Scientific Publications, 1993.

59. Heedle N. The efficiency of leukodepletion to improve platelet transfusion response: A critical appraisal of clinical studies. Trans Med Reviews 8:15, 1994.

60. Lindahl-Kiessling K, Safwenberg J. Inability of UV-irradiated lymphocytes to stimulate allogeneic cells in mixed lymphocyte culture. Int Arch Allergy 41:670, 1971.

61. Deeg HJ, Bazar L, Sigaroudinia M, Cottler-Fox M. Ultraviolet B light inactivates bone marrow T lymphocytes but spares hematopoietic precursor cells. Blood 73:369, 1989.

62. Lau H, Reemtsma K, Hardy MA. Pancreatic islet allograft prolongation by donor-specific blood transfusions treated with ultraviolet irradiation. Science 221:754, 1983.

63. Deeg HJ, Aprile J, Graham TV, Appelbaum FR, Storb R. Ultraviolet irradiation of blood prevents transfusion-induced sensitization and marrow graft rejection in dogs. Blood

67:537, 1986.

64. Oluwole SF, Iga C, Lau H, Reemtsma K, Hardy MA. Prolongation of rat heart allografts by donor-specific transfusion treated with ultraviolet irradiation. Heart Transplant 4:385, 1985.

65. Slichter SJ, Deeg HJ, Kennedy MS. Prevention of platelet alloimmunization in dogs with systemic cyclosporine and by UV-irradiation or cyclosporine-loading of donor platelets. Blood 69:414, 1987.

66. Baadsgaard O, Fox DA, Cooper KD. Human epidermal cells from ultraviolet light exposed skin preferentially activate autoreactive CDR+2H4+suppressor-inducer lymphocytes and CD8+ suppressor/cytotoxic lymphocytes. J Immuno 140:1738, 1988.

67. Hersey P, Haran G, Hasic E, Edwards A. Alteration of T cell subsets and induction of suppressor T cell activity in normal subjects after exposure to sunlight. J Immunol 131:171, 1983.

68. Ullrich SE. Suppression of the immune response to allogeneic histocompatibility antigens by a single exposure to ultraviolet radiation. Transplantation 42:287, 1986.

69. Ullrich SE. The effect of ultraviolet radiation-induced suppressor cells on T-cell activity. Immunology 60:353, 1987.

70. Greene MI, SY MS, Kripke M, Benacerraf B. Impairment of antigen presenting cell function by ultraviolet radiation. Proc Natl Acad Sci USA 76:6591, 1979.

71. Jakway JP, Shevach EM. Stimulation of T-cell activation by UV-treated, antigen-pulsed macrophages: Evidence for a requirement for antigen processing and interleukin-1 secretion. Cellular Immunol 80:151, 1983.

72. Everson MP, Spalding DM, Koopman WJ. Exquisite sensitivity of dendritic cells to ultraviolet radiation and temperature changes. Transplantation 48:666, 1989.

73. Crow NK, Kunkel HG. Human dendritic cells: Major stimulators of the autologous and allogenic mixed leukocyte reactions. Clin Exp Immunol 49:338, 1982.

74. Gromo G, Inverardi L, Geller RL, Alter BJ, Bach FH. The step wise activation of cytotoxic T lymphocytes. Immunol Today 8:259, 1987.

75. Tominaga A, Lefort S, Mizel SB, et al. Molecular signals in antigen presentation. I. Effects of interleukin 1 and 2 on radiation treated antigen presenting cells in vivo and in vitro. Clin Immunol Immunolpathol 29:282, 1983.

76. Slater LM, Murray S, Liu J, Hudelson B. Dissimilar effects of ultraviolet light on HLA-D and HLA-DR antigens. Tissue Antigens 15:431, 1980.

77. Gruner S, Volk HD, Noack F, Meffert H, von Baehr R. Inhibition of HLA-DR antigen expression and of the allogeneic mixed leukocyte reaction by photochemical treatment. Tissue Antigens 27:147, 1986.

78. Czernielewski J, Viagot P, Asselineau D, Prunieras M. In vitro effect of UV radiation on immune function and membrane markers of human Langerhans' cells. J Invest Dermatol 83:62, 1984.

79. Aprile J, Deeg HJ. Ultraviolet irradiation of canine dendritic cells prevents mitogen-induced cluster formation and lymphocyte proliferation. Transplantation 42:653, 1986.

80. Andre G, Perrot JY, Pirenne F, Bocaccio C. The effect of ultraviolet light on antigen-presenting cells: Implications for transfusion-induced sensitization. Semin Hematol 29:122, 1992.

81. Menitove JE, Kagen LR, Aster RH. Alloimmunization is decreased in platelets receiving UV-B irradiated platelet concentrates and leukocyte-depleted red cells. Blood (Suppl 1)76:1607, 1990.

82. Pamphillon DH. Personal communication.

83. Andreu G. Personal communication.

CHAPTER 8

ROLE OF DONOR LEUKOCYTES AND LEUKODEPLETION IN TRANSFUSION-ASSOCIATED VIRAL INFECTIONS

Michael P. Busch, Tzong-Hae Lee

SUMMARY

Research over the past decade has led to increasing appreciation of the importance of donor leukocytes in the transmission of blood-borne viruses. Donor leukocytes are directly involved in transmission of herpes viruses and retroviruses, agents which exist primarily as latent infections in lymphocytes of asymptomatic carriers. Controlled clinical studies have now established that filter-leukodepletion can prevent transmission of cytomegalovirus, and in vitro data suggests possible reduction in transmission of several retroviruses. Recent evidence also suggests that the immunological activation events that occur following transfusion of allogeneic donor leukocytes may both facilitate transmission of donor viral infections to recipients and precipitate reactivation of pre-existing recipient viral infections.

This chapter reviews each of the major classes of transfusion-associated viruses (TAV), with particular consideration of whether circulating leukocytes represent significant vectors for transmission by transfusion. Evidence suggesting that leukocyte reduction, achievable with state-of-the-art leukodepletion filters, can reduce the risk of transmission of each virus is then presented. The growing body of data on the less widely appreciated, but probably more common effect of transfused donor leukocytes on reactivation of latent recipient infections, is then reviewed, and the potential impact of leukodepletion on the prevention of such reactivation considered.

Clinical Benefits of Leukodepleted Blood Products, edited by Joseph Sweeney, M.D. and Andrew Heaton, M.D. © 1995 R.G. Landes Company.

DUAL ROLE
OF DONOR LEUKOCYTES
IN TRANSMISSION OF VIRUSES

Donor leukocytes may facilitate primary infection of recipients by transfusion-associated viruses (TAVs) by several mechanisms. First, several of the major TAVs are highly lymphotropic, and persist in circulating donor lymphocytes as latent or low-level chronic infections.[1-3] Transfusion of blood components containing large numbers of donor leukocytes, some of which may harbor a TAV, therefore increases the probability that the virus will be transmitted to the recipient. Second, transfusion of allogeneic donor leukocytes incites an immunological activation response in the recipient, somewhat analogous to an in vitro mixed lymphocyte reaction.[4] Activation of donor leukocytes harboring a TAV can trigger a latent virus infection into an active infection, thereby enhancing its infectivity and facilitating transmission to the recipient. Activation of recipient immune cells results in enhanced susceptibility to infection.

DONOR LEUKOCYTES AS RESERVOIRS OF TRANSFUSION-ASSOCIATED VIRUSES

Blood donors are routinely screened for signs and symptoms of symptomatic (acute

and chronic) viral infections, and persons with clinically apparent infections are deferred from donation. Laboratory screening tests directed at viral antigens or antibodies are also employed to detect asymptomatic carriers of the more important TAVs. Although highly accurate, these tests are not perfect, and infections continue to be transmitted, due both to donations by recently infected persons lacking detectable antigens or antibodies, and test failure attributable to either biological (i.e. variant viruses or immunosilent infections) or technical reasons (e.g. errors in performing the test). Estimates for the residual risk of the major transfusion-transmitted viruses (TTV) are given in Table 8.1.

For purposes of the present discussion on viremia in screened blood donors we will focus on the compartmentalization of TTVs in the circulation of persons in either the preseroconversion window phase of infection, or in the asymptomatic carrier stage. From this perspective, the major TAVs can be considered as belonging to one of three groups: (1) those harbored exclusively in leukocytes, with no significant cell-free (plasma) component; (2) those harbored exclusively in plasma, with no significant cell-associated component, and (3) those with both significant cell-associated and cell-free components (Table 8.2).

The group 1 (cell-associated only) viruses include the major human herpes viruses, all of which establish life-long infections associated with intermittent periods of latency and reactivation. The most important herpes virus from the transfusion medicine perspective is cytomegalovirus (CMV).[1] Although the exact reservoirs of CMV in blood and tissues are not fully established,[5] data suggests that CMV is harbored primarily in T lymphocytes during asymptomatic (latent) phases of infection,[6,7] while the majority of virus is present in granulocytes during periods of reactivation viremia.[8] In addition to CMV, attention has recently increased with regard to transfusion transmission of Epstein-Barr virus (EBV) and Human Herpes Virus, type 6 (HHV-6), particularly in the con-

Table 8.1. Estimated risk of acquiring the major transfusion-associated viruses from screened blood transfusions

AGENT	Risk per unit
Retroviruses	
HIV-1	1 in 225,000
HIV-2	<1 in 20,000,000
HTLV-I	<1 in 70,000
HTLV-II	1 in 70,000
Hepatitis Viruses	
HBV	1 in 200,000
HCV	1 in 5,000

(Adapted from information appearing in the *New England Journal of Medicine,* Dodd RY. Editorial. N Engl J Med 327:419, 1992, with permission)

text of immunocompromised transplant recipients.[9,10] Group 1 also includes the human T cell leukemia viruses types I and II (HTLV-I/II).[3] These retroviruses have never been isolated from plasma of asymptomatic carriers, nor is there any evidence for their transmission by cell-free blood components or plasma derivatives (see below). Group 1 viruses are clearly the most amenable to complete removal by leukodepletion.

Group 2 (cell-free only) viruses include the major transfusion-transmitted hepatitis viruses, hepatitis B virus (HBV)[11] and hepatitis C virus (HCV).[12] These viruses circulate in the blood stream primarily as free viral particles in plasma. Although there are occasional reports of detection of leukocyte-associated HBV and HCV nucleic acids using polymerase chain reaction (PCR),[13,14] the replication competency of these leukocyte-associated "infections" is doubtful. Moreover, the levels of leukocyte-associated HBV and HCV appear to be very low compared to cell-free virus concentrations, and therefore they probably represent insignificant fractions of total viremia. Two other viruses that are occasionally transmitted by transfusions also belong to group 2. Hepatitis A virus, which is transmitted primarily by the fecal-oral route and causes acute hepatitis without establishing a chronic carrier state, has reportedly been transmitted by transfusions on 10 occasions over the past 10 years; all of these cases were attributed to donors who donated during the viremic phase immediately preceding the onset of symptoms (personal communication, William Fricke, Food and Drug Administration). Parvovirus B19, which causes fifth disease in children, transient aplastic crises in patients with congenital or acquired anemias, and, rarely, hydrops fetalis, is also best classified in group 2, although this virus infects erythroid precursors and, as such, may also be associated with circulating red blood cells.[15] Since group 2 viruses can be readily transmitted by cell-free plasma, leukodepletion is unlikely to diminish transmission rates to a significant extent.

Table 8.2. Transfusion-associated viruses grouped according to their compartmentalization in blood of asymptomatic donors

I. Cell-Associated Viruses
   Cytomegalovirus (CMV)
   Epstein-Barr Virus (EBV)
   Human Herpes Virus Type 6 (HHV-6)
   Human T-Lymphotropic Virus Type I
   (HTLV-I)
   Human T-Lymphotropic Virus Type II
   (HTLV-II)

II. Cell-Free Viruses
   Hepatitis A Virus (HAV)
   Hepatitis B Virus (HBV)
   Hepatitis C Virus (HCV)
   Human Parvovirus B19

III. Cell-Associated and Cell-Free Viruses
   Human Immunodeficiency Virus Type 1
   (HIV-1)
   Human Immunodeficiency Virus Type 2
   (HIV-2)

The human immunodeficiency viruses (HIV-1 and HIV-2) are the most important members of group 3 (cell-associated and cell-free viruses). The HIVs have significant leukocyte and plasma reservoirs throughout the course of infection,[16] and in particular during the acute preseroconversion phase of infection missed by donor anti-HIV screening.[17] Since virus can be recovered from, and is efficiently transmitted by transfusion of, cell-free plasma and plasma derivatives,[18,19] leukodepletion will clearly never play a definitive role in reducing HIV transmission. On the other hand, both sexual and transfusion transmission appear to be most efficient when large numbers of infected leukocytes are present in the inoculum.[20,21] Moreover, there is in vitro[22-24] as well as some clinical data[18] to suggest that significant, albeit incomplete, reduction in HIV-infectivity of blood components following leukodepletion (see below).

DONOR LEUKOCYTES ENHANCE SUSCEPTIBILITY OF RECIPIENTS TO VIRAL TRANSMISSION

Allogeneic blood transfusions, and particularly those containing viable donor leukocytes, lead to activation of the recipient's immune system. In 1972 Schechter et al[4] first demonstrated that during the first week after blood transfusion, there is a rise in the concentration of atypical lymphocytes and DNA-synthesizing mononuclear cells in the circulation of patients who received moderate amounts of blood. The increases in these parameters were greatest in patients transfused with fresh blood, while those transfused with blood stored more than 5 days showed modest activation, and those given leukocyte- and platelet-depleted red cells prepared by the glyc-erol-freezing method had no detectable responses (Fig. 8.1). In subsequent cytogenetic studies, Schechter et al[25] showed that the majority of transfusion-induced, spontaneously dividing mononuclear cells in a recipient's circulation were recipient cells. Occasional donor cells were also detected in the spontaneously dividing cell population at one week post-transfusion, an observation that has recently been confirmed by Adams, et al[26] using PCR directed at Y chromosome genetic sequences.

We recently extended this line of investigation. Using quantitative allele-specific PCR directed at donor HLA and Y chromosome sequences, we found that donor lymphocytes proliferated transiently following transfusions of immunocompetent humans and dogs (Fig. 8.2).[27] Thus,

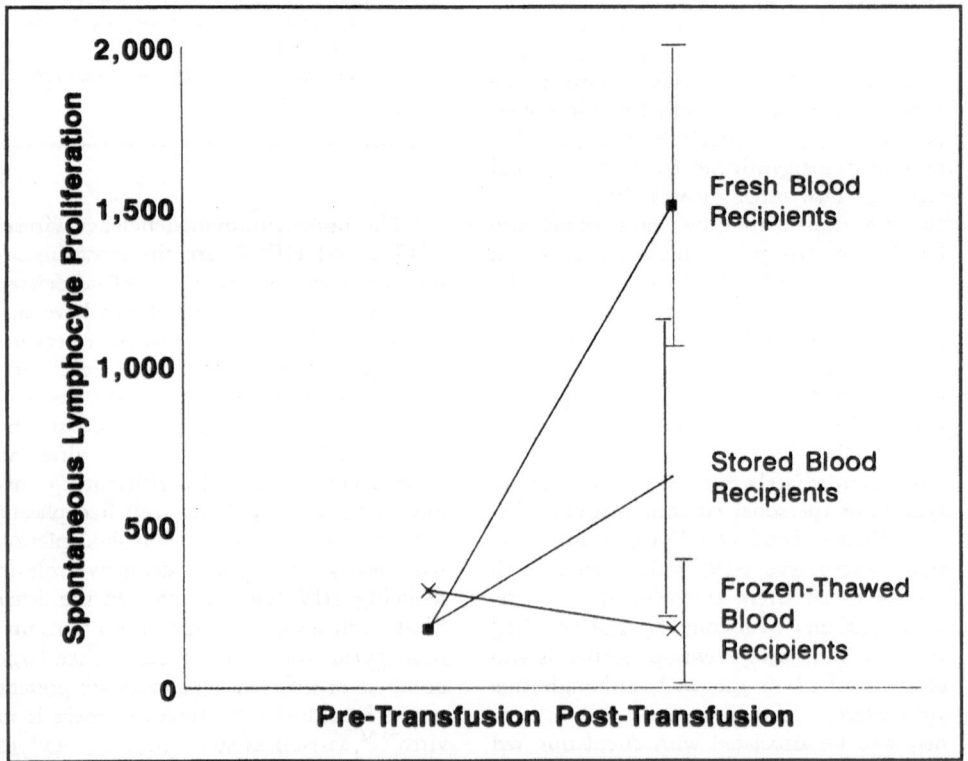

Fig. 8.1. Effect of transfusion of fresh, stored, and frozen RBC components on appearance of spontaneously proliferating lymphocytes in the circulation of recipients 5 days post-transfusion. Proliferation was determined by ^{3}H-thymidine incorporation. (From Schechter GP, Soehnlen F, McFarland W. N Engl J Med 287:1169, 1972, with permission.)

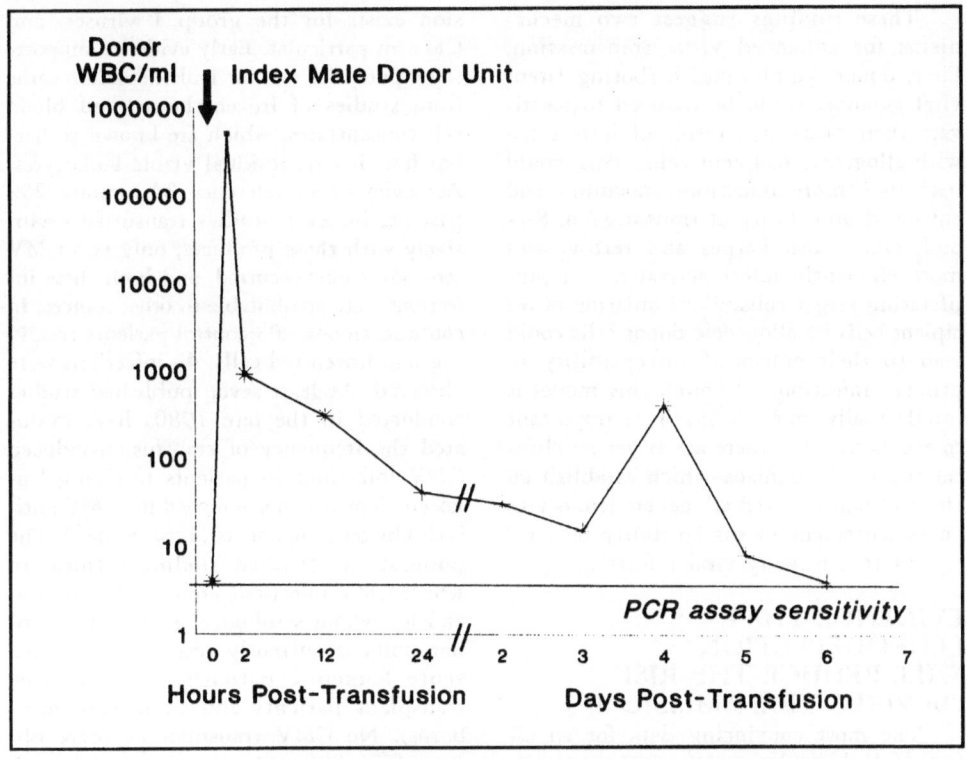

Fig. 8.2. Results of tracing male donor leukocytes transfused into a female orthopedic surgery patient using human Y chromosome allele-specific PCR. Note that following initial clearance of infused donor leukocytes, there is a 1 log increase on day 4 post-transfusion. Similar results were seen in five additional recipients and in a canine model. Gamma irradiation prevented donor cell expansion in transfused dogs, indicating that it results from proliferation. (From Lee T-H, Donegan E, Slichter S, Busch MP. Abstract #S-195. Blood, 1995, in press.)

introduction of allogeneic leukocytes into a transfusion recipient leads to a mixed-lymphocyte proliferative response analogous to an in vitro MLC.[28] This typically eventuates in complete clearance of the infused donor leukocytes, often associated with development of alloimmunization. In contrast, in immunosuppressed recipients or in situations where HLA homozygous donor cells are transfused into haplotype-identical recipients, the expanding donor lymphocyte proliferation may go unchecked and fatal graft versus host disease evolve.[29,30]

There are several lines of evidence suggesting that the activation of donor and recipient leukocytes following allogeneic transfusion increases the probability of transmission of donor viral infections to

recipients.[31] In studies conducted using murine CMV and inbred mice as a model system, Cheung and Lang[32] compared the rate of virus transmission following infusion of blood from mice harboring latent CMV into uninfected allogeneic and syngeneic recipients. After a latent period of days to weeks, virus was detected invariably in allogeneic but only rarely in syngeneic recipients (Fig. 8.3). Similarly, in in vitro studies on the effect of allogeneic leukocytes on HIV-1 reactivation and transmission, we[33] showed that coculture of mononuclear cells from two allogeneic donors prior to virus inoculation resulted in enhanced susceptibility to lower doses of virus, relative to the susceptibility of target cells that had not been stimulated by allogeneic cells (Fig. 8.4).

These findings suggest two mechanisms for enhanced virus transmission. First, donor lymphocytes harboring latent viral genomes could be induced to reactivate their virus as a result of interaction with allogeneic recipient cells. This would lead to a more infectious inoculum and enhanced probability of transmission. Second, since both herpes and retroviruses more efficiently infect activated and proliferating target cells,[2,31] stimulation of recipient cells by allogeneic donor cells could lead to their enhanced susceptibility to primary infection. Although this model is intellectually compelling, it is important to emphasize that there are as yet no clinical studies in humans which establish an effect of non-infected allogeneic leukocytes on enhancement of susceptibility of a recipient to a primary viral infection.

EVIDENCE THAT LEUKODEPLETION WILL REDUCE THE RISK OF VIRUS TRANSMISSION

The most convincing data for an effect of leukodepletion on virus transmission exists for the group 1 viruses, and CMV in particular. Early evidence supporting a potential role for leukodepletion came from studies of frozen-thawed red blood cell concentrates, which are known to harbor few, if any, residual viable leukocytes. As reviewed in reference 34, among 252 patients in seven studies transfused exclusively with these products, only two CMV seroconversions occurred, and both these infections were attributable to other sources. In contrast, among 203 control patients receiving non-frozen red cells, 43 infections were observed. At least seven published studies conducted in the late 1980s have evaluated the frequency of transfusion-induced CMV infections in patients receiving leukocyte-depleted (not screened for CMV antibody) blood components (Table 8.3).[34-41] The populations studied included those in whom CMV infections are most significant, and for whom serological screening of donor units is currently recommended (i.e., acute leukemia patients, bone marrow transplant patients and premature newborns). No CMV transmissions were observed in 200 patients supported with

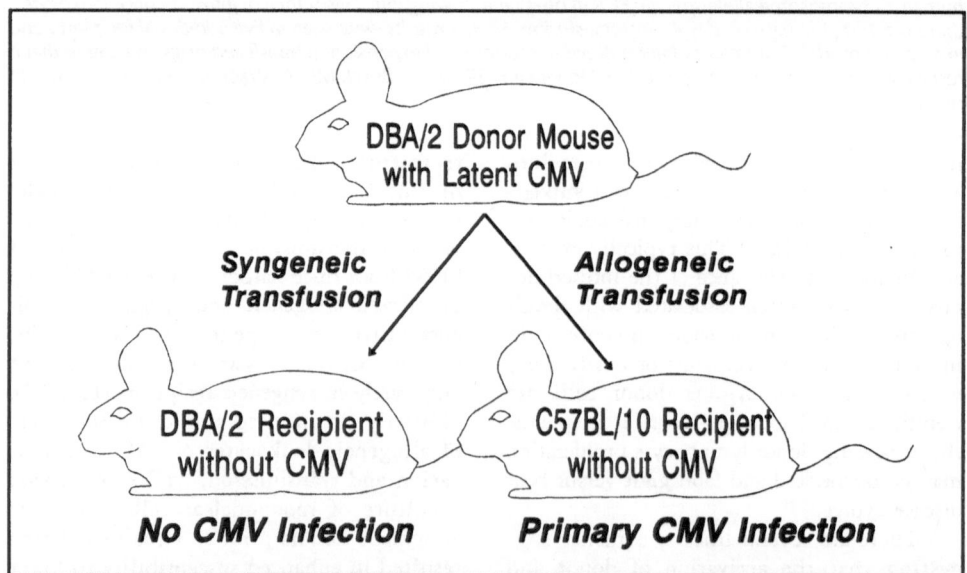

Fig. 8.3. Effect of MHC compatibility of donor and recipient on transmission of CMV by transfusion in murine model system. Transmission is significantly enhanced if donor and recipient are MHC-mismatched (i.e. allogeneic). (Adapted from Cheung K-S, Lang DJ. J Inf Dis 135:841, 1977, with permission.)

leukodepleted blood, whereas 17% of control patients receiving nonleukodepleted products were infected. These impressive results were obtained with filters that achieved only 2 to 3 log reductions in leukocytes. A multicenter, randomized study using contemporary 3 to 4 log leukodepletion filters has just been completed in the

Table 8.3. Frequency of transfusion-induced CMV infection in patients receiving leukocyte-depleted red blood cells and platelet concentrates

Authors [Ref]	Number of Patients	Diagnosis	CMV seroconversion: Control	Number & (%) Leukocyte-poor
Gilbert et al, 1989 [36]	72	Newborns	9/42 (21%)	0/30 (0%)
Murphy et al, 1988 [37]	20	Hematologic malignancy	2/9 (22%)	0/11 (0%)
DeGraan-Hentzen et al, 1989 [38]	145	Hematologic disease/ cardiac surgery	10/86 (12%)	0/59 (0%)
Bowden et al, 1989 [39]	65	Allo- and auto-BMT	7/30 (23%)	0/35 (0%)
Verdonck et al, 1987 [40]	29	BMT		0/29 (0%)
DeWitte et al, 1990 [41]	28	Hematologic malignancy		0/28 (0%)
Andreu, 1991 [35]	8	Acute leukemia		0/8 (0%)

BMT = bone marrow transplantation
(Modified from Andreu G. Sem Hematol 28:26, 1991, with permission)

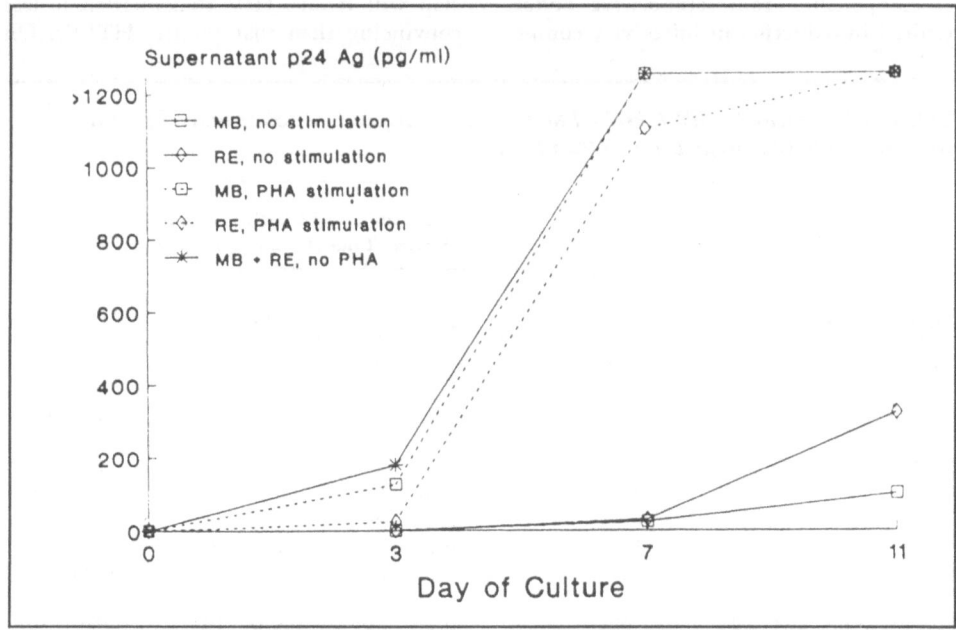

Fig. 8.4. Allogeneic leukocyte interaction facilitates acute HIV-1 infection of PBMC. Prior coculture of heterologous PBMC, (MB + RE, no PHA) increased kinetics of HIV-1 replication relative to unstimulated cells (MB, no stimulation; RE, no stimulation). The stimulatory effect of allogeneic cells was quantitatively similar to that seen after PHA-induced activation of either PBMC population (MB, PHA-stimulation; RE, PHA-stimulation). (Adapted from Busch MP, Lee T-H, Heitman J. Blood 80:2128, 1992, with permission.)

Seattle and Minneapolis regions which, based on a preliminary report, corroborates the efficacy of filtration in prevention of transfusion-transmitted CMV.[42]

Evidence for reduction in HTLV-I/II transmission by leukodepletion is more circumstantial. Studies from Japan, the Caribbean and the United States, in which recipients of anti-HTLV positive blood components were traced and tested, have each documented complete absence of transmission of HTLVs by plasma and plasma derivatives.[3,43] These studies have also shown virtual elimination of infectivity of red cells stored at 4°C for more than two weeks. Representative data (from the U.S. Transfusion Safety Study)[43] on infectivity of HTLV types I and II by component type and length of storage is shown in Table 8.4. A group in Japan has recently studied the effects of 3-log depletion filters on HTLV-I viral burden in vitro using quantitative PCR and viral culture techniques. Filtration of red cell and platelet components from seropositive donors resulted in reduction in infectivity compa-

rable to the overall levels of leukodepletion, although residual virus was demonstrable by PCR (personal communication, T. Takahashi). Because the frequency of transmission of HTLV-I/II from anti-HTLV-I screened blood in the U.S. is now exceedingly low (0.0016%/unit transfused),[44,45] it is unlikely that studies proving an effect of filtration on further reduction in risk are possible in either Japan or the United States. Although a controlled study comparing HTLV-transmission rates in filtered versus anti-HTLV screened blood would be of interest, such a study would need to be conducted in an area such as the Caribbean, where seroprevalence among donors is high and serological screening not yet routine. Were such a study conducted and the results convincing, perhaps anti-HTLV screening could be discontinued were routine leukodepletion implemented, thereby partially offsetting the cost of leukodepletion.

The data suggesting that leukodepletion will reduce HIV transmission is less convincing than that for the HTLVs. On

Table 8.4. Infectivity of HIV-1, HTLV-I and HTLV-II seropositive donor units, by component type and length of storage prior to transfusion

Component Type	Storage (Days)	Recipient's post-transfusion serostatus positive/total and unit infectivity (%)					
		HIV-1		HTLV-I		HTLV-II	
Cryoprecipitate/FFP	NA	16/18	(89)	0/8	(0)	0/9	(0)
Platelets	≤ 5	20/21	(95)	6/7	(86)	9/13	(69)
Red Cells	≤ 5	14/14	(100)	1/1	(100)	1/2	(50)
	6–10	17/18	(94)	2/7	(29)	6/11	(55)
	11–20	35/38	(92)	0/1	(0)	0/16	(0)
	21–25	6/7	(86)	0/0	(0)	1/4	(25)
	≤ 26	4/8	(50)	0/1	(0)	0/11	(0)
Frozen/Washed Red Cells	NA	0/2	(0)	0/0	(0)	0/4	(0)
Overall		112/126	(88)	9/25	(36)	17/70	(24)

(Compiled from Donegan E et al, and the Transfusion Safety Study Group, Transfusion 30:851, 1990; and Donegan E et al and the Transfusion Safety Study Group Transfusion 34; 478-483, 1994 with permission)

the negative side, fresh-frozen plasma from anti-HIV-1 positive donors transmits the virus at an approximately 90% rate, similar to that for fresh red cell and platelet components (Table 8.4).[18,43] Moreover, factor concentrates derived from unscreened plasma donations in the early 1980s were highly infectious, as evidenced by the approximately 50% rate of HIV infection among treated hemophiliacs,[19] with rates approaching 100% among those who received frequent, high doses of factor VIII (personal communication, James W. Mosley, TSS, University of Southern California). On the other hand, frozen-thawed and washed RBC, as well as RBC components stored greater than 3 weeks at 4°C, are associated with significantly lower (< 50%) transmission rates (Table 8.4).[18] Laboratory studies have also shown marked reduction in the number of infected leukocytes in units either spiked in vitro with infected cells or drawn from HIV seropositive donors, following leukodepletion using three to four log reduction filters (Table 8.5).[22,24] Current leukodepletion filters do not appear to impact free virus concentrations in plasma.[23,24]

As with HTLVs, clinical studies demonstrating reduction in HIV transmission by filtration are unlikely to be conducted in the United States, in part because the low residual risk of antibody screened blood (0.0004%/unit)[44,45] would necessitate a study including millions of recipients. A study comparing filtration with anti-HIV screening in third world countries where anti-HIV screening is not routine would

be academically interesting, but is probably unethical given the excellent performance of anti-HIV tests and the anticipated marginal effect and high cost of filtration. Nonetheless, several groups continue to investigate a role for leukodepletion, combined with other antiviral modalities, on reduction of HIV infectivity of blood collected from donors in the antibody-negative window phase of infection. In recent studies in our lab toward this objective, we made the surprising discovery that platelets have high levels of HIV particles adsorbed to them.[46,47] This is true both pre- and post-seroconversion. Although we have not yet established that platelet-associated HIV is infectious, these results further indicate that leukodepletion alone is unlikely to play a major role in safeguarding the blood supply from HIV.

DONOR LEUKOCYTE-INDUCED REACTIVATION OF RECIPIENT VIRAL INFECTIONS

As discussed above, donor leukocytes in transfused blood trigger an allograft-related mixed lymphocyte reaction involving donor and recipient leukocytes. Activation and subsequent proliferation of recipient cells can then trigger reactivation of a latent virus. An effect of donor leukocytes on reactivation of recipient infections was first described in the murine cytomegalovirus model (Fig. 8.5).[31,32] Infusion of blood from allogeneic, CMV-negative mice into mice harboring latent CMV infections leads to reactivation of CMV replication (i.e. ability to recover virus from blood and rise in

---

Table 8.5. In vitro studies of effects of leukocyte filtration on cell-associated HIV burden in donor blood

Experimental Conditions	Filter	Level of Depletion of Infected Cells (Log$_{10}$)	Reference
HIV-IIIB-infected H9 cells	RC100	5.4 – ≥ 5.5	Rawal et al, 1989 [22]
Naturally infected PBMC *	RC100	1.6 – 2.2	Rawal et al, 1989 [22]
in vitro HIV-infected PBMC	NPBI OC	2.5 – 2.9	Bruisten et al, 1990 [24]
Naturally infected PBMC *	NPBI OC	2.4 – ≥ 2.5	Bruisten et al, 1980 [24]

* PBMC derived from seropositive blood donor units

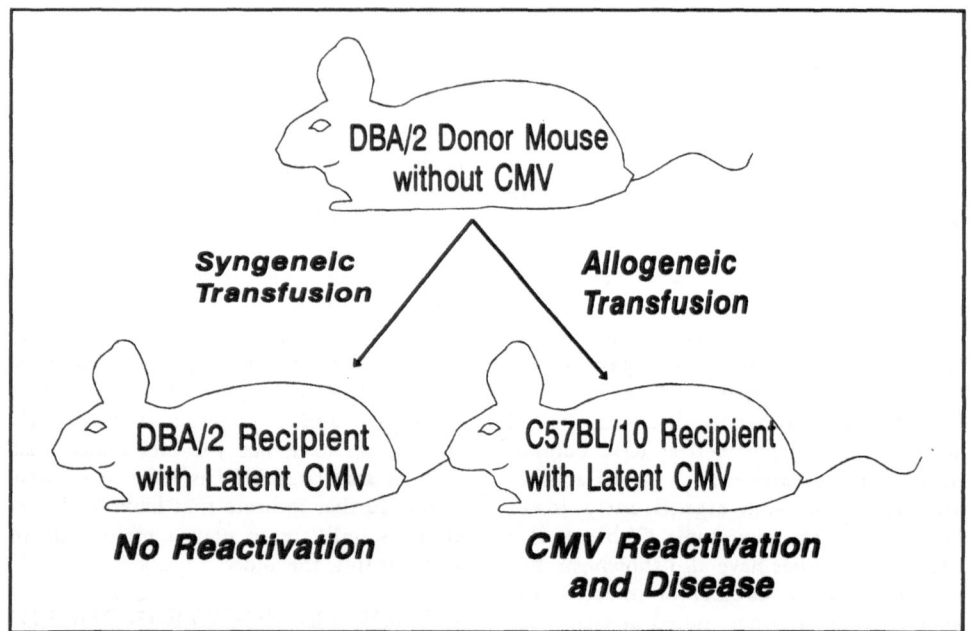

Fig. 8.5. Effect of MHC compatibility of donor and recipient on transfusion-induced reactivation of CMV in recipient mice. MHC-mismatched (allogeneic) transfusions induced reactivation, whereas MHC-identical (syngeneic) transfusions did not. (Adapted from Cheung K-S, Lang DJ. J Inf Dis 135:841, 1977, with permission.)

anti-CMV titers) days-to-weeks following transfusion. In humans, an effect of allogeneic blood transfusions on inducing reactivation of latent CMV infections is also well documented but not widely appreciated. Studies which contain this evidence were actually designed to determine whether there is a benefit to transfusion of CMV-seronegative blood into CMV-seropositive recipients. The answer was unequivocally no, since virtually identical infection rates (ranging from 7 to 30% in different study populations) were observed among seropositive recipients irrespective of the CMV status of donor blood (reviewed in reference 48). A low rate (1% or less) of reinfection could not be appreciated above the high level of background reactivation of recipient CMV. This data is often cited (appropriately) to argue that seropositive recipients will not benefit from CMV-screened blood. What has been frequently overlooked is the fact that the 13% rate of CMV viremia among transfused seropositive patients is very high relative

to spontaneous reactivation rates among seropositive donors (<1%) or non-transfused patients (<3%).[48] Thus, allogeneic transfusions appear to increase the rate of CMV reactivation 5- to 10-fold (Table 8.6). Although reactivation CMV infections are often asymptomatic and generally not as serious as primary infections,[1,48] if the pa-

Table 8.6. Rate of CMV infection and reactivation following allogeneic transfusion relative to CMV status of the donor and recipient

Serostatus of		Rate of
Recipient	Donor	CMV Viremia
−	+	< 1 – 7%
−	−	0
+	+	7 – 30%
+	−	7 – 30%

(Compiled from Tegtmeier GE. Arch Pathol Lab Med 113:236, 1989, with permission)

tient is immunosuppressed (e.g. bone marrow and organ transplant recipients and AIDS patients) the clinical consequences may be serious and even fatal.[1,49]

We recognized that giving an allogeneic blood transfusion to an HIV-1-infected patient is analogous to the current in vitro methodology for isolating HIV-1, in which mononuclear cells from an infected person are cocultured with PHA-stimulated cells from an allogeneic blood donor.[50] To pursue this hypothesis, we conducted a series of in vitro experiments to determine whether transfusion of cellular blood components (particularly those containing leukocytes) might activate HIV-1

in infected recipient cells, and thereby facilitate viral dissemination and disease progression.[33] We cocultured peripheral blood mononuclear cells (PBMC) from anti-HIV-1-positive individuals with serial dilutions of allogeneic PBMC, as well as purified populations of donor lymphocytes, monocytes, granulocytes, platelets, red blood cells (RBC), and plasma. Allogeneic donor PBMC, lymphocytes, monocytes, and granulocytes, but not platelets, red blood cells, or plasma, induced reactivation of HIV-1 in patient PBMC. The induction was dose-dependent, and enhanced by prior activation of the donor lymphocytes by phytohemagglutinin (PHA) (Fig. 8.6).

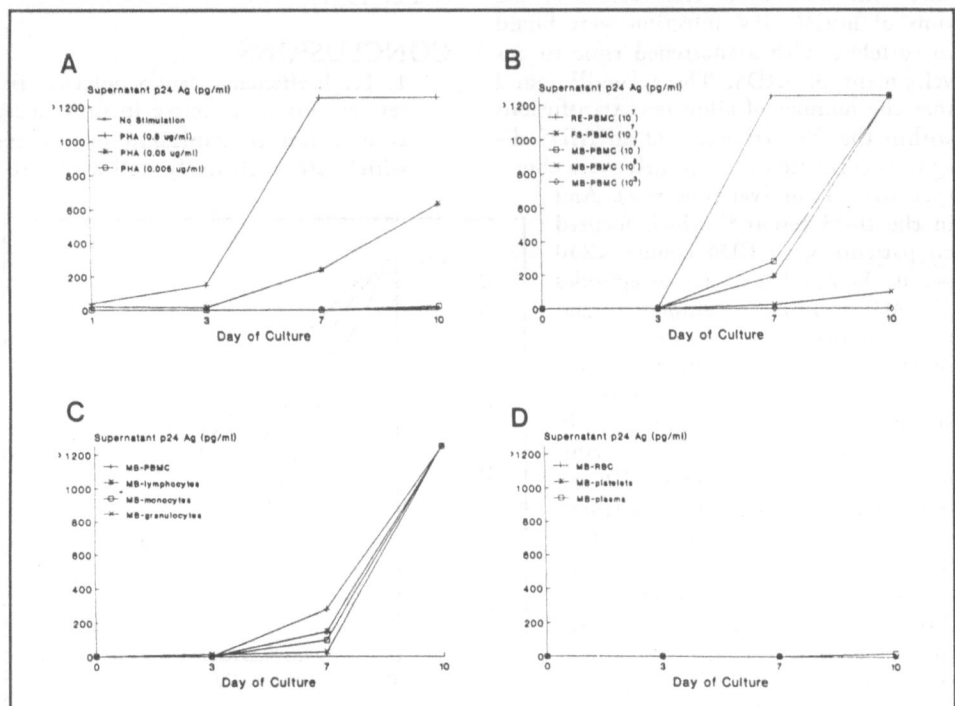

Fig. 8.6. Effect of allogeneic donor blood constituents on HIV replication in PBMC of a seropositive individual. No detectable viral antigen was observed when infected patient PBMC were cultured under conditions of minimal stimulation (5% serum and no supplemental IL-2 or PHA), whereas PHA stimulation of PBMC resulted in a dose-dependent induction of HIV-1 p24 antigen in culture supernatants (A). Coculture of PBMC from three normal donors (RE, FS, and MB) with patient PBMC induced p24 antigen expression in a dose-dependent manner (B). Induction of HIV p24 antigen expression was also observed after coculture of infected patient PBMC with allogeneic donor lymphocytes, monocytes, and granulocytes (C), whereas heterologous donor RBC, platelets, and plasma showed no effect (D). (Adapted from Busch MP, Lee T-H, Heitman J. Blood 80:2128, 1992, with permission.)

Careful kinetic studies using quantitative PCR and immunocytochemistry showed a biphasic pattern: an initial up-regulation of viral gene expression in in vivo infected cells was followed by dissemination to previously uninfected patient cells.

These in vitro results suggest that transfusion of allogeneic leukocytes, but not therapeutic blood constituents (RBC, platelets, plasma), may lead to up-regulation of HIV-1 expression and replication in infected PBMC, thereby accelerating further viral dissemination and cell death and accelerating the disease course. Three retrospective observational studies have recently documented just such a negative impact of transfusion on course of HIV infection. In one,[51] the number of transfusions at the time of initial HIV infection were found to correlate with a shortened time to development of AIDS. The second[52] found that the number of allogeneic transfusions within the first trimester of an AIDS diagnosis correlated significantly with shortened overall survival (Fig. 8.7). And in the third report,[49] which focused on patients with CD4 counts <250 per µl, the number of serious episodes of CMV retinitis, pneumonitis and gastroenteritis increased in proportion to the number of transfusions received. In a follow-up laboratory investigation to this study, we recently obtained preliminary data showing induction of CMV viremia in HIV infected patients following transfusion of red blood cell components (Fig. 8.8).

Is there any clinical evidence that directly implicates donor leukocytes in this viral reactivation, or which shows that use of leukodepleted blood would reduce or eliminate this problem? Unfortunately, the recent prospective study[1,42] which demonstrated that leukodepletion can prevent CMV transmission was restricted to seronegative recipients, so an effect of leukodepletion on CMV reactivation could not be evaluated. However, a small study involving cardiac trans-

plant patients recently reported by Thompson et al[53] in abstract form includes intriguing preliminary data suggesting that leukodepletion may prevent CMV reactivation (Table 8.7). The rate of CMV-reactivation-related disease in seropositive recipients was reduced from 33% (11/33) to 0 (0/15) by use of leukodepleted blood components. The National Heart, Lung and Blood Institute recently announced plans to conduct a prospective multicenter study to determine the impact of allogeneic transfusion on HIV and CMV viral burden and disease course. Patients will be randomized to receive leukodepleted, gamma irradiated, or standard transfusions. Definitive data should be available by the end of 1997.

CONCLUSIONS

1. High-efficiency leukodepletion filters are highly effective in preventing transfusion transmission of viruses which are exclusively cell-associated

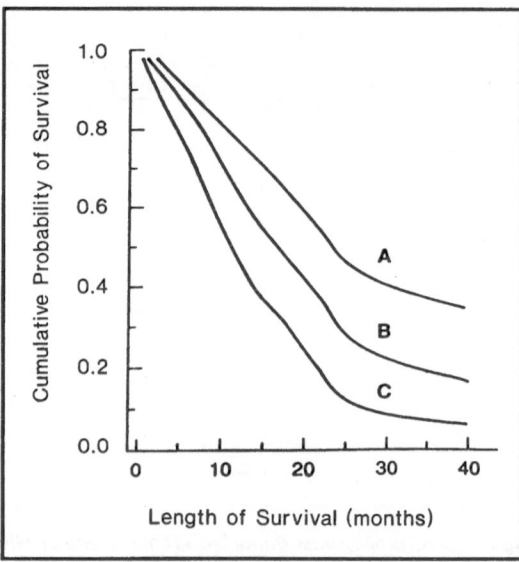

Fig. 8.7. Transfusions decrease survival of HIV-infected AIDS patients. Theoretical construction of survivor functions for untransfused (A), lightly transfused (B), and heavily transfused (C) AIDS patients who otherwise have the most favorable prognostic attributes to illustrate the effect of blood transfusion. (Adapted from Vamvakas E, Kaplan HS. Transfusion 33:111, 1993, with permission.)

(e.g. CMV and possibly HTLV-I and HTLV-II).

2. Allogeneic transfusions containing leukocytes induce immune activation of recipient and donor lymphocytes. This may facilitate virus transmission by activation of latent virus in donor cells and/or enhancing susceptibility of recipient cells to infection.

3. Allogeneic donor leukocytes may trigger reactivation of pre-existing recipi-

ent viral infections. Preliminary data suggest that leukodepletion may prevent this complication.

4. Since donor leukocytes harbor transfusion-associated viruses and may induce reactivation of recipient infections, routine exclusion of leukocytes from allogeneic blood transfusions should be considered a long-term goal.

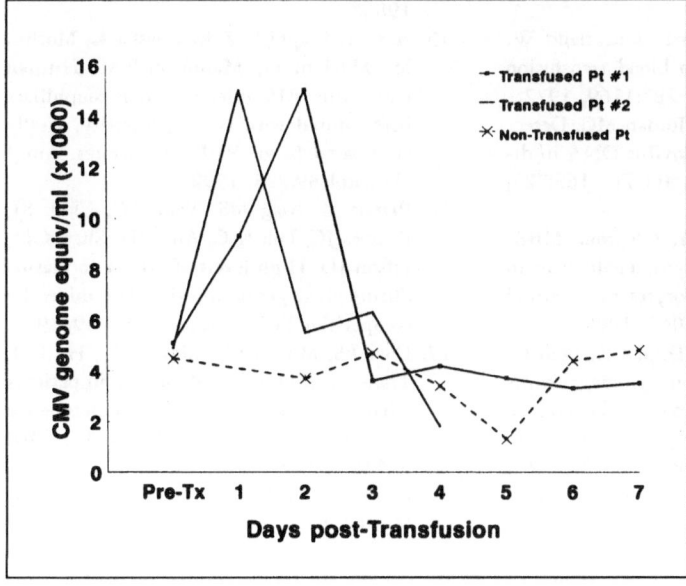

Fig. 8.8. Induction of CMV viremia by allogeneic RBC transfusion (non-leukodepleted) of HIV-positive patients. CMV-DNA signal amplification assay (Branched DNA; Chiron Corp.) was used to quantitate CMV DNA in plasma collected serially pre- and post-transfusion. As a control a non-transfused HIV-positive patient with similar CD4 cell count was sampled on a daily basis.

Table 8.7. Rate of CMV infection in heart transplant patients receiving leukodepleted versus non-leukodepleted transfusions

CMV Serostatus		Transfused Components	
Recipient	Heart	Non-filtered	Filtered *
neg	neg	0/4 (0)	0/8
neg	pos	-	2/7
pos	neg	1/13 (8%)	0/5
pos	pos	10/20 (50%)	0/15

* Pall RC100 and PL100 filters
(Modified from Reference 53, with permission)

REFERENCES

1. Bowden RA. Cytomegalovirus: transmission by blood components and measures of prevention. Chapter 7 in Nance SJ, Blood Safety: Current Challenges. Amer Assn of Blood Banks, Bethesda MD, 1992.

2. Pantaleo G, Graziosi C, Fauci AS. The immunopathogenesis of human immunodeficiency virus infection. N Engl J Med 328:327, 1993.

3. Sandler SG, Fang CT, Williams AE. Human T-cell lymphotropic virus type I and II in transfusion medicine. Transfus Med Rev 5:93, 1991.

4. Schechter GP, Soehnlen F, McFarland W. Lymphocyte response to blood transfusion in man. N Engl J Med 287:1169, 1972.

5. Collins T, Pomeroy C, Jordan MC. Detection of latent cytomegalovirus DNA in diverse organs of mice. J Inf Dis 168:725, 1993.

6. Schrier RD, Nelson JA, Oldstone MBA. Detection of human cytomegalovirus in peripheral blood lymphocytes in a natural infection. Science 230:1048, 1985.

7. Bitsch A, Kirchner H, Dupke R, Bein G. Failure to detect human cytomegalovirus DNA in peripheral blood leukocytes of healthy blood donors by the polymerase chain reaction. Transfusion 32:612, 1992.

8. Bitsch A, Kirchner H, Dupke R, Bein G. Cytomegalovirus transcripts in peripheral blood leukocytes of actively infected transplant patients detected by reverse transcription-polymerase chain reaction. J Inf Dis 167:740, 1993.

9. Drobyski WR, Dunne WM, Burd EM, Knox KK, Ash RC, Horowitz MM, Flomenberg N, Carrigan DR. Human herpesvirus-6 (HHV-6) infection in allogeneic bone marrow transplant recipients: evidence of a marrow-suppressive role for HHV-6 in vivo. J Inf Dis 167:735, 1993.

10. Hanto DW, Frizzera G, Gajl-Peczalska J, Simmons RL. Epstein-Barr virus, immunodeficiency, and B cell lymphoproliferation. Transplantation 39:461, 1985.

11. Hoofnagle JH. Posttransfusion hepatitis B. (editorial) Transfusion 30:384, 1990.

12. Gill P. Transfusion-associated Hepatits C: Reducing the risk. Transfus Med Reviews

7:104, 1993.

13. Casarin C, Ruvoletto MG, de Moliner L, et al. HCV DNA in serum, peripheral blood mononuclear cells (PBMC) and liver of patients with chronic hepatitis C treated with alpha interferon. Abstract 106. IV Intl Symposium on HCV, Tokyo, May:93, 1993.

14. Noonan CA, Yoffe B, Mansell PWA, Melnick JL, Hollinger FB. Extrachromosomal sequences of hepatitis B virus DNA in peripheral blood mononuclear cells of acquired immune deficiency syndrome patients. Proc Natl Acad Sci USA, 83:5698, 1986.

15. Azzi A, Ciappi S, Zakvrzewska K, Morfini M, Mariani G, Mannucci PM. Human parvovirus B19 infection in hemophiliacs first infused with two high-purity, virally attenuated factor VIII concentrates. Am J Hematol 39:228, 1992.

16. Piatak M, Saag MS, Yang LC, Clark SJ, Kappes JC, Luk K-C, Ahn BH, Shaw GM, Lifson JD. High levels of HIV-1 in plasma during all stages of infection determined by competitive PCR. Science 259:1749, 1993.

17. Daar ES, Moudgil T, Meyer RD, Ho DD. Transient high levels of viremia in patients with primary human immunodeficiency virus type 1 infection. N Engl J Med 324:961, 1991.

18. Donegan E, Lenes BA, Tomasulo PA, Mosley JW, and the Transfusion Safety Study Group. Transmission of HIV-1 by component type and duration of shelf storage before transfusion. Transfusion 30:851, 1990.

19. Kim HC, Nahum K, Raska K, Jr., Gocke DJ, Kosmin M, Karp GI, Saidi P. Natural history of acquired immunodeficiency syndrome in hemophilic patients. Amer J Hematol 24:168, 1987.

20. Anderson DJ, Politch JA, Martinez A, van Voorhis BJ. White blood cells and HIV-1 in semen from vasectomised seropositive men. Lancet 338:573, 1991.

21. Transfusion Safety Study, represented by Busch MP. Clinical and virological factors influencing transmission of HIV-1 by transfusion. Abstract S-214. Transfusion 32 (Suppl):56-S, 1992.

22. Rawal BD, Busch MP, Endow R, et al.

Reduction of human immunodeficiency virus-infected cells from donor blood by leukocyte filtration. Transfusion 26:460, 1989.

23. Rawal B, Yen TSB, Vyas GN, Busch M. Leukocyte filtration removes infectious particulate debris but not free virus derived from experimentally lysed HIV-infected cells. Vox Sang, 60:214, 1991.

24. Bruisten SM, Tersmette M, Wester MR, Vos AHV, Koppelman MHGM, Huisman JG. Efficiency of white cell filtration and a freeze-thaw procedure for removal of HIV-infected cells from blood. Transfusion 30:833, 1990.

25. Schechter GP, Whang-Peng J, McFarland W. Circulation of donor lymphocytes after blood transfusion in man. Blood 49:651, 1977.

26. Adams PT, Davenport RD, Reardon DA, Roth MS. Detection of circulating donor white blood cells in patients receiving multiple transfusions. Blood 80:551, 1992.

27. Lee T-H, Donegan E, Slichter S, Busch MP. Transient increase in circulating in immunocompetent recipients compatible with donor cell proliferation. Blood 1994/5, in press.

28. Dzik WH, Jones KS. The effects of gamma irradiation versus leukocyte reduction on the mixed lymphocyte reaction. Transfusion 33:493, 1993.

29. Ferrara JLM, Deeg HJ. Graft-versus-host disease (review). New Engl J Med 324:667, 1991.

30. Petz LD, Calhoun L, Yam P, et al. Transfusion-associated graft-versus-host disease in immunocompetent patients: report of a fatal case associated with transfusion of blood from a second-degree relative, and a survey of predisposing factors. Transfusion 33:742, 1993.

31. Oldstone MBA, Molecular Basis of Viral Persistence. AIDS Research and Human Retroviruses 3:207, 1987.

32. Cheung K-S, Lang DJ. Transmission and activation of cytomegalovirus with blood transfusion: a mouse model. J Inf Dis 135:841, 1977.

33. Busch MP, Lee T-H, Heitman J. Allogeneic leukocytes but not therapeutic blood elements induce reactivation and dissemi-

nation of latent HIV-1 infection: Implications for transfusion support of infected patients. Blood 80:2128, 1992.

34. Sniecinski I. Prevention of immunologic and infectious complications of transfusion by leukocyte depletion. Cptr 18 in Clinical Application of Leukocyte Depletion. (Proceedings of the 3rd Hokkaido Symposium on Transfusion Medicine) S. Sekiguchi, ed. 1993:202. Blackwell Scientific Publ, Oxford U.K.

35. Andreu G. Role of leukocyte depletion in the prevention of transfusion-induced cytomegalovirus infection. Sem Hematol 28:26, 1991.

36. Gilbert GL, Hayes K, Hudson IL, James I, and the Neonatal Cytomegalovirus Infection Study Group. Prevention of transfusion-acquired cytomegalovirus infection in infants by blood filtration to remove leukocytes. Lancet i:1228, 1989.

37. Murphy MF, Grint PCA, Hardiman AE, Lister TA, Waters AH. Use of leukocyte-poor blood components to prevent primary cytomegalovirus (CMV) infection in patients with acute leukemia. Br J Haematol 70:253, 1988.

38. DeGraan-Hentzen YC, Gratama JW, Mudde GC, et al. Prevention of primary cytomegalovirus infection in patients with hematologic malignancies by intensive white cell depletion of blood products. Transfusion 29:757, 1989.

39. Bowden RA, Sayers MH, Cays M, Slichter SJ. The role of blood product filtration in the prevention of transfusion associated cytomegalovirus (CMV) infection after marrow transplant. Abstract #205-S. Transfusion 29(suppl):57-S, 1989.

40. Verdonck LF, DeGraan-Hentzen YC, Dekker AW, Mudde GC, DeGast GC. Cytomegalovirus seronegative platelets and leukocyte-poor red blood cells from random donors can prevent primary cytomegalovirus infection after bone marrow transplantation. Bone Marrow Transplant 2:73, 1987.

41. DeWitte T, Schattenberg A, van Dijk BA, Galama J, Olthuis H, van der Meer JWW, Kunst VAJM. Prevention of primary cytomegalovirus infection after allogeneic bone marrow transplantation by using leukocyte-

poor random blood products from cytome-galovirus-unscreened blood-bank donors. Transplantation 50:964, 1990.

42. Bowden RA, Cays M, Schoch G, Sayers M, et al. Comparison of filtered blood (FB) to seronegative blood products (SB) for prevention of cytomegalovirus (CMV) infection after marrow transplant. Abstract #800. Blood 82(10-Suppl 1):204, 1993.

43. Donegan E, Lee H, Operskalski EA, Shaw GM, Kleinman SH, Busch MP, Stevens CE, Schiff ER, Nowicki MJ, Hollingsworth CG, Mosley JW and the Transfusion Safety Study Group. Transfusion transmission of retroviruses: human T-lymphotopic viruses types I and II compared with human immunodeficiency virus type 1. Transfusion 34: 478-483, 1994.

44. Nelson KE, Donahue JG, Munoz A, et al. Transmission of retroviruses from seronegative donors by transfusion during cardiac surgery; a multicenter study of HIV-1 and HTLV-I/II infections. Ann Int Med 117:554, 1992.

45. Dodd RY. The risk of transfusion-transmitted infection (editorial). N Engl J Med 327:419, 1992.

46. Lee T-H, StrombergRR, Henrard D, Busch MP. Effect of platelet-associated virus ·on assays of HIV-1 in plasma. (comments on Piatak, et al.) Science, 262:1585-1586, 1993.

47. Lee T-H, Heitman J, Stromberg RR, Busch MP. Distribution of HIV in Units of Blood from Infected Donors. Abstract S-257. Transfusion 33(9 suppl):67-S, 1993.

48. Tegtmeier GE. Posttransfusion cytomegalovirus infections. Arch Pathol Lab Med 113:236, 1989.

49. Sloand EM, Kumar P, Merritt S, Klein H, Sacher R. Transfusion of blood components to persons infected with HIV: Relationship to opportunistic infection. Transfusion 34:48, 1994.

50. Busch MP, Rajagopalan MS, Gantz DM, Fu S, Steimer KS, Vyas GN. In situ hybridization and immunocytochemistry for improved assessment of human immunodeficiency virus cultures. Am J Clin Path 88:673, 1987.

51. Ward JW, Bush TJ, Perkins HA, et al. The natural history of transfusion-associated infection with human immunodeficiency virus. N Engl J Med 321:947, 1989.

52. Vamvakas E, Kaplan HS. Early transfusion and length of survival in acquired immune deficiency syndrome: experience with a population receiving medical care at a public hospital. Transfusion 33:111, 1993.

53. Thompson KS, Plapp FV, Long ND, Heenan TA. CMV infection in transplant recipients. Abstract #S-249 Transfusion 32(suppl):65-S, 1992.

CHAPTER 9

LEUKOCYTE DEPLETION AND TRANSFUSION–INDUCED IMMUNOMODULATION

Darrell J. Triulzi, Neil Blumberg

SUMMARY

The paradigm related to the immunologic consequences of allogeneic blood transfusions has been extended from humoral allosensitization to the effects of transfusion on cellular immune function. This includes down-regulation of effector cells, activation of latent viral infection, and the prolonged circulation of donor immunocompetent cells, as seen in graft-versus-host disease (GVHD).

In addition, there are now extensive data showing conclusively that allogeneic transfusions are associated with enhanced renal allograft tolerance, increased risks of cancer recurrence rates (about 80% in colorectal cancer) and postoperative bacterial infections (as much as 200-1000% in some studies). Whether these last two associations are causal or not remains in doubt although convincing animal data exist for all three outcomes. These associations are most likely in part due to immune modulation caused by transfusion, perhaps augmented by the effects of hemorrhage, anesthesia, and surgical stress.

The most likely mechanism underlying transfusion-induced immunosuppression is anergy due to presentation of large amounts of antigen through the intravenous route. This favors presentation of antigen by "non-professional" antigen presenting cells, a situation that usually leads to anergy or tolerance rather than immune activation. For some years it has been thought that transfused allogeneic white cells are the major mediator of transfusion induced immunomodulation. Results from animal and clinical studies strongly support this possibility. Results of some initial interventional studies, employing autologous transfusions or leuko-depletion of allogeneic donor blood suggest that relatively simple, cost-

Clinical Benefits of Leukodepleted Blood Products, edited by Joseph Sweeney, M.D. and Andrew Heaton, M.D. © 1995 R.G. Landes Company.

effective strategies to ameliorate these complications may be suitable for application in the near future.

INTRODUCTION

The concept that transfusions modulate the immune system is not a new one. Sentinel work in animal models by Medawar, Billingham, and others in the 1940s and 50s showed that large antigenic challenges in the form of transfusion were capable of inducing donor specific sensitization as well as donor specific tolerance. It was not until 1973 that the immunomodulating effect of transfusion was conclusively demonstrated in humans when Opelz and Terasaki reported that pretransplant transfusions prolonged renal allograft survival.[1] The dichotomy in immune response to transfusion observed in animals studies was also observed in humans since sensitization occurred in 30% of transfused renal transplant candidates.[2] Confirmation of the "transfusion effect" in renal transplantation led investigators to examine the immunosuppressive effect of transfusion in other clinical settings. The first, and probably most controversial effect, was the adverse association of transfusion with colon cancer recurrence originally reported by Burrows and Tartter in 1982.[3] This was followed by a proliferation of studies examining the effect of transfusion not only in the area of tumor recurrence, but in numerous other clinical settings such as postoperative bacterial infection, and most recently, reactivation and progression of viral infections.

To this day the mechanism by which transfusion mediates one or more of these effects remains obscure. The observation that the effect is donor specific in transplantation and nonspecific in the setting of cancer recurrence and postoperative bacterial infection, makes it unlikely that only one mechanism is operative. Nonetheless, mounting evidence implicates the transfused leukocyte as the central actor. This does not preclude an additional role for stored plasma since leukocytes break down during storage, releasing membrane fragments and

cytokines into the supernatant. In addition, while class I and class II antigens are most strongly expressed on leukocytes, large amounts of soluble HLA antigen also are found in plasma. Studies of transfusion immunomodulation with leukocyte depleted blood components have provided insight into the mechanism of the transfusion effect and a potential method for altering the adverse outcomes associated with transfusion. The data regarding the effect of leukocyte depletion on transfusion immunomodulation in the setting of transplantation, postoperative bacterial infection, cancer recurrence, and viral infection will be reviewed.

TRANSPLANTATION

Blood components which were leukocyte depleted by washing were widely recommended for dialysis dependent chronic renal failure patients in the 1960s to prevent sensitization. Transfusion practices eventually changed completely after Opelz and Terasaki reported that renal allograft survival was prolonged by transfusion.[1] Numerous studies confirmed the benefit of pretransplant transfusion and some demonstrated that leukocyte depleted blood products were less effective then whole blood or packed cells in prolonging allograft survival.[4] Transplant centers abandoned washed red cells and liberalized transfusion practice with the development of deliberate random donor or donor specific transfusion protocols. This remained accepted practice for more than a decade despite a continuing risk of sensitization of approximately 30% in unconditioned patients and 5-10% in patients treated with azathioprine concomitant with transfusion.[2]

The adoption of cyclosporine containing regimens in the early 1980s led to a decline in the benefit of pretransplant transfusions. The graft survival advantage conferred by transfusions has progressively declined for a multitude of reasons including better immunosuppression, better treatment of rejection, and improved patient care.[5] Additionally, current red cell concentrates often contain less than 10% of the plasma and 5% of the leukocytes present in red cell concentrates from the 1970s. Thus the disappearing transfusion effect may also be due in part to the decreasing leukocyte and plasma content of pretransplant transfusions. In 1991, for the first time, the UCLA and UNOS transplant registries reported that renal transplant recipients who were not transfused had superior graft survival rates to transfused recipients of either cadaveric or living related renal transplants.[6] Furthermore, transfused patients were more likely to be sensitized.[6] These data have produced a full circle reversal in most transplant centers away from deliberate transfusions and back to leukocyte depleted blood products to reduce the risk of alloimmunization.

Leukocyte depleted blood products are also increasingly used to reduce the risk of alloimmunization in candidates for other solid organs including heart and heart-lung transplants. Data in heart transplant recipients show that the degree of alloimmunization, as assessed by the percent of panel reactive antibody, correlates with the risk of acute and chronic heart allograft rejection.[7,8] A similar relationship appears to exist in heart-lung transplant recipients[9] and is suspected in lung transplant recipients, although published data in this group are lacking. There is little evidence to support leukocyte depleted blood products for liver transplant candidates since HLA alloimmunization appears to play little if any role in liver allograft rejection.[10] However, alloimmunized patients appear to require more intraoperative blood products, particularly platelet transfusions.[11] These data suggest that the strategy for transfusion support of solid organ transplant candidates should be to avoid transfusions when possible and use leukocyte depleted blood when transfusion is necessary prior to transplantation.

POSTOPERATIVE BACTERIAL INFECTION

A review of this topic several years ago showed that the preponderance of animal data and 11 of 12 clinical studies found transfusion to be an independent risk factor for postoperative bacterial infection.[12] A total of 34 clinical studies are summarized in Table 9.1. These comprise eleven studies in gastrointestinal surgery,[13-22,46] seven in trauma patients,[23-29] five in cardiac/vascular surgery,[30-34] four in head and neck surgery,[35-38] four in orthopedic surgery,[39-42] one in burn patients[43] and two with a mixed patient population.[44,45] Thirty of 34 studies have found transfusion to be associated with postoperative bacterial infection using univariate statistical analysis. In the 30 studies which used multivariate analysis to account for covariates, transfusion was an independent predictor of infection in 28 studies.

Table 9.1. Clinical studies: transfusion and postoperative bacterial infection

Patients	# Studies	#Prospective/ #Retrospective	Transfusion as a Predictor of Increased Infection Rates*	
			#Univariate	#Multivariate
Colon/GI[13-22,46]	11	8/3	10	9
Trauma[23-29]	7	3/4	7	6
Cardiovascular[30-34]	5	1/4	5	5
Head/Neck[35-38]	4	2/2	3	1
Orthopedic[39-42]	4	2/2	3	4
Burn[43]	1	0/1	1	1
Mixed[44,45]	2	1/1	1	2
TOTALS	34	17/17	30	28

* Number of studies finding transfusion to be a significant predictor of increased infection rates by univariate and/or multivariate analysis.

Despite the overwhelming clinical data demonstrating the adverse effect of transfusion in this setting, the criticism that transfusion may be merely a surrogate for other risk factors (i.e. surgical difficulty, tissue destruction or contamination) persists. While there is little evidence for such a "surrogacy" effect in the observational studies, tightly controlled studies were lacking. This problem has been addressed by three recent prospective randomized studies, two of which show a protective effect of autologous or leukocyte depleted transfusions.[19,20,46] Jensen and colleagues[19] studied 197 patients undergoing elective colorectal surgery (Fig. 9.1). Patients requiring transfusion were randomized to receive whole blood or whole blood leukocyte depleted by bedside filtration using Pall filters. The postoperative infection rate in the untransfused group (2%), and the group receiving filtered whole blood (2%), was significantly lower than the infection rate in the group receiving standard whole

blood (23%, p < 0.01). Their clinical observation was supported by in vitro immunologic data showing that patients receiving unfiltered whole blood had depressed NK cell activity 1 to 4 weeks postoperatively. Quantitative decreases in NK cells have been previously been reported in surgical patients who received allogeneic, but not autologous blood.[42] The clinical and surgical characteristics of the patients receiving unfiltered vs. filtered whole blood were similar except for more patients with fecal loaded bowel in the unfiltered whole blood group (8 of 56 versus 2 of 48). This did not correlate with infection since only 2 of the 10 patients with fecal loaded bowel developed infection. This study provides strong evidence that transfusion is an independent risk factor for infection, and that the effect is mediated by allogeneic leukocytes and not plasma.

The only negative prospective randomized study was performed by Busch and associates.[20] Four hundred and twenty-three

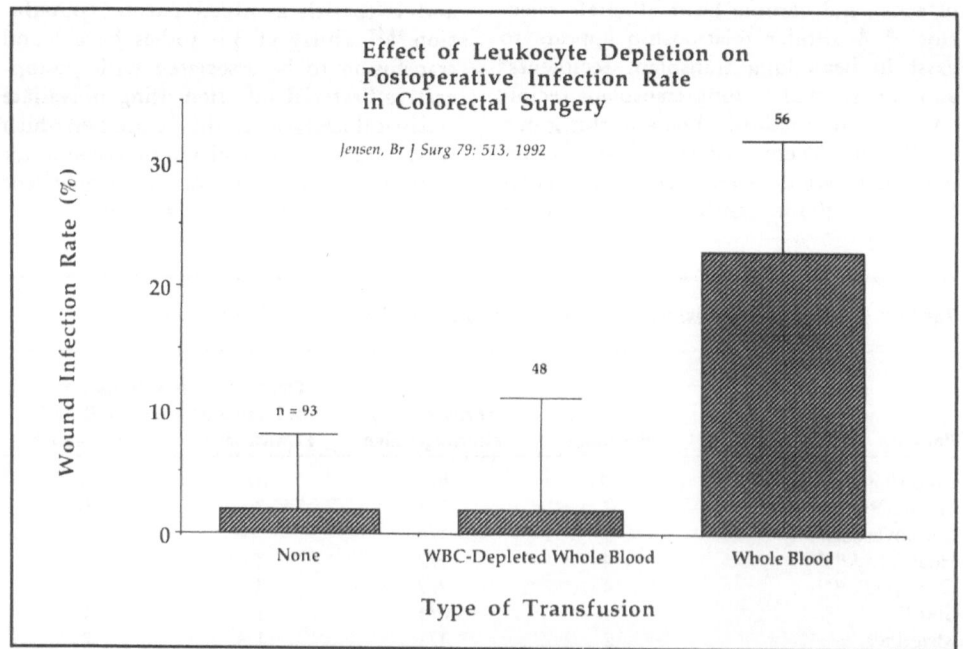

Fig. 9.1. *The results of a study of transfusion induced enhancement of postoperative infections in colorectal surgery are shown.[19] Recipients of allogeneic blood had significantly higher infection rates than recipients of leukocyte depleted allogeneic transfusions or no transfusions.*

patients undergoing curative resection of colorectal cancers were randomized to donate two units of autologous blood or receive allogeneic banked blood. The postoperative infection rate in the group receiving allogeneic blood (25%) was not different from the infection rate of 27% in the autologous group, but detailed analysis has not yet been published of these findings. There are two important methodologic concerns regarding this study. First, patients who received both autologous and allogeneic blood were grouped with the autologous only recipients in calculating the infection rate. Second, standard blood components in the Netherlands have the buffy coat removed during processing and thus are about 65-70% leukocyte depleted. Thus this study probably compared moderately leukocyte depleted allogeneic transfusions with autologous transfusions. The study by Jensen[19] suggests that leukocyte content of the transfusion is an important determinant in the immunosuppressive effect of transfusion as regards postoperative infection. In another study that compared standard red cell allogeneic transfusions (not leukocyte reduced in any manner) with autologous transfusions, the recipients of autologous blood had lower infection rates.[46]

The immunomodulating effect of allogeneic leukocytes in reducing resistance to bacterial infection is supported by observational clinical studies demonstrating that autologous transfusion is not associated with the increased risk of postoperative infection seen after allogeneic transfusions.[40-42,44,46] Animal models using whole blood transfusion and a bacterial challenge have been conflicting with some[47-51] but not all[52-55] showing that allogeneic transfusion is associated with an impaired resistance to infection compared to controls receiving syngeneic transfusion or saline. The only animal study to date that examined the relative effects of different blood components found that the leukocyte fraction of allogeneic blood most impaired bacterial clearance and survival.[51] While the mechanism of the immunomodulating effect of transfusion on postoperative infection is still under investigation, the role of the transfused leukocyte is emerging as the central actor. Additional prospective randomized clinical studies of leukocyte depleted blood components in surgical patients are needed before leukocyte depleted blood can be routinely recommended for this indication.

CANCER RECURRENCE

The most controversial association between transfusion, altered host immune function and clinical outcome is that for earlier tumor recurrence in transfused patients. Early animal studies actually demonstrated a protective effect of transfusion in one setting.[56] Later animal studies have largely shown that transfusion from allogeneic sources accelerates tumor growth, increases the number of metastases or leads to more rapid death. Of 23 studies, 18 found an enhancing effect of allogeneic transfusion on tumor growth as compared with either syngeneic transfusions and/ or saline control infusions.[56-78] However, in one instance, stored syngeneic transfusions have been shown to accelerate tumor progression as well.[63] In a few instances, transfusion has inhibited tumor take or progression.[56,70]

While this evidence seems overwhelmingly supportive of the hypothesis that transfusion impairs host resistance to tumor or accelerates tumor growth, or both, there are important caveats. Animal models are quite different from spontaneously arising human tumors in many important biologic characteristics. In most models, transfusions are given prior to tumor challenge, the opposite of the clinical situation. The transfusions given are often with heparin anticoagulant rather than the clinically used citrate anticoagulant-preservative. Heparin may have tumor inhibiting properties of its own.[79] The transfusions in animal models are not stored for days to weeks prior to use, as are clinical transfusions. Thus while most animal models support the notion that transfusion enhances tumor progression, the extrapolation to the clinical setting remains one of informed speculation rather than certainty.

Because of the early studies demonstrating a possible tumor enhancing effect of allogeneic transfusions, retrospective studies of transfused patients with a variety of tumors were performed, beginning with that of Burrows and Tartter in colorectal cancer in 1982.[3] The single largest number of studies has been performed in patients with this tumor, but putative transfusion effects have been reported in multiple other tumors (see reviews 3, 80-84). Of 40 studies in colorectal cancer[20,85-123] slightly less than 70% (27 out of 40) demonstrate a statistically significant deleterious effect of transfusion. Almost all the rest demonstrate a poorer outcome in transfused patients that either fails to achieve statistical significance, or becomes statistically insignificant in multivariate analysis. Meta-analyses of these studies[84,124,125] demonstrate a certain association between transfusion and increased risks of recurrence or death that vary from 37% to 90% (Fig. 9.2). Thus the issue is no longer whether transfusion is associated with colorectal cancer recurrence or death. Transfusion is clearly associated with poor prognosis, but is the effect due to cause and effect?

The major criticism of the retrospective studies to date, including the meta-analyses, is that perhaps transfusion is merely acting as a surrogate measure of other prognostic factors that are in reality the true causes of earlier tumor recurrence. The only uniformly accepted prognostic factor in colorectal cancer is histopathologic or clinical stage. However, it is not always the case that transfused patients have more advanced disease, and in some studies, transfused patients were comparable to non-transfused patients in this respect. One approach to determining whether transfusion is likely causal in cancer recurrence is to perform multivariate analyses on factors likely to predict transfusion (e.g. anemia, duration of surgery, estimated blood loss, age, type of operation, location of tumor, gender), as well as the known prognostic factor of disease stage, and determine whether transfusion has any independent

influence. If transfusion is acting independently it should be more significant than these other factors or remain significant even whether the other factors are controlled for. Most studies have not performed such thorough analyses, but many have analyzed at least some of these factors.

Of the 28 studies examining the role of stage, 24 (86%) found it to be a significant predictor of poorer outcome. In a handful of studies transfusion was actually a better predictor of recurrence or death than stage. Of six studies examining histologic differentiation, five (83%) found this factor to be significant. However, when traditionally accepted prognostic factors such as type of operation (1 of 4; 25%) or tumor location (rectum versus colon) (5 of 12; 42%) were analyzed, most studies did not find these factors to be significant predictors of clinical outcome, as compared with transfusion (27 of 40; 68%). Prognostic factors which predict transfusion, and for which transfusion might be acting as a surrogate marker, usually have not been found to be predictors of increased recurrence and death in studies examining these variables: anemia (1 of 13; 8%), duration of surgery (0 of 5); estimated blood loss (0 of 5); gender (1 of 11; 9%); age (5 of 15; 33%). Thus while most studies have not examined the factors that might confound the proposed effect of transfusion on recurrence, those that have done so provide virtually no evidence that the variables that lead to transfusion have any effect on cancer outcome. Given that 12 studies that examined both stage and transfusion in Cox regressions found transfusion to be an independent predictor of recurrence or death,[86,88,90,91,102,103,106,107,110,116,119] it seems likely that in some circumstances transfusion is causally involved with earlier tumor recurrence in colorectal cancer. Currently there is no other explanation supported by the data, although it is possible that transfusion is confounded with some unknown factor yet to be identified.

In earlier work our group found that transfusion of whole blood was associated with particularly poor outcome in patients with colorectal, cervical or prostate tumors, and proposed that plasma or stored blood supernatant contained substances that inhibited immune function or facilitated tumor growth.[126-128] Others have confirmed this observation in varying degrees, with each study finding poorer outcome in recipients of whole blood or plasma components.[102,103,129] The logical clinical trial, use of washed red cell transfusions in cancer surgery, has yet to be performed. Because of the evidence from the renal allograft literature in animals, white cells have strongly been suspected as mediators of immunomodulation after transfusion. Recent evidence in two animal models from Blajchman and his colleagues strongly support this concern about white cells.[62,130]

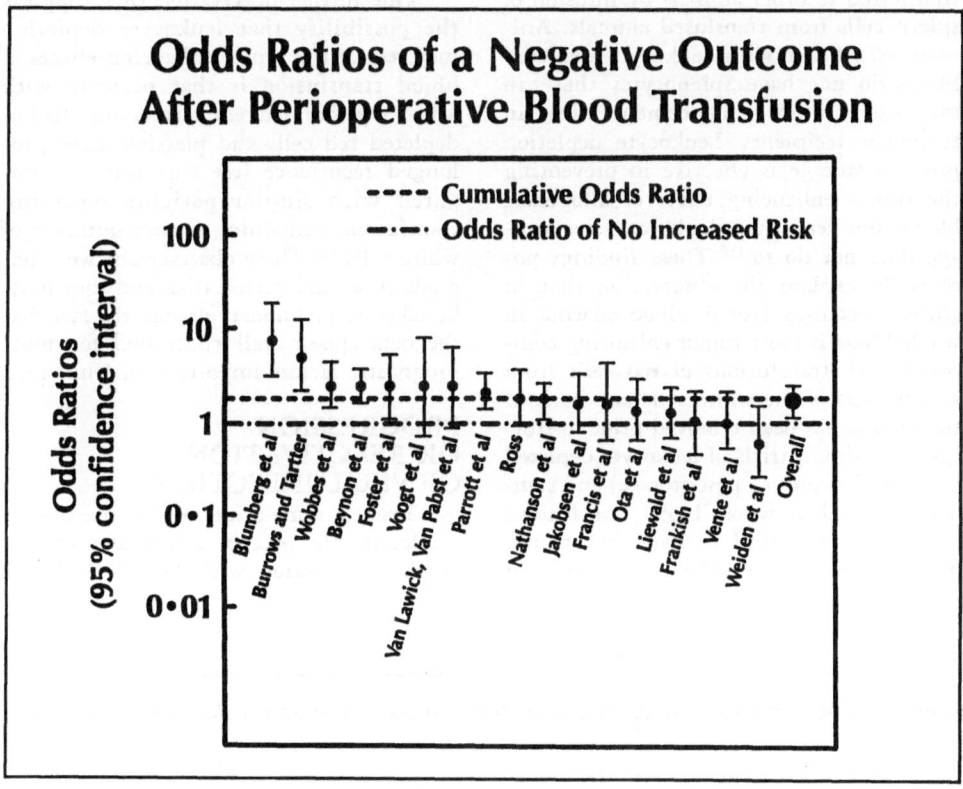

Fig. 9.2. The results of a meta-analysis of retrospective studies of colorectal cancer recurrence or death after transfusion or no transfusion are shown.[84] The odds ratio (an approximation of the risk ratio) expresses the likelihood of a recurrence or death in transfused patients versus that in non-transfused patients. The overall ratio at far right is a mathematical combination of the studies in a proportional manner, demonstrating an estimated 80% excess of adverse events in the transfused patients. Virtually all the individual studies have odds ratios above 1.0, suggesting that the differences between studies represent quantitative rather than qualitative differences. That is, even in the "negative" studies, transfusion is indeed associated with adverse outcomes, but biologic variability and small sample size led to the potentially misleading (but not incorrect) acceptance of the null hypothesis that there was no association between transfusion and cancer recurrence. The positive and negative studies probably reflect different points in a continuous spectrum reflecting transfusion's association with increased cancer deaths and recurrences. The 95% confidence intervals are for the individual studies, except for that at far right. The upper dashed line represents the pooled, point estimate for increased risk (80% or an odds ratio of 1.8) and the lower dash/dot line is the risk ratio of 1.0 (0% increased risk). The overall estimate's 95% confidence limits do not overlap a risk ratio of 1.0, demonstrating that the association of transfusion with recurrence and death is likely correct, although causality is not proven.

In both an inbred mouse model and an outbred rabbit model, this group has demonstrated convincingly that allogeneic blood transfusion leads to increased numbers of pulmonary metastases compared with syngeneic or saline control transfusion. Furthermore, this effect is abrogated by leukocyte depletion of the transfused allogeneic blood. (Table 9.2).[62] The effect is almost certainly immunologic as it can be transferred to other animals by infusion of spleen cells from transfused animals. Animals transfused with leukocyte depleted blood do not have splenocytes that can mediate a tumor enhancement effect in syngeneic recipients. Leukocyte depletion prior to storage is effective in preventing the tumor enhancing effect of allogeneic blood, but leukocyte depletion after storage does not do so.[130] These findings potentially explain the observation that in clinical settings stored blood plasma in whole blood is more tumor enhancing compared with transfusions of red cells from which some of the white cells and most of the plasma has been removed prior to storage. No clinical trials of leukocyte depleted blood (either pre- or post-storage) and standard red cell or whole blood transfusions have been performed to date, but would be of great interest. The initial trials of autologous transfusions to reduce colorectal cancer recurrence have yielded conflicting results with one trial finding a benefit, and the other no benefit.[20,131] Given the strong evidence for reduced postoperative infections with autologous transfusions, and the absence of any adverse effects to date, this modality is one which should be considered for suitable patients undergoing elective colorectal cancer resections.

One further observation that supports the possibility that leukocyte depletion may reduce the tumor enhancing effects of blood transfusion is that patients with acute myeloid leukemia receiving leukodepleted red cells and platelets have prolonged recurrence free survivals as compared with similar patients receiving transfusions containing greater numbers of white cells.[132] These observations were not made in a randomized trial, and thus must be taken as preliminary despite the fact that the data appear well controlled for most prognostic factors important in leukemia.

PROGRESSION OR REACTIVATION OF VIRAL INFECTION

There is some evidence that transfusion accelerates the pace or exacerbates the severity of infection with HIV-1[133-135] and

Table 9.2. Effect of syngeneic or allogeneic heparinized blood transfusions on metastasis in a mouse model

Type of Transfusion	% of Animals with Mets	Median No. Mets
Syngeneic	18 of 22	1
Allogeneic	30 of 34	5
Leukodepleted Allogeneic	25 of 34	1

The results of a study of transfusion induced enhancement of pulmonary metastases in a mouse model are shown.[62] Recipients of allogeneic blood had significantly greater numbers of metastases than recipients of either syngeneic blood or leukocyte depleted allogeneic blood.

CMV,[136-140] respectively. This effect is probably multifactorial. The data to date are perhaps explained by two possibilities, not necessarily mutually exclusive: (1) patients requiring transfusion are sicker and thus progress to AIDS or death more rapidly due to their underlying severity of disease and (2) transfusion is immunomodulatory and both reactivates latent viral infection and impairs host defenses against virus spread. Evidence for reactivation of viral infection in vitro by exposure to allogeneic white cells exists,[141,143] and transfusion also appears to impair important antiviral defenses such as natural killer cell function.[19,142] There is preliminary evidence in both animals and patients that the effect of transfusion on viral infection severity may be reduced in the case of CMV by use of leukocyte depleted blood.[139,140] Similar studies in HIV-1 infected patients are urgently needed.

CONCLUSIONS

1. Allogeneic blood transfusions cause perturbations in host immune function.
2. These perturbations are associated with improved allograft survival in animal models and patients suggesting down regulation of immune function.
3. While the transfusion induced renal allograft enhancement effect no longer is of clinical significance in cadaveric, unrelated transplants, allogeneic transfusions are epidemiologically linked to increased rates of solid tumor recurrence, increased rates of postoperative infection and increased severity of viral infection.
4. These deleterious effects of transfusion induced immunomodulation have not been proven to be cause and effect, but the bulk of animal experimental data and multivariate clinical analysis suggest a high likelihood of a cause and effect relationship accounting for some of the association.
5. Preliminary data from prospective and interventional studies in both animals and humans support the possibility that use of autologous transfusions or leukocyte depleted transfusions may avoid the morbidity associated with allogeneic transfusions.
6. Further data will be needed before widespread adoption of leukocyte depleted transfusions in settings other than hematologic malignancies and transplantation.

REFERENCES

1. Opelz G, Sengar DPS, Mickey MR, Terasaki PI. Effect of blood transfusions on subsequent kidney transplants. Transplant Proc 5:253, 1973.
2. Glass NR, Miller DT, Sollinger HW, et al. Comparative analysis of the DST and Immuran-plus-DST protocol for live donor renal transplantation. Transplantation 36:636, 1983;.
3. Burrows L, Tartter P. Effect of blood transfusions on colonic malignancy recurrence rate (letter). Lancet 2:662, 1982.
4. Horimi T, Terasaki PI, Chia D, Sasaki N. Factors influencing the paradoxical effect of transfusions on kidney transplants. Transplantation 35:320, 1983.
5. Opelz G. The role of HLA matching and blood transfusions in the cyclosporine era. Transplant Proc 21:609, 1989.
6. Ahmed Z, Terasaki P. Effect of Transfusions. In: Terasaki PI, Cecka JM (eds): Clinical Transplants 1991. Los Angeles, CA, UCLA Tissue Typing Laboratory; 305, 1992.
7. Kormos RL, Colson YL, Hardesty RL, et al. Immunologic and blood group compatibility in cardiac transplantation. Transplant Proc 20:741, 1988.
8. Lavee J, Kormos RL, Duquesnoy RJ, et al. Influence of panel-reactive antibody and lymphocytotoxic crossmatch on survival after heart transplantation. J Heart Lung Transplant 10:921, 1991.
9. Festenstein H, Banner N, Smith J, et al. The influence of HLA matching and lymphocytotoxic antibody status in heart-lung allograft recipients receiving cyclosporine and azathioprine. Transplant Proc 21:797, 1989.

10. Gordon RJ, Fung JJ, Markus B, et al. The antibody crossmatch in liver transplantation. Surgery 100:705, 1986.

11. Marino IR, Weber T, Esquivel CO, Kang YG, Starzl TE, Duquesnoy RJ. Intraoperative blood transfusion requirements and deficient hemostasis in highly alloimmunized patients undergoing liver transplantation. Transplant Proc 20:1087, 1988.

12. Triulzi DJ, Blumberg N, Heal JM. Association of transfusion with postoperative bacterial infection. CRC Crit Rev Clin Lab Sci 28:95, 1990.

13. Tartter PI, Driefuss RM, Malon AM, Heimann TM, Aufses AH. Relationship of postoperative septic complications and blood transfusions in patients with Crohn's disease. Am J Surg 155:43, 1988.

14. Tartter PI. Blood transfusion and infectious complications following colorectal cancer surgery. Br J Surg 75:789, 1988.

15. Jensen LS, Andersen A, Fristrup SC, et al. Comparison of one dose versus three doses of prophylactic antibiotics, and the influence of blood transfusion, on infectious complications in acute and elective colorectal surgery. Br J Surg 77:513, 1990.

16. Wobbes T, Bemelmans BLH, Kuypers JHC, Beerthuizen GIJM, Theeuwes AGM: Risk of postoperative septic complications after abdominal surgical treatment in relation to perioperative blood transfusion. Surg Gynecol Obstet 171:59, 1990.

17. Pinto V, Baldonedo R, Nicolas C, Barez A, Perez A, Aza J. Relationship of transfusion and infectious complications after gastric carcinoma operations. Transfusion 31:114, 1991.

18. Braga M, Vignali A, Radaelli G, Gianotti L, Di Carlo V. Association between perioperative blood transfusion and postoperative infection in patients having elective operations for gastrointestinal cancer. Eur J Surg 158:531, 1992.

19. Jensen LS, Andersen AJ, Christiansen PM, et al. Postoperative infection and natural killer cell function following blood transfusion in patients undergoing elective colorectal surgery. Br J Surg 79:513, 1992.

20. Busch ORC, Hop WCJ, Hoynck van Papendrecht MAW, Marquet RL, Jeekel J. Blood transfusions and prognosis in colorectal cancer. N Engl J Med 328:1372, 1993.

21. Ford CD, VanMoorleghem G, Menlove RL. Blood transfusions and postoperative wound infection. Surgery 113:603, 1993.

22. George SM, Fabian TC, Voeller GR, Kudsk KA, Mangiante EC, Britt LG. Primary repair of colon wounds A prospective trial in nonselected patients. Ann Surg 209:728, 1989.

23. Dellinger EP, Oreskovich MR, Wertz MJ, Hamasaki V, Lennard ES. Risk of infection following laparotomy for penetrating abdominal injury. Arch Surg 119:20, 1984.

24. Nichols RL, Smith JW, Klein DB, et al. Risk of infection after penetrating abdominal trauma. N Engl J Med 311:1065, 1984.

25. Dawes LG, Aprahamian C, Condon RE, Malangoni MA. The risk of infection after colon injury. Surgery 100:796, 1986.

26. Rosemurgy AS, Hart MB, Murphy CG, et al. Infection after injury: Association with blood transfusion. Am Surgeon 58:104, 1992.

27. Agarwal N, Murphy JG, Cayten CG, Stahl WM. Blood transfusion increases the risk of infection after trauma. Arch Surg 128:171, 1993.

28. Edna T-H, Bjerkeset T. Association between blood transfusion and infection in injured patients. J Trauma 33:659, 1992.

29. Nichols RL, Smith JW, Robertson GD, et al. Prospective alterations in therapy for penetrating abdominal trauma. Arch Surg 128:55, 1993.

30. Miholic J, Hudec M, Domanig E, et al. Risk factors for severe bacterial infections after valve replacement and aortocoronary bypass operations: Analysis of 246 cases by logistic regression. Ann Thorac Surg 40:224, 1985.

31. Ottino G, DePaulis R, Pansini S, et al. Major sternal wound infection after open-heart surgery: a multivariate analysis of risk factors in 2579 consecutive operative procedures. Ann Thorac Surg 44:173, 1987.

32. Loop FD, Lytle BW, Cosgrove DM, et al. Sternal wound complications after isolated

coronary artery bypass grafting: Early and late mortality, morbidity, and cost of care. Ann Thorac Surg 49:179, 1990.

33. Verwaal VJ, Wobbes T, Koopman-van Gemert AWMM, Buskens FGM, Theeuwes AGM. Effect of perioperative blood transfusion and cell saver on the incidence of postoperative infective complications in patients with an aneurysm of the abdominal aorta. Eur J Surg 158:477, 1992.

34. Murphy PJ, Connery C, Hicks GL,Jr, Blumberg N. Homologous blood transfusion as a risk factor for postoperative infection after coronary artery bypass graft operations. J Thorac Cardiovasc Surg 104: 1092, 1992.

35. Böck M, Grevers G, Koblitz M, Heim MU, Mempel W. Influence of blood transfusion on recurrence, survival and postoperative infections of laryngeal cancer. Acta Otolaryngol (Stockholm) 110:155, 1990.

36. Robbins KT, Favrot S, Hanna D, Cole R. Risk of wound infection in patients with head and neck cancer. Head and Neck 12:143, 1990.

37. von Doersten P, Cruz RM, Selby JV, Hilsinger RL,Jr. Transfusion, recurrence, and infection in head and neck cancer surgery. Otolaryngol Head Neck Surg 106:60, 1992.

38. Weber RS, Hankins P, Rosenbaum B, Raad I. Nonwound infections following head and neck oncologic surgery. Laryngoscope 103:22, 1993.

39. Dellinger EP, Miller SD, Wertz MJ, et al. Risk of infection after open fracture of the arm or leg. Arch Surg 123:1320, 1988.

40. Murphy P, Heal JM, Blumberg N. Infection or suspected infection after hip replacement surgery with autologous or homologous transfusions. Transfusion 31:212, 1991.

41. Fernandez MC, Gottlieb M, Menitove JE. Blood transfusion and postoperative infection in orthopedic patients. Transfusion 32:318, 1992.

42. Triulzi DJ, Vanek K, Ryan DH, Blumberg N. A clinical and immunologic study of blood transfusion and postoperative bacterial infection in spinal surgery. Transfusion 32:517, 1992.

43. Graves TA, Cioffi WG, Mason Jr AD, et al. Relationship of transfusion and infection in a burn population. J Trauma 29:948, 1989.

44. Mezrow CK, Bergstein I, Tartter PI. Postoperative infections following autologous and homologous blood transfusions. Transfusion 32:27, 1992.

45. Chiu P, Roy PD, Marshall JC. Blood transfusion is a risk factor for ICU-acquired infection and the multiple organ dysfunction syndrome. Critical Care Med 21(Supplement): S226, 1993-(Abstract).

46. Heiss MM, Mempel W, Jauch KW, Delanoff C, Mayer G, Mempel M, Eissner H-J, Schildberg FW. Beneficial effect of autologous blood transfusion on infectious complications after colorectal cancer surgery. Lancet 342:1328, 1993.

47. Waymack JP, Gallon L, Barcelli U, etal. Effect of blood transfusions on immune function. Arch Surg 122:56, 1987.

48. Waymack JP, Warden GD, Alexander JW, et.al. Effect of blood transfusion and anesthesia on resistance to bacterial peritonitis. J Surg Res 42:528, 1987.

49. Waymack JP, Miskell P, Gonce S. Alterations in host defense associated with inhalation anesthesia and blood transfusion. Anesth Analg 69:163.1989.

50. Gianotti L, Pyles T, Alexander JW, Babcock GF, Carey MA. Impact of blood transfusion and burn injury on microbial translocation and bacterial survival. Transfusion 32:312, 1992.

51. Gianotti L, Pyles T, Alexander JW, Fukushima R, Babcock GF. Identification of the blood component responsible for increased susceptibility to gut-derived infection. Transfusion 33:458, 1993.

52. Goldman M, Frame B, Singal DP, Blajchman MA. Effect of blood transfusion on survival in a mouse bacterial peritonitis model. Transfusion 31:710, 1991.

53. Cué JI, Peyton JC, Malangoni MA. Does blood transfusion or hemorrhagic shock induce immunosuppression? J Trauma 32:613, 1992.

54. Brunson ME, Ing R, Tchervenkov JI, Alexander JW. Variable infection risk following allogeneic blood transfusions. J Surg

Res 48:308, 1990.

55. George CD, Pietsch JD, Byck DC, Shields RE, Polk HC. Effect of blood transfusion on host susceptibility to bacterial infection. Br J Surg 74:537, 1987 (Abstract).

56. Oikawa T, Hosokawa M, Imamura M, et al. Anti-tumour immunity by normal allogeneic blood transfusion in rat. Clin Exp Immunol 27:549, 1977.

57. Parrott NR, Lennard TWJ, Proud G, et al. Blood transfusion and surgery: the effect on growth of a syngeneic sarcoma. Ann R Coll Surg Engl 72:77, 1990.

58. Waymack JP, Fernandes G, Yurt RW, et al. Effect of blood transfusions on immune function Part VI Effect on immunologic response to tumor. Surgery 108:172, 1990.

59. Shirwadkar S, Blajchman MA, Frame B, Singal DP. Effect of allogeneic blood transfusion on solid tumor growth and pulmonary metastases in mice. J Cancer Res Clin Oncol 118:176, 1992.

60. Jones RDM, Moore GJ, Bacon-Shone J. An investigation of the enhancement of tumour growth by blood transfusion. Med Sci Res 20:423, 1992.

61. Domasu S, Terada N, Sano H, Kodama M. The effect of blood transfusion on immunological response in mice. Nippon Geka Gakkai Zasshi 93:1, 1992.

62. Blajchman MA, Bardossy L, Carmen R, Sastry A, Singal DP. Allogeneic blood transfusion-induced enhancement of tumor growth: two animal models showing amelioration by leukodepletion and passive transfer using spleen cells. Blood 81:1880, 1993.

63. Ichikura T, Tamakuma S, Ito H, Tomimatsu S, Valeri CR. Effects of syngeneic preserved blood cells on metastatic growth of the Lewis lung carcinoma. Nippon Geka Gakkai Zasshi-Journal of the Japanese Surgical Society 92:734, 1991.

64. Nakano K, Sagara N, Inufusa H, et al. The effect of blood transfusion on tumor growth and metastasis formation. Hum Cell 2:304, 1989.

65. Waymack JP, Chance WT. Effect of blood transfusions on immune function. IV. Effect on tumor growth. J Surg Oncol 39:159,

1988.

66. Ninomiya M. Study on the induction of immunologic suppression by blood transfusion. J Japan Surg Soc (Nippon Geka Gakkai Zasshi) 87:1380, 1986.

67. Singh SK, Marquet RL, Westbroek DL, Jeekel J. Abrogation of the tumor promoting effect of allogeneic blood transfusion by polyadenylic-polyuridylic acid (poly A-poly U). Cancer Immunol Immunother 25:242, 1986.

68. Jakóbisiak M, Wlodarski K, Lasek W, Górecki D, Plodziszewska M. Transfusions of syngeneic blood do not seem to induce suppressive effects on antitumor or transplantation immunity in mice. Arch Immunol Therap Exper 33:543, 1985.

69. Clarke PJ, Tarin D. Effect of preoperative blood transfusion on tumour metastases. Br J Surg 74:520, 1987.

70. Judson RT, Robb L, D'Apice AJF. Blood transfusion and tumour growth: an experimental study. Aust N Z J Surg 55:503, 1985.

71. Singh SK, Marquet RL, Westbroek DL, Jeekel J. Enhanced growth of artificial tumor metastases following blood transfusion: the effect of erythrocytes, leukocytes and plasma transfusion. Eur J Cancer Clin Oncol 23:1537, 1987.

72. Horimi T, Kagawa S, Ninomiya M, Yoshida E, Hiramatsu S, Orita K. Possible induction by blood transfusion of immunological tolerance against growth of transplanted tumors in mice. Acta Med Okayama 37:259, 1983.

73. Francis DMA, Shenton BK. Blood transfusion and tumour growth: evidence from laboratory animals. Lancet ii 871, 1981 (Letter).

74. Marquet RL, de Bruin RWF, Dallinga RJ, Singh SK, Jeekel J. Modulation of tumor growth by allogeneic blood transfusion. J Cancer Res Clin Oncol 111:50, 1986.

75. Francis DMA, Burren CP, Clunie GJA. Acceleration of B16 melanoma growth in mice after blood transfusion. Surgery 102:485, 1987.

76. Lenhard V, Scholler P, Zeller W. Transfusion-induced T suppressor cell activity and experimental tumor growth. Transplant Proc

21:580, 1989.

77. Francis DMA, Shenton BK, Proud G, Taylor RMR. Tumor growth and blood transfusion. J Exp Clin Cancer Res 1:121, 1982.

78. Lieberman MD, Shou J, Sigal RK, Yu J, Goldfine J, Daly JM. Transfusion-induced immunosuppression results in diminished host survival in a murine neuroblastoma model. J Surg Res 48:498, 1990.

79. Hilgard P, Thornes RD. Anticoagulants in the treatment of cancer. Eur J Cancer 12:755, 1976.

80. Blumberg N, Heal JM. Transfusion and host defenses against cancer recurrence and infection. Transfusion 29:236, 1989.

81. Tartter PI. Does blood transfusion predispose to cancer recurrence? Am J Clin Oncol 12:169, 1989.

82. Blumberg N, Triulzi DJ, Heal JM. Transfusion-induced immunomodulation and its clinical consequences. Transf Med Rev IV. 24, 1990.

83. Francis DMA. Relationship between blood transfusion and tumour behaviour. Br J Surg 78:1420, 1991.

84. Chung M, Steinmetz OK, Gordon PH. Perioperative blood transfusion and outcome after resection for colorectal carcinoma. Br J Surg 80:427, 1993.

85. Burrows L, Tartter P, Aufses A. Increased recurrence rates in perioperatively transfused colorectal malignancy patients. Cancer Detect Prev 10:361, 1987.

86. Blumberg N, Agarwal M, Chuang C. Relation between recurrence of cancer of the colon and blood transfusion. Br Med J 290:1037, 1985.

87. Foster RS,Jr., Costanza MC, Foster JC, et al. Adverse relationship between blood transfusions and survival after colectomy for colon cancer. Cancer 55:1195, 1985.

88. Corman J, Arnoux R, Peloquin A, et.al. Blood transfusions and survival after colectomy for colorectal cancer. Can J Surg 29:325, 1986.

89. Parrott NR, Lennard TWJ, Taylor RMR, et al. Effect of perioperative blood transfusion on recurrence of colorectal cancer. Br J Surg 73:970, 1986.

90. Voogt PJ, Van de Velde CJH, Brand A, et al. Perioperative blood transfusion and cancer prognosis Different effects of blood transfusion on prognosis of colon and breast cancer patients. Cancer 59:836, 1987.

91. Creasy TS, Veitch PS, Bell PR. A relationship between perioperative blood transfusion and recurrence of carcinoma of the sigmoid colon following potentially curative surgery. Ann R Coll Surg Engl 69:100, 1987.

92. Ota D, Alvarez L, Lichtiger B, et al. Perioperative blood transfusions in patients with colon carcinoma. Transfusion 25:392, 1985.

93. Weiden PL, Bean MA, Schultz P. Perioperative blood transfusion does not increase risk of colorectal cancer recurrence. Cancer 60:870, 1987.

94. Frankish PD, McNee RK, Alley PG, Woodfield DG. Relation between cancer of the colon and blood transfusion (letter). Br Med J 290:1827, 1985.

95. Francis DMA, Judson RT. Blood transfusion and recurrence of cancer of the colon and rectum. Br J Surg 74:26, 1987.

96. Nathanson SD, Tilley BC, Schultz L, Smith RF. Perioperative allogeneic blood transfusions—survival in patients with resected carcinomas of the colon and rectum. Arch Surg 120:734, 1985.

97. Ross WB. Blood transfusion and colorectal cancer. J R Coll Surg Edinb 32:197, 1987.

98. Waymack JP, Moomaw CJ, Popp MB. The effect of perioperative blood transfusions on long-term survival of colon cancer patients. Milit Med 154:515, 1989.

99. Mecklin JP, Jarvinen HJ, Ovaska JT. Blood transfusion and prognosis in colorectal carcinoma. Scand J Gastroenterol 24:33, 1989.

100. Vente JP, Wiggers TH, Weidema WF, et al. Perioperative blood transfusions in colorectal cancer. Eur J Surg Oncol 15:371, 1989.

101. Beynon J, Davies PW, Biol. M, et al. Perioperative blood transfusion increases the risk of recurrence in colorectal cancer. Dis Colon Rectum 32:975, 1989.

102. Wobbes T, Joosen KHG, Kuypers HHC, Beerthuizen GIJM, Theeuwes AGM: The effect of packed cells and whole blood trans-

effect of packed cells and whole blood transfusions on survival after curative resection for colorectal carcinoma. Dis Colon Rectum 32:743, 1989.

103. Marsh J, Donnan PT, Hamer-Hodges DW. Association between transfusion with plasma and the recurrence of colorectal carcinoma. Br J Surg 77:623, 1990.

104. Modin S, Karlsson G, Wählby L. Blood transfusion and recurrence of colorectal cancer. Eur J Surg 158:371, 1992.

105. Jahnson S, Andersson M. Adverse effects of perioperative blood transfusion in patients with colorectal cancer. Eur J Surg 158:419, 1992.

106. Tartter PI. The association of perioperative blood transfusion with colorectal cancer recurrence. Ann Surg 216:633, 1992.

107. Liewald F, Wirsching RP, Zülke C, Demmel N, Mempel W. Influence of blood transfusions on tumor recurrence and survival rate in colorectal carcinoma. Eur J Cancer 26:327, 1990.

108. Crowson MC, Hallissey MT, Kiff RS, Kingston RD, Fielding JWL. Blood transfusion in colorectal cancer. Br J Surg 76:522, 1989.

109. Jakobsen EB, Eickhoff JH, Andersen J, Lundvall L, Stenderup JK. Perioperative blood transfusion and recurrence and death after resection for cancer of the colon and rectum. Scand J Gastroenterol 25:435, 1990.

110. Onodera H, Maetani S, Tobe T. Effect of blood transfusion on prognosis of colorectal cancer patients. J Japan Surg Soc (Nippon Geka Gakkai Zasshi) 90:1890, 1989.

111. Bentzen SM, Balslev I, Pedersen M, et al. Blood transfusion and prognosis in Dukes' B and C colorectal cancer. Eur J Cancer 26:457, 1990.

112. Van Lawick van Pabst WP, Langenhorst BLAM, Mulder PGH, Marquet RL, Jeekel J. Effect of perioperative blood loss and perioperative blood transfusions on colorectal cancer survival. Eur J Cancer Clin Oncol 24:741, 1988.

113. Cheslyn-Curtis S, Fielding LP, Hittinger R, Fry JS, Phillips RKS. Large bowel cancer: the effect of perioperative blood transfusion

on outcome. Ann R Coll Surg Engl 72:53, 1990.

114. Werner C, Nielsen J, Ottesen SS. The significance of blood transfusion for recurrence after colorectal cancer surgery. Ug Laeger 150:3182, 1988.

115. Zimmerman T, Dobroschke J, Borowek U, Padberg W. Effect of perioperative allogenic blood transfusion on prognosis of colorectal cancer. Zent bl Chir 116:1125, 1991.

116. Tang R, Wang JY, Chien CRC, Chen JS, Lin SE, Fan HA. The association between perioperative blood transfusion and survival of patients with colorectal cancer. Cancer 1993;72:341-348.

117. Fuhrman GM, Davidson BS, Larach SW, Williamson PR. Analysis of local recurrence of midrectal cancer after low anterior resection and stapled anastomosis. Southern Med J 85:502, 1992.

118. Kjems E, Schydlowski P, Sqndergaard JO. The influence of blood transfusions upon the recurrence rate of colorectal cancer. Rev Med Chir Soc Med Nat IASI 95:265, 1991.

119. Arnoux R, Corman J, Péloquin A, Smeesters C, St-Louis G. Adverse effect of blood transfusions on patient survival after resection of rectal cancer. Can J Surg 31:121, 1988.

120. Faenza A, Cunsolo A, Selleri S, Lucarelli S, Farneti PA, Gozzetti G. Correlation between plasma or blood transfusion and survival after curative surgery for colorectal cancer. Int Surg 77:264, 1992.

121. Fernández Fernández L, Sanz Anquela M, Ratia T, et al. Transfusión de sangre perioperatoria y pronóstico en el cáncer colorrectal.Análisis de una serie. Rev Esp Enf Digest 82:317, 1992.

122. Pellicer Franco EM, Olmo G, Parilla Paricio P, Morales Cuenca G, y Prieto A. La transfusión sanguínea ensombrece el pronóstico del cáncer colorrectal Estudio preliminar en una serie de 717 casos. Rev Esp Enf Digest 77:189, 1990.

123. Elorza Orúe JL, Palomar de Luis M, y Tubía Landaberea J. Recidiva del cáncer colorrectal y transfusión sanguínea. Rev Esp Enf Digest 82:150, 1992.

124. Vamvakas E, Moore SB. Perioperative blood

transfusion and colorectal cancer recurrence: A qualitative statistical overview and meta-analysis. Transfusion 33:754, 1993.

125. Amato A, Butti A. Do patients with less advanced colorectal cancers recur more when perioperatively transfused? J Surg Oncol 48[Supplement 2]:169, 1993-abstract.

126. Blumberg N, Heal JM, Murphy P, et al. Association between transfusion of whole blood and recurrence of cancer. Br Med J 293:530, 1986.

127. Blumberg N, Heal JM, Chuang C, et al. Further evidence supporting a cause and effect relationship between blood transfusion and cancer recurrence. Ann Surg 207:410, 1988.

128. Blumberg N, Chuang-Stein C, Heal JM. The relationship between blood transfusion, tumor staging and cancer recurrence. Transfusion 30:291, 1990.

129. Hermanek P Jr., Guggenmoos-Holzmann I, Schricker KT, et al. The influence of blood and hemoderivatives on the prognosis of colorectal carcinoma. Langenbecks Arch Chir 374:118, 1989.

130. Bordin JO, Bardossy L, Singal DP, Blajchman MA. Lack of efficacy of post-storage leukodepletion of allogeneic blood transfusions in preventing growth enhancement of animal tumors. Blood 82 [Supplement 1]:392a, 1993-abstract.

131. Heiss MM, Jauch KW, Delanoff C, Mempel W, Schildberg FW. Blood transfusion modulated tumor recurrence: a randomized study of autologous vs. homologous blood transfusion in colorectal cancer. Proc Annu Meet Am Soc Clin Oncol 11:A503, 1992-Abstract.

132. Oksanen K, Elonen E. Impact of leukocyte-depleted blood components on the haematological recovery and prognosis of patients with acute myeloid leukaemia. Br J Haematol 84:639, 1993.

133. Blumberg N, Heal JM. Evidence for plasma-mediated immunomodulation-transfusions of plasma-rich blood components are associated with a greater risk of acquired immunodeficiency syndrome than transfusions of red blood cells alone. Transplant Proc 20:1138, 1988.

134. Ward JW, Bush TJ, Perkins HA, et al. The natural history of transfusion-associated infection with human immunodeficiency virus. Factors influencing the rate of progression to disease. N Engl J Med 321:947, 1989.

135. Vamvakas E, Kaplan HS. Early transfusion and length of survival in AIDS: experience with a population receiving medical care at a public hospital. Transfusion 33:111, 1993.

136. Preiksaitis JK, Brown L, McKenzie M. The risk of cytomegalovirus infection in seronegative transfusion recipients not receiving exogenous immunosuppression. J Infect Dis 157:523, 1988.

137. Adler SP, McVoy MM. Cytomegalovirus infections in seropositive patients after transfusion The effect of red cell storage and volume. Transfusion 29:667, 1989.

138. Cheung KS, Lang DJ. Transmission and activation of cytomegalovirus with blood transfusion: a mouse model. J Infect Dis 135:841, 1977.

139. Lang DJ, Ebert PA, Rodgers BM, Boggess HP, Rixse RS. Reduction of postperfusion CMV infections following the use of leukocyte depleted blood. Transfusion 17:391, 1977.

140. Thompson KS, Plapp FV, Long ND, Heenan TA. CMV infection in heart transplant recipients. Transfusion 32(Supplement): 65S, 1992 Abstract.

141. Busch MP, Lee T-H, Heitman J. Allogeneic leukocytes but not therapeutic blood elements induce reactivation and dissemination of latent HIV-1 infection: implications for transfusion support of infected patients. Blood 80:2128, 1992.

142. Ford CD, Warnick CT, Sheets S, et al. Blood transfusions lower natural killer cell activity. Transplant Proc 9:1456, 1987.

143. Bruggeman CA. Reactivation of latent CMV in the rat. Transplant Proc 23 (Supplement 3): 22,1991.

CHAPTER 10

THE ROLE OF LEUKOCYTE DEPLETION IN PREVENTION OF TRANSFUSION-RELATED ACUTE LUNG INJURY

Mark A. Popovsky

SUMMARY

Transfusion related acute lung inquiry (TRALI) is a pulmonary complication attributed to blood transfusion which clinically resembles adult respiratory distress syndrome. The frequency of occurrence of TRALI is unknown, as it is likely that many cases go undiagnosed. TRALI is thought to be due to an interaction between granulocytes (most often of host, but possibly of donor origin) and anti-granulocyte antibodies (most often of donor but, sometimes of recipient origin) in which activated complement components participate in alveolar damage. Prognosis is generally good, although prompt and aggressive respiratory support is required.

The vast majority of cases are related to the presence of antileukocyte antibodies in donor plasma. Some cases (approximately 10%) may be mediated by intact donor granuloyctes or substances generated during in vitro storage of leukocytes. The impact of leukodepletion (preferably prestorage) in reducing the frequency of TRALI is considered to be only slight.

The paucity of attention given by standard textbooks of medicine and surgery to pulmonary complications of transfusion might suggest that the respiratory system is a rare target of injury from hemotherapy. When pulmonary problems are noted at all, it is usually in the context of circulatory overload from hypertransfusion or anaphylactic transfusion

Clinical Benefits of Leukodepleted Blood Products, edited by Joseph Sweeney, M.D. and Andrew Heaton, M.D. © 1995 R.G. Landes Company.

reactions. Pulmonary edema from hyper-transfusion may occur as frequently as 1:3000 transfusion episodes[1] while anaphylactic transfusion reactions are extremely rare, estimated at 1:20,000 transfusions.[2] It is only in the last decade that another complication, acute lung injury, has been recognized as an important complication of transfusion. One of the reasons for the lack of earlier recognition of this transfusion reaction was that there were so few case reports and these utilized several terms to describe the same entity. The transfusion-related acute lung injury (TRALI) syndrome has previously been referred to as "pulmonary leukoagglutinin reaction,"[3] allergic pulmonary edema,"[4] and "hypersensitivity reaction,"[5] but these terms obscure the clinical picture and underlying mechanism.

CLINICAL DESCRIPTION

Transfusion-related acute lung injury (TRALI) is a life-threatening complication which is clinically indistinguishable from the adult respiratory distress syndrome (ARDS) resulting from causes (i.e. sepsis, toxin inhalation, or aspiration) other than transfusion. Like ARDS, TRALI is characterized by acute respiratory distress; severe, bilateral pulmonary edema; and severe hypoxemia (arterial oxygen tensions of 30-50 torr are frequent).[6] The respiratory distress may first present as dyspnea or cyanosis. The edema may first be confined to the lower lung fields, but over several hours usually involves the entire lung. Roengenograms classically demonstrate "white out" by interstitial and alveolar infiltrates.[7] Other manifestations include fever and mild to moderate hypotension.[6-8] When hypotension occurs, it frequently is unresponsive to fluid administration. These symptoms arise in the setting of recent transfusion of plasma-containing blood components, always within 1-6 hours, and usually within 1-2 hours. In contrast to other causes of pulmonary edema, patients with TRALI have normal central venous pressure and normal or low pulmonary wedge pressure.

TRALI differs from the adult respiratory distress syndrome (ARDS) in important ways. Unlike ARDS with its attendant high morbidity and mortality (death rate of 50%),[9] in approximately 80% of cases TRALI improves both clinically and physiologically within 48-96 hours of the original onset, provided there is prompt and vigorous respiratory support. While in many ARDS patients, the lung injury is irreversible, in TRALI the pulmonary lesion is most typically transient. Roengenograms document the rapid clearing of the edema fluid. In a report by Popovsky and Moore involving 36 cases, 100% of patients required oxygen support, while 72% required short-term mechanical ventilation. There is a subset of patients, however, with a slightly prolonged course. In about one-fifth of cases, pulmonary infiltrates persist for at least 7 days, but even in these patients it is believed that there are no permanent sequelae.[8] Although there are limited data, it would appear that approximately 5% of patients die from complications related to the pulmonary insult. In an analysis of causes of 256 transfusion-associated deaths in the United States reported to the Food and Drug Administration from 1976 to 1985, acute pulmonary edema was implicated in 12.1% (31 cases).[9] In this study acute pulmonary injury was the second most common cause of death from transfusion, more frequent than death due to bacterial contamination or anaphylaxis.[10] For obvious reasons, TRALI is an important clinical diagnosis.

FREQUENCY

The incidence of TRALI is unknown. In one study from the mid-1980s, one in 5000 plasma-containing transfusions was associated with this reaction.[6] Since this study took place during the period in which blood banks in the United States were converting to red cell components containing significantly less plasma (decreasing from an average of 100 cc to approximately 50 cc), one might assume that the frequency has decreased. On the other hand the number of reports in the literature has increased dramatically. Prior to 1985, there were only 31 case reports.[3-7,11-22] Since then, descriptions of more than 55 recipient reactions have appeared in the literature and the author is aware of at least an additional 50 unpublished cases.[6,8,9,23-31] The relative abundance of recent reports may reflect increased awareness, rather than a change in incidence.

There is reason to believe that TRALI may be significantly underdiagnosed. In a series of 40 patients with pulmonary edema in the operative setting, Cooperman and Price found that 50% of cases were attributed to circulatory overload or an unknown cause. It is conceivable that some of these cases represented TRALI.[32] Culliford and colleagues described a type of noncardiogenic pulmonary edema in three patients following cardiopulmonary bypass that is consistent with TRALI but tests which might have confirmed the diagnosis were not performed.[33]

IMPLICATED BLOOD PRODUCTS

As stated previously, TRALI is associated with the transfusion of blood products containing plasma. These products include whole blood, red blood cells (prepared in CPD, CPDA-1 as well as protein-poor anticoagulant-preservative solutions such as AS-1), granulocytes collected by apheresis, platelets collected by apheresis, and cryoprecipitate.[3-9,11-31] In most instances the implicated blood product contains more than 60 cc of plasma, but it is apparent that in some instances smaller quantities (i.e. cryoprecipitate contains only 10-15 cc of plasma) are sufficient to initiate the pulmonary events previously described.[15] It is noteworthy that commercially available plasma derivatives, such as albumin, plasma protein fraction, and gamma globulin, which are manufactured by fractionation procedures, have not been associated with any case reports.

PATHOGENESIS

Although the precise mechanism of TRALI is unknown, there are sufficient

clues to assume that it is an immune-mediated event. Unlike most immunologically-triggered transfusion reactions, the pathologic antibodies are typically of donor, rather than recipient origin. Numerous reports have documented the presence of HLA-specific or leukoagglutinating antibodies in the plasma of the donors of implicated blood components.[3,6-8,12,16,18,23-26,29] Popovsky and Moore found such antibodies in 89% (of 36) of cases. In about half of the cases studied, the HLA-A or -B antibodies of the implicated donor corresponded with one or more HLA epitopes of the recipient.[8] Popovsky et al, Goeken and coworkers, as well as others have confirmed these findings.[7,14,25] In other cases, neutrophil specific antibodies (anti-NA2, anti-5b, and anti-NB2) have been identified in the serum of implicated units.[13,23,24] These antibodies are usually found in the blood of multiparous female donors. On the other hand, in 5% of reported cases, similar specificities of antibodies are found in the pretransfusion serum of the transfusion recipient.[3,5,8] Finally, in 5-10% of cases no antibody has been identified in either the patient or donor(s).

The likely explanation for antibodies in the donor, rather than antibodies in the recipient, as the causative agent is that the "substrate" with which the white cell (WBC) antibodies can react namely, the recipient's entire circulating and marginated pool of WBCs, is far larger than the quantity of donor WBCs present in a single transfused component. It appears that TRALI begins with passive transfer of antibody from donor's plasma to the recipient.[6]

What do these antibodies have to do with TRALI? Much of current understanding is gleaned from studies of the adult respiratory distress syndrome. Although the mechanisms involved in the development of ARDS are complex, there is considerable evidence to support a major role for complement activation and neutrophil influx into the lung causing damage to the pulmonary microvasculature. When complement is activated, C5a promotes neutrophil aggregation, margination and sequestration in microvasculature of the lung,[34,35] which is at least partially related to increased granulocyte adhesion.[36] Experimental studies in rabbits as well as observations in ARDS patients, suggest that when complement-activated neutrophils release their proteases, acidic lipids, and oxygen radical contents, the underlying pulmonary vascular endothelium is damaged, with subsequent extravasation of protein-laden fluid into the adjacent interstitium and alveoli.[37,38] Larsen et al demonstrated that C5 fragments consistently produced lung inflammation characterized by neutrophil accumulation and edema.[39] In all likelihood, these pathologic changes account for the radiographic and clinical findings seen in TRALI. Brittingham noted that when 50 ml of blood known to contain leukoagglutinins was transfused to a normal person, the result was a severe pulmonary reaction characterized by hypoxemia, pulmonary edema, hypotension, and fever.[18] This study suggested that passive transfer of leukocyte antibodies may play an important, if not decisive, role in triggering the reaction. As lymphocytotoxic (i.e. HLA) antibodies readily fix complement, passive transfusion of these antibodies probably account for complement activation and the sequence of events described above.

Seeger et al recently provided a powerful model for understanding the relationship between donor antibodies and the development of TRALI.[40] Using an ex vivo rabbit lung model, these investigators found that acute lung injury characterized by severe lung edema resulted from the infusion of an admixture of complement, anti-5b antibody and 5b-positive human neutrophils. These changes were seen within 3-6 hours after infusion, which parallels the clinical presentation in humans. If complement, anti-5b antibody or 5b-positive granulocytes antigen were deleted, no pathologic changes occurred. While these data suggest that the correspondence of antibody specificity for a recipient epitope is important in the pathogenesis of the respiratory decompensation seen in TRALI, cases in which the HLA or neutro-phil-specific antibody do not share epitopes with the recipient are left unexplained.

Silliman et al recently identified a cohort of TRALI patients in whom no HLA or leukocyte antibodies were found.[30] Rather, they described the presence of a neutrophil priming agent, a lipid, in the blood components given to the patients who developed TRALI. They postulated that this lipid develops during routine storage of blood components and that it primes polymorphonuclear oxidase. As this is the first description of an alternative, non-antibody mediated model of TRALI, further studies are needed to confirm or refute this finding.

DIAGNOSIS

TRALI is a diagnosis of exclusion. Acute respiratory distress in the setting of transfusion is grounds for its clinical consideration. One must rule out cardiogenic as well as other causes of pulmonary edema. The identification of lymphocytotoxic, HLA-specific or granulocyte-specific antibodies in an implicated donor or plasma-containing blood component provides strong support for the diagnosis of TRALI.[6,8] Conversely, in the correct clinical setting, the presence of such antibodies in the pre-transfusion serum of the patient is equally diagnostic.

AT RISK POPULATION

Although it would be clearly useful to identify which patients are at risk for the development of TRALI, current understanding does not allow for such a profile. Cases have been described in both very young as well as elderly transfusion recipients. No disease associations have been identified. Approximately 1-2% of blood donors have HLA-specific antibodies; yet TRALI is an infrequent result of transfusion.[7] This suggests that other factors such as the character of the antibody, the nature and distribution of the related antigen, the extent of complement activation, and the immune status of the recipient are all important variables which determine the final clinical response.[41,42]

ROLE OF LEUKOCYTE DEPLETION

Is there a role for the leukocyte depletion of blood components in the prevention of TRALI? Based on the preponderance of evidence that passive transfer of antibody from donor to recipient is at play, the removal of white blood cells from blood components would not be expected to significantly impact on the incidence of these reactions. For the 5-10% of patients in which recipient, rather than donor antibody is identified, leukocyte depletion might be beneficial. Thus, routine leukocyte reduction of cellular blood components would be anticipated to have a modest effect in reducing the incidence of TRALI. If a patient with a history of TRALI is shown to have a granulocyte or HLA-specific antibody in their plasma and needs subsequent transfusions of cellular products, leukocyte-depleted blood components would be justifiable. Based on the lack of available data, stronger recommendations would be premature.

CONCLUSION

1. TRALI is a serious, infrequent, but life-threatening complication of transfusion.
2. The etiology and pathogenesis need to be further defined, but passive transfer of antibodies which activate complement and/or agglutinate granulocytes appears to play an important role.
3. There is a limited role for leukocyte reduction of blood components in decreasing the frequency of this complication.

REFERENCES

1. Popovsky MA, Taswell HF. Circulatory overload: an underdiagnosed consequence of transfusion (abstract). Transfusion 25:469, 1985.
2. Bjerrum OJ, Jerslid C. Class-specific anti-IgA associated with severe anaphylactic transfusion reactions in a patient with pernicious anaemia. Vox Sang 21:411, 1971.
3. Ward HN. Pulmonary infiltrates associated with leukoagglutinin transfusion reactions. Ann Intern Med 73:689, 1970.
4. Kernoff PB, Durrant IJ, Rizza CR, Wright FW. Severe allergic pulmonary oedema after plasma transfusion. Br J Haematol 23:777, 1972.
5. Wolf CFW, Canale VC. Fatal pulmonary hypersensitivity reaction to HL-A incompatible blood transfusion: report of a case and review of the literature. Transfusion 16:135, 1976.
6. Popovsky MA, Chaplin HC Jr, Moore SB. Transfusion-related acute lung injury: a neglected, serious complication of hemotherapy. Transfusion 32:589, 1992.
7. Popovsky MA, Abel MD, Moore SB. Transfusion-related acute lung injury associated with passive transfer of antileukocyte antibodies. Am Rev Respir Dis 128:185, 1983.
8. Popovsky MA, Moore SB. Diagnostic and pathogenetic considerations in transfusion-related acute lung injury. Transfusion 25:573, 1985.
9. Sazama K. Reports of 355 transfusion-associated deaths: 1976 through 1985. Transfusion 30:583, 1990.
10. von dem Borne AEG Kr, Simsek S, van der Schoot CE, Goldschmiding R. Platelet and neutrophil alloantigens: their nature and role in immune-mediated cytopenias. In: Immunobiology of Transfusion Medicine. Ed. George Garratty. Marcel Dekker, 1994, New York.
11. Thompson JS, Severson CD, Parmely MJ, Marmorstein BL, Simmons A. Pulmonary "hypersensitivity": reactions induced by transfusion of non-HL-A leukoagglutinins. N Engl J Med 284:1120, 1971.
12. Andrews AT, Zmijewski CM, Bowman HS, Reihart JK. Transfusion reaction with pulmonary infiltration associated with HL-A-specific leukocyte antibodies. Am J Clin Pathol 66:483, 1976.
13. Yomtovian R, Kline W, Press C, Clay M, Engman H, Hammerschmidt D, McCullough J. Severe pulmonary hypersensitivity associated with passive transfusion of a neutrophil-specific antibody. Lancet i:244, 1984.
14. Goeken NE, Schulak JA, Nghiem DD, Knox LB, Reynolds LS, Corry RJ. Transfusion reactions in donor-specific blood transfusion patients resulting from transfused

maternal antibody. Transplantation 38:306, 1984.

15. Reese EP Jr., McCullough JJ, Craddock PR. An adverse pulmonary reaction to cyroprecipitate in a hemophiliac. Transfusion15:583, 1975.

16. Ward HN. Pulmonary infiltrates associated with leukoagglutinin transfusion reactions. Ann Intern Med 73:689, 1970.

17. Ward HN, Lipscomb TS, Cawley LP. Pulmonary hypersensitivity reaction after blood transfusion. Arch Intern Med 122:362, 1968.

18. Brittingham TE. Immunologic studies on leukocytes. Vox Sang 2:242, 1957.

19. Felbo M, Jensen KG. Death in childbirth following transfusion of leukocyte-incompatible blood. Acta Haematol (Basel) 27:113, 1962.

20. Campbell DA Jr, Swartz RD, Waskerwitz JA, Haines RF, Turcotte JG. Leukoagglutination with interstitial pulmonary edema: a complication of donor-specific transfusion. Transplantation 34:300, 1982.

21. Carilli AD, Ramanamurty MV, Chang Y-S, Shin D, Sethi V. Noncardiogenic pulmonary edema following blood transfusion. Chest 74:310, 1978.

22. DuBois M, Lotze MT, Diamond WJ, Kim YD, Flye MW, Macnamara TE. Pulmonary shunting during leukoagglutinin-induced noncardiac pulmonary edema. JAMA 244:2186, 1980.

23. Nordhagen R, Conradi M, Dromtorp SM. Pulmonary reaction associated with transfusion of plasma containing anti-5b. Vox Sang 51:102, 1986.

24. Van Buren NL, Stroncek DF, Clay ME, McCullough J, et al. Transfusion-related acute lung injury caused by an NB2 granulocyte-specific antibody in a patient with thrombotic thrombocytopenic purpura. Transfusion 30:42, 1990.

25. Eastlund T, McGrath PC, Britten A, Propp R. Fatal pulmonary transfusion reaction to plasma containing donor HLA antibody. Vox Sang 57:63, 1989.

26. Eastlund DT, McGrath PC, Burkart P. Platelet transfusion reaction associated with interdonor HLA incompatibility. Vox Sang 55:157, 1988.

27. O'Connor JC, Strauss RG, Goeken NE, Knox LB. A near-fatal reaction during granulocyte transfusion of a neonate. Transfusion 28:173, 1988.

28. Levy GJ, Shabot MM, Hart ME, Mya WW, Goldfinger D. Transfusion-associated noncardiogenic pulmonary edema: report of a case and a warning regarding treatment. Transfusion 26:278, 1986.

29. DeWolf AM, Van Den Berg BW, Hoffman HJ, Van Zundert AA. Pulmonary dysfunction during one-lung ventilation caused by HLA-specific antibodies against leukocytes. Anesth Analg 66:463, 1987.

30. Silliman C, Pitman J, Thurman G, Ambruso D. Neutrophil (PMN) priming agents develop in patients with transfusion-related acute lung injury (Abstract). Blood 80:(Suppl 1)261a, 1992.

31. Dann EJ, Gillis S, Cohen E, Ilan Y. Transfusion-related acute lung injury. Harefuah 124(1):12, 1993.

32. Cooperman LH, Price HL. Pulmonary edema in the operative and postoperative period: a review of 40 cases. Ann Surg 172:883, 1970.

33. Culliford AT, Thomas S, Spencer FC. Fulminating noncardiogenic pulmonary edema: a newly recognized hazard during cardiac operations. J Thorac Cardiovasc Surg 80:868, 1980.

34. Malouf M, Granville AR. Blood transfusion related adult respiratory distress syndrome. Anaesth Intens Care 21:44, 1993.

35. Jacob HS, Craddock PR, Hammerschmidt DE, Moldow CF. Complement-induced granulocyte aggregation: an unsuspected mechanism of disease. N Eng J Med 302:789, 1980.

36. Craddock PR, Hammerschmidt DE, Moldow CF, Yamada O, Jacob HS. Granulocyte aggregation as a manifestation of membrane interactions with complement: possible role in leukocyte margination, microvascular occlusion, and endothelial damage. Semin Hematol 16:140, 1979.

37. Shasby DM, VanBenthuysen KM, Tate RM, Shasby SS, McMurtry I, Repine JE. Granulocytes mediate acute edematous lung injury in rabbits and in isolated rabbit lungs perfused with phorbol myristate acetate: role

of oxygen radicals. Am Rev Respir Dis 125:443, 1982.

38. Sznajder JI, Fraiman A, Hall JB, et al. Increased hydrogen peroxide in the expired breath of patients with acute hypoxemic respiratory failure. Chest 96:606, 1989.

39. Larsen GL, McCarthy K, Webster RO, Henson J, Henson PM. A differential effect of C5a and C5a des Arg in the induction of pulmonary inflammation. Am J Pathol 100:179, 1980.

40. Seeger W, Schneider U, Kreusler B, Witzleben EV, Walmrath D, Grimminger F, Neppert J. Reproduction of transfusion-related acute lung injury in an ex vivo lung model. Blood 76:1438, 1990.

41. Westaby S. Mechanisms of membrane damage and surfactant depletion in acute lung injury. Intensive Care Med 12:2, 1986.

42. Gans ROB, Duurkens VAM, van Zundert AA, Hoorntje SJ. Transfusion-related acute lung injury. Intensive Care Med 14:654, 1988.

CHAPTER 11

THE ROLE OF LEUKOCYTE DEPLETION IN THE PREVENTION OF REPERFUSION INJURY ASSOCIATED WITH OPEN HEART SURGERY

Terry Gourlay, Kenneth M. Taylor

SUMMARY

Reperfusion injury (RI) is a term used to describe tissue injury associated with revascularization after a period of ischaemia. This phenomenon may occur in open heart surgery and result in considerable morbidity. The mechanism of RI is thought to be an interaction between activated leukocytes, and reperfused endothelium, resulting in the release of variety of substances, such as activated oxygen species or proteolytic enzymes, with potential for parenchymal damage.

Leukocyte activation occurs during cardiopulmonary bypass and strategies to minimize RI include minimizing organ underperfusion, improving the surfaces of the extracorporeal circuit so as to reduce cellular and protein activation, pharmacological agents such as steroids, radical scavengers or enzymes which remove activated oxygen species and leuko-depletion of re-infused blood.

Leukodepletion of re-infused autologous blood or transfused allogeneic blood has become possible using in-line filtration. Leukodepletion of autologous blood can be achieved in both the extracorporeal perfusion circuit and the cardioplegia delivery system. Several early clinical studies indicated benefit of this approach in reducing postoperative morbidity, length of stay in the intensive care unit (ITU/ICU) and ventilation times.

INTRODUCTION

Reperfusion injury, as the name implies, describes the sequence of pathological events which occurs after blood flow is restored to an organ

Clinical Benefits of Leukodepleted Blood Products, edited by Joseph Sweeney, M.D. and Andrew Heaton, M.D. © 1995 R.G. Landes Company.

or tissue after a period of flow reduction or cessation.[1] In this regard, reperfusion injury, as such, is not restricted to cardiac surgery, but may be associated with many surgical specialties involving the application of tourniquets or indeed crush injury.[2] Leukocytes are considered to be important in the mediation of reperfusion injury.

Despite the uneventful progress of most patients undergoing open heart surgery, there remain a number of patients who exhibit a profound adverse reaction to the procedure, which is particularly apparent in the postoperative recovery phase. Reperfusion injury has been recognized for some time as a significant factor in the morbidity of such patients undergoing open heart surgical procedures. The cellular dysfunction attributed to this phenomenon ranges from mild neurological disruption[3-6] to moderate sequelae such as the "wet lung" syndrome to, in extreme cases, death due to severe cardiopulmonary injury.[7] These sequelae were observed even in the very early days of cardiac surgery. Cleland et al published their observations describing an increase in extravascular fluid and pulmonary insufficiency in patients who had undergone cardiopulmonary bypass procedures in 1966.[8] In cardiac surgical practice, the wide ranging spectrum of adverse events associated with this injurious mechanism are known as the postperfusion syndrome reflecting the major importance of cardiopulmonary bypass in its etiology. Before considering the various methods, both pharmacological and mechanical, which have evolved to reduce or limit the adverse clinical reactions associated with reperfusion injury, it is important to understand the pathogenesis of the reperfusion injury syndrome as it exists in the cardiac surgical field.

As already stated, reperfusion injury occurs when blood flow is restored to a region of tissue after a period of low or no-flow. This is in contrast to ischemic injury which may be characterized as cell death mediated by long term deprivation of nutrients under conditions of reduced or eliminated blood flow. This nutrient starvation results in cell death due to a reduction in metabolism leading to an accumulation of toxic metabolites. Reperfusion injury is thought to be the consequence of activated leukocytes attacking otherwise healthy tissues by the uncontrolled release of mechanisms normally employed as a host defense system. In this regard, reperfusion injury differs from ischemic injury. Reperfusion injury does not require a reduction or elimination of cellular metabolism as is the case in ischemic injury. However the ischemic phenomenon and the release of toxins and mediators are essential prerequisites for the reperfusion syndrome. Gorlick[1] elegantly described the difference between ischemic cell death and reperfusion injury as being a passive mechanism versus an active and violent one. What is clear from the literature is that the leukocyte (in particular the neutrophil) has a very important role to play in the development of reperfusion injury and that flow restriction following periods of no flow or reduced flow is necessary for the development of the syndrome. It is essential, therefore, to characterize why the conditions present during cardiopulmonary bypass offer the required combination of leukocyte activating processes and altered hemodynamics required for this phenomenon to occur.

HEMODYNAMICS DURING CARDIOPULMONARY BYPASS

The cardiac surgical patient is placed on a cardiopulmonary support system which performs the function of the patient's heart and lungs during the operative procedure. This is essential in order that the surgical team can operate on a static heart. The use of cardiopulmonary bypass (CPB) has been associated with an increase in peripheral vascular resistance index (PVRI) (Fig. 11.1) indicating a reduction in perfusion to peripheral tissues.[9] The use of "core cooling" to reduce the metabolic requirements of the tissues during the perfusion period and the vasoconstriction associated with hypothermia compound this phenomenon.[10] A reduction in tissue oxygen uptake during this phase of the operation has been demonstrated in patients undergoing open heart surgery together with an increase in tissue acidosis, suggesting that ischemic conditions may exist.[11] Reduced tissue perfusion and the potential for the development of regional ischemia represent precisely those conditions required for reperfusion injury to occur. The subsequent re-establishment of improved peripheral perfusion associated with the re-warming phase of the operation together with re-establishment of perfusion to the previously isolated heart and lungs presents the second hemodynamic requirement for the reperfusion injury event, the re-establishment of oxygenated blood flow to a previously ischemic tissue.

LEUKOCYTE ACTIVATION DURING CARDIOPULMONARY BYPASS

The extracorporeal perfusion circuit employed during open heart surgery consists of several major prosthetic components, including a large surface area membrane lung, PVC and/or Silastic rubber circuit tubing, various filters for arterial, cardiotomy and transfusion blood and several roller pumps (Fig. 11.2). The surface area of even the simplest perfusion circuit is several square meters. This circuit provides the ideal medium for contact activation of leukocytes. It has been demonstrated that blood undergoes a number of changes when it is exposed to large foreign surfaces.

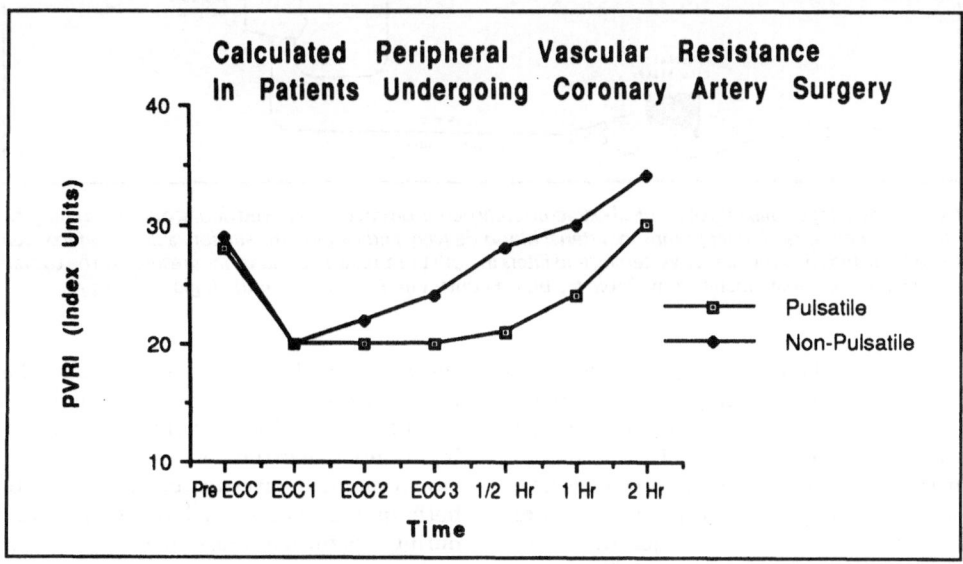

Fig. 11.1. Peripheral vascular resistance index (PVRI) in patients undergoing elective coronary artery bypass surgery. PVRI is assessed in the following manner:

$$PVRI = \frac{Pa - Pv}{Q}$$

Where: Pa = Arterial Pressure
Pv = Venous Pressure
Q = Blood Flow/m²

The PVRI measured during the open heart surgical procedure is shown under pulsatile and non-pulsatile flow conditions. ECC1 to 3 represent the perfusion period with calculations being made at the beginning middle and end of the perfusion. In the non-pulsatile group there is an initial rise in PVRI which continues during the post-operative period. Under pulsatile flow conditions there is a more stable profile with little rise in PVRI during the perfusion period followed by a rise in PVRI post-operatively. The PVRI under pulsatile flow conditions is consistently lower than that measured during non-pulsatile perfusion.

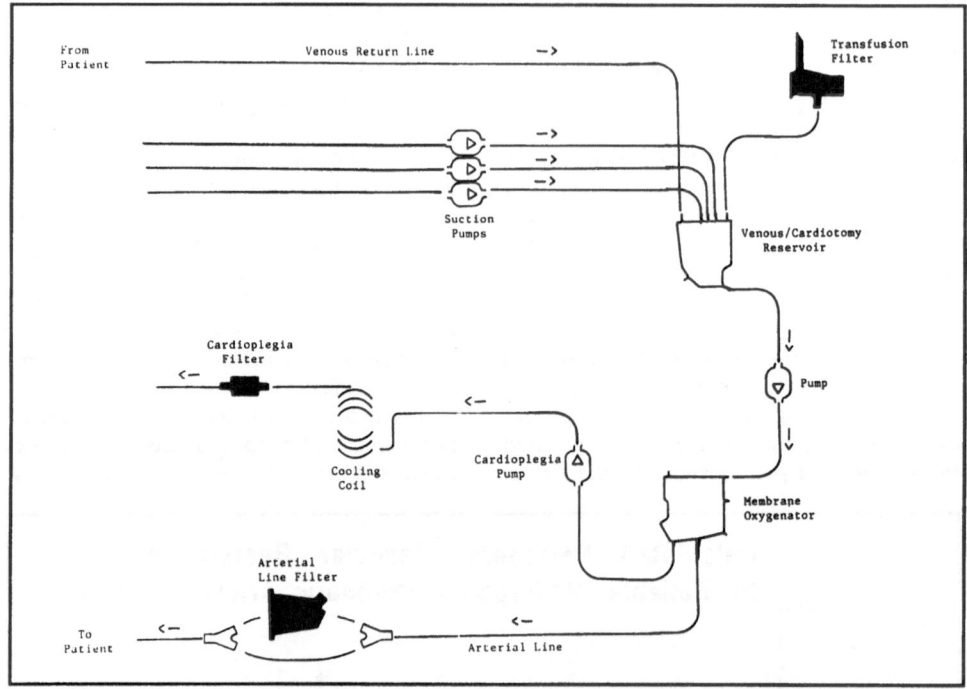

Fig. 11.2. Schematic diagram of a typical extracorporeal perfusion circuit employed during open heart surgery. The system consists of roller pumps for arterial blood delivery and cardiotomy suction, a large surface area membrane blood oxygenator, PVC tubing and filters in both the arterial line and venous reservoir. The overall surface area of foreign materials available for blood contact in this circuit is in the region of 7 sq m.

Such hematological change has also been shown in the less challenging circumstances of hemodialysis. Studies carried out on patients undergoing hemodialysis have confirmed short-term neutropenia associated with temporary pulmonary dysfunction related to complement activation in the initial stages of the procedure.[13] These significant sequelae occur in renal dialysis despite the relatively small foreign material interfaces present in the hemodialysis perfusion systems employed. Significantly, the phenomenon observed in the hemodialysis patients was associated with the initial contact period. The complement system seems to be activated by exposure of plasma to foreign surfaces.[14-17] Complement components, specifically C5a and C3a, have been shown to be responsible for the activation of leukocytes. The ultimate consequence of this sequence of events is

the release of free radical species and the release of proteolytic enzymes.[18] The digestive action of proteolytic enzymes and the highly reactive nature of superoxide anions have prompted investigators to implicate both in the type of cell death observed during reperfusion injury. It is known that complement activation of the neutrophil stimulates membrane bound NADPH-oxidase which is part of the energy conversion system required for cell function. In neutrophils, an electron is shuttled to the extracellular space when NADPH-oxidase removes an electron from NADPH. These electrons are added to dissolved oxygen in the extracellular space to form the superoxide anion.[19,20] The superoxide anion, which contains an unpaired electron, is known as a free radical and is extremely unstable and highly reactive. Subsequent additions of electrons result in the production of hydrogen peroxide and by addition of a further electron the hydroxyl anion, another free radical species. With the addition of another electron-water and oxygen are produced. The presence of hydrogen peroxide and other free radical species is believed to play a substantial part in the cellular disruption associated with reperfusion injury. Peroxide is known to be capable of oxidizing many substances including the lipid components of cell membranes. Due to their ability to be measured easily using spectrophotometry, the products of this lipid peroxidation (conjugated dienes) are used as markers of oxidative cell injury by researchers. In the presence of myeloperoxidase, a neutrophil-derived enzyme, hydrogen peroxide can react with chloride ions to produce hypochlorous acid another highly reactive substance which can react with secondary amines in the extracellular fluid to produce chloramines, another highly reactive oxidant. Although all of these oxidants may be sufficient to produce the damage observed in the reperfusion injury state, there are other factors involved in this complicated scenario. As already mentioned, neutrophils in the activated state release a number of proteolytic enzymes from cytoplasmic granules. Elastase, collagenase and gelatinase, in particular, have been shown to be capable of destroying the extracellular matrix responsible for maintaining cellular integrity. This cellular destruction is consistent with the type of damage observed in reperfusion injury.

Much of the hypothesis implicating the neutrophil in reperfusion injury is, to say the least, speculative. There is a case for stating that the highly reactive substances released upon activation of the neutrophil are unlikely to survive long enough in plasma to cause any damage whatsoever. Certainly, the free radical species involved are so highly reactive that they are, due to the presence of a high concentration of oxidizable material in plasma, unlikely to survive long enough in a free circulating state to cause any harm at all. The proteolytic enzymes are also highly reactive;

elastase for example is neutralized in plasma by specific enzyme inhibitors, and alpha-1-antiprotease is present in high concentration in plasma and binds readily with elastase, neutralizing its proteolytic action.

There is however some evidence that free radicals and proteolytic enzymes may act in concert in a self-regulatory manner to cause the injury associated with reperfusion. Elastase, inhibited by alpha-1-antiproteases can be disinhibited by HOCl and chloramines reacting with the enzyme inhibitor. It has been demonstrated that under these conditions the half-life of elastase may be prolonged from half of a millisecond to up to one and a half seconds.[21] This reaction is by no means unique. It also occurs with other proteolytic enzymes and free radical species. Much work is required in this area to unravel the complex mechanisms involved in reperfusion injury and to offer new methods of protection and prevention.

The fact that reperfusion injury and ischemic injury are inextricably linked is further compounded by the so called "no re-flow" phenomenon. One of the properties of the activated leukocyte, in addition to the well documented release of reactive oxidants and enzymes, is that they are also attracted to the endothelial cell layer lining the vasculature.[22,23] In the activated state therefore, leukocytes may form microaggregates which, due to their relatively large size, can occlude the smallest capillary vessels.[24] Under these conditions, it is possible for regions of local ischemia to exist, resulting in further ischemic and reperfusion injury.

PREVENTING REPERFUSION INJURY

Theoretically, reperfusion injury could be attenuated either by preventing or minimizing the period or duration of reduced blood flow, or by preventing or minimizing leukocyte activation.

IMPROVED BLOOD FLOW

In recent years, steps have been taken to address the poor peripheral perfusion associated with cardiopulmonary bypass

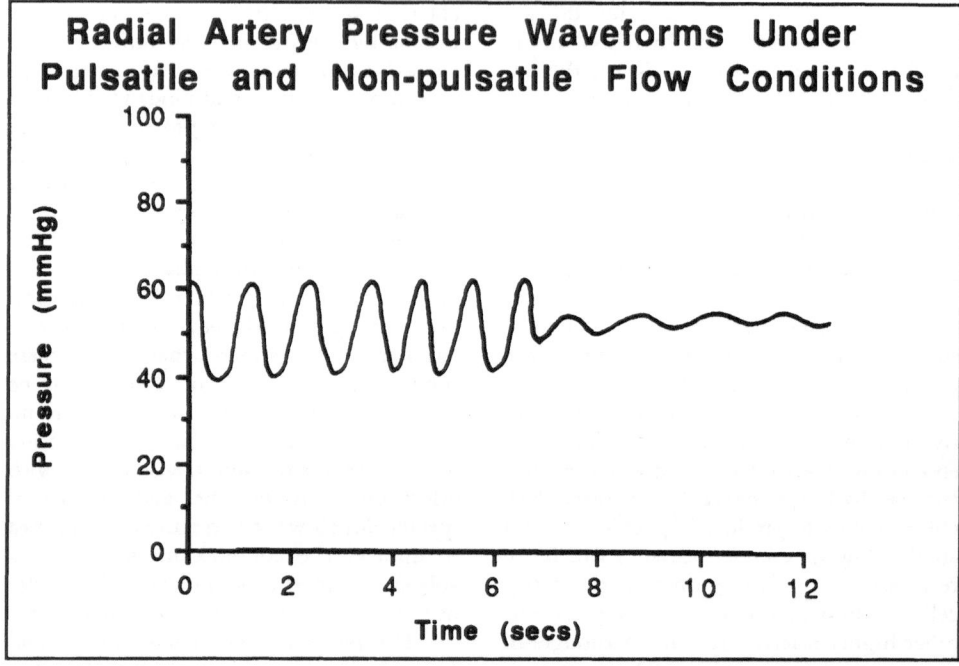

Fig. 11.3. Radial artery pressure tracings from the same patient undergoing firstly, non-pulsatile flow and secondly, pulsatile flow. Both pressure profiles were generated by the same pump (Cobe/Stockert, Cobe Laboratories, Gloucester, England), employing a PFC2 flow controller to generate pulsatile flow.

during open heart surgery. One of the most successful in this regard has been the development of pulsatile perfusion systems which offer a more physiological form of perfusate delivery. The most widely used systems of this type are modified roller pumps which generate pulsatility by accelerating and decelerating the pump head. This technology has been well accepted by the cardiothoracic surgical community because of its inherent familiarity, in that the pumps employed are essentially similar to those traditionally employed to deliver a non-pulsatile flow pattern (Fig. 11.3). This simple innovation has been associated with a reduction in peripheral vascular resistance, increased oxygen uptake, and improved organ blood flow in clinical use[25-29] together with a measurable reduction in both patient mortality and morbidity. Recent advances in the other devices employed in the extracorporeal perfusion circuit have supported the advances in per-

fusate delivery. The oxygenators employed during the perfusion phase of the operation to perform the function of the isolated lungs, have evolved into high performance gas exchange devices which are capable of supporting the increased oxygen demand made by the well perfused tissues.[30-32] This improvement in device performance, both in terms of blood and oxygen delivery and an increased confidence on the part of the users regarding the consistency and safety margin associated with their performance, has led to a resurgence in interest in recent years in the use of normothermia during cardiac surgical procedures. This development may eliminate the last remaining hurdle in eliminating the increased PVRI traditionally associated with induced hypothermia during cardiopulmonary bypass procedures. These improvements in technology go some way to eliminating the conditions required for the generation of reperfusion injury by reducing the low perfusion state which is required for the development of the syndrome.

IMPROVED MATERIAL TECHNOLOGY

Advances in material technology offer further advances in the prevention or reduction of reperfusion injury. It has been demonstrated that contact activation of the complement cascade results in the activation of leukocytes, subsequent generation of free radicals and release of proteolytic enzymes. This contact activation by blood/plastic interfaces may be reduced by coating the plastic with more physiologically acceptable substances. The focus of much of the early work in this area was the treatment of circuitry materials with a bonded heparin complex which would, at the very least, inhibit blood-to-plastic contact, thus reducing foreign material contact activation of complement. Although initial studies are promising in this area in terms of reducing complement activation,[33-35] this treatment of materials deals solely with the contact activation phenomenon which takes place in the early stages of the surgical procedure, but will have little or no effect on circumstances leading to reperfusion injury associated with local areas of stasis leading to regional ischemia. In addition to dealing with only one aspect of the inflammatory response to cardiac surgery, surface treatment with heparin complexes is an extremely expensive process resulting in a significant increase in the cost of the products employed in the perfusion circuitry.

USE OF PHARMACOLOGICAL AGENTS

Another approach is necessary which will address both the contact activation mechanism and the phenomenon associated with the release of endotoxins and mediators from the ischemic tissues upon release of the aortic cross clamp and from peripheral tissues during the rewarming phase of the procedure. Two techniques are currently undergoing study in this area. Pharmacological inhibition of the inflammatory response to surgery by employing pharmacological agents which either inhibit free radicals or degranulation of leukocytes have

been the focus of many animal studies.[36,37] These agents were found to be effective to a limited extent in the animal model,[38,39] but were found to be less effective clinically. This may be due to the complex mechanism involved in the inflammatory response to open heart surgery. The utilization of corticosteroids as both a single dose pre-operatively and during the operative period has been shown to offer some improvement in post-op patient status.[40-42] Studies have shown a reduction in non-infective fever in the postoperative period, reduced fluid administration requirements, and improved microcirculatory perfusion.[43,44] The use of free radical scavengers during heart-lung transplantation and during routine open heart surgical procedures, particularly in the cardioplegia delivery system, appears to be extremely promising.[45] Several drug cocktails have been employed in his area, but the principal agents employed include superoxide dismutase (SOD) and catalase (CAT) which degrade superoxide anion and hydrogen peroxide respectively. The aim in using these particular agents is to eliminate these reactive oxygen metabolites under the extreme conditions encountered during the ischemic or reperfusion phases when the generation of the radical species overwhelms the ability of naturally occurring enzymes to eliminate them. Other agents have been studied in this regard, particularly dimethyl-thiourea (DMTU) and mannitol cardioplegia solution.[46] Initial results are extremely promising. However, problems remain regarding the definition of optimal dosage and timing together with concern over harmful side effects.

REDUCTION IN LEUKOCYTE ASSAULT ON THE MICROCIRCULATION

The final and most recent development aimed at addressing the reperfusion injury syndrome is to prevent the leukocyte mediated aspect of the problem by removing neutrophils during the perfusion procedure rather than to attempt to prevent their activation. An increasing number of studies have demonstrated that the pathological effects of activated leukocytes may be reduced by physically eliminating leukocytes. It has been demonstrated that the deleterious effects of activated leukocytes, such as the release of oxygen free radicals, microvascular occlusions and the release of other toxic agents can be reduced by utilizing leukocyte depleted blood in the reperfusion phase after extended hypothermic storage of organs for transplantation.[47] Animal models have been employed to demonstrate that the use of leukocyte depletion reduces the incidence of postoperative pulmonary insufficiency, increased extravascular lung water and increased pulmonary vascular resistance in the perfused bovine model.[48] Although leukocyte depletion is not new in general medical practice, products have only recently been developed which will remove free circulating activated leukocytes from the various blood delivery sites of the extracorporeal perfusion system employed in open heart surgery (Fig. 11.4). There are three main intervention points available in this circuitry. All three are of some importance if the benefits of leukodepletion are to be maxi-mized in terms of protection from leukocyte mediated tissue damage. These three intervention sites include the major arterial and venous return lines, the cardioplegia delivery line and the blood transfusion lines. Of the three intervention sites, two are new in terms of the application of leukodepletion technology. Leukodepletion of transfused blood has been available for many years. However leukodepletion of the extracorporeal perfusion circuit and the cardioplegia delivery system employed during cardiac surgery are new areas for the application of this technology. It is necessary to characterize individually these different areas for the application of leukodepletion in order that the potential overall importance of the combined effect of these different functional applications can be understood.

LEUKODEPLETION OF THE EXTRACORPOREAL CIRCUIT

Much of the early research in this area focused on the animal transplant model. Leukocyte depletion was investigated in vitro and in vivo on both isolated heart

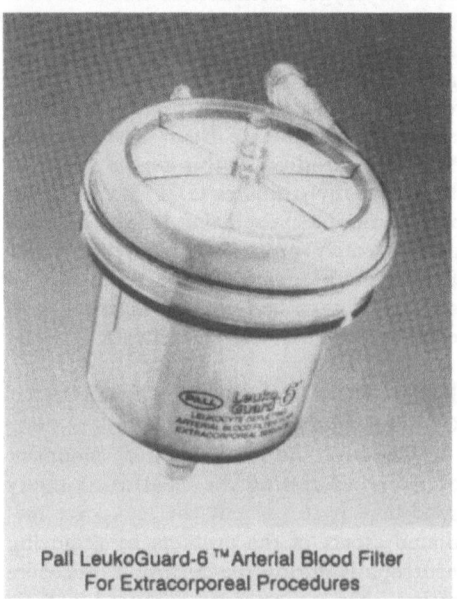

Pall LeukoGuard-6 ™ Arterial Blood Filter
For Extracorporeal Procedures

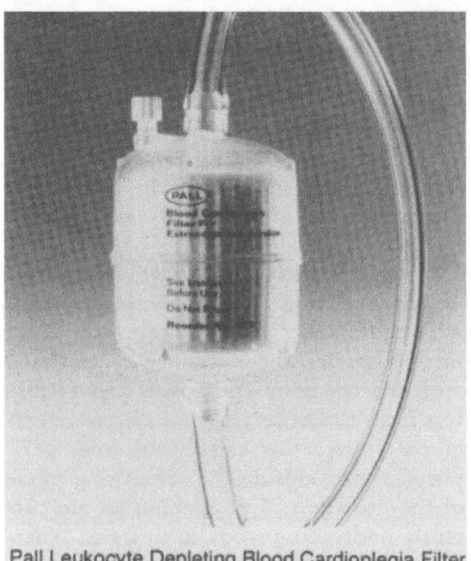

Pall Leukocyte Depleting Blood Cardioplegia Filter

Fig. 11.4. Leukocyte depleting filters for use in the arterial and cardioplegia delivery lines of the extracorporeal circuit employed during open heart surgery.

preparations and conventional extracorporeal circulation.[40,50-53] The results of these studies in the 1980s and early 1990s have been extremely promising and confirmed that organ damage normally associated with cold ischemic storage of organs for transplantation could be reduced and the storage time extended by employing this relatively simple technique. The positive outcome of this work stimulated the development of filters for routine clinical application. An in-line arterial filter has been developed by the Pall Corporation (Leukoguard LG6 leukocyte depleting arterial line filter. Pall Biomedical Ltd., Portsmouth, United Kingdom) which is intended to replace the arterial return line filter in the extracorporeal circuit and offer the additional function of leukodepletion. The removal of neutrophils is facilitated by a medium present on the filter surface upstream of the filter screen. The efficiency of the filter at removing neutrophils has been demonstrated in the laboratory environment employing fresh heparinized bovine blood.[54,55] (Fig. 11.5) These laboratory studies demonstrated that the filter removed neutrophils whilst sparing lymphocytes (Figs. 11.6 and 11.7) and offered no additional potentially deleterious effects in terms of either platelet depletion or hemolysis. Whilst the development of this filter has been a fairly recent innovation in this field, early clinical trials have demonstrated specific advantages associated with its use in routine clinical practice. Allen et al,[56] in a recent presentation to the Scandinavian Society for Extracorporeal Technology, demonstrated that postoperative neutrophilia was attenuated together with a substantial reduction in extracorporeal bypass related morbidity. Palanzo et al[57] showed in a more recent study that postoperative lung function was improved with the use of leukodepletion, and that ITU (ICU) stay and ventilation times were reduced. Gu et al[58] demonstrated that systemic depletion of leukocytes resulted in a reduction in inflammatory damage. These results are clearly promising in terms of

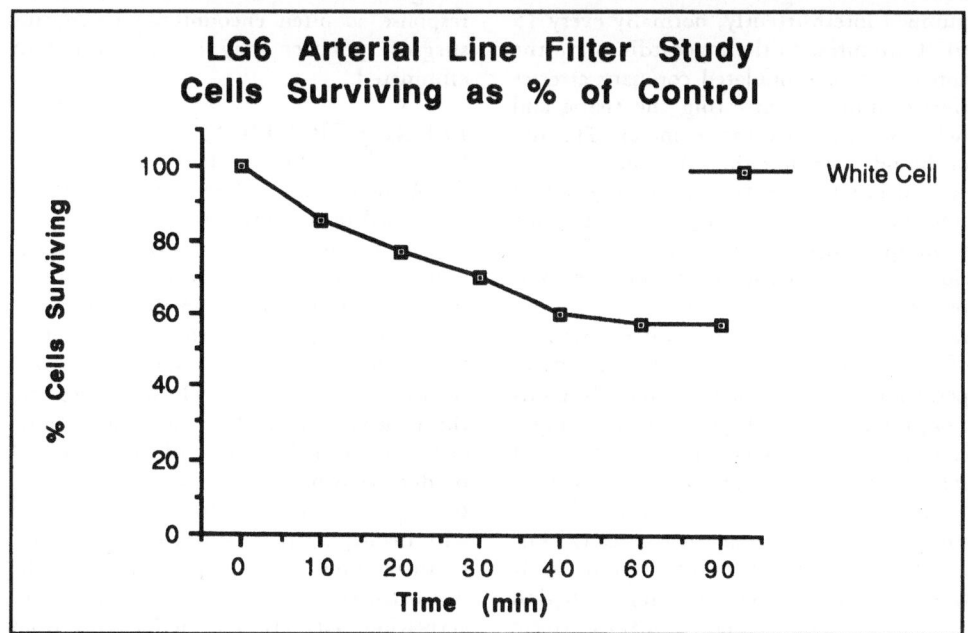

Fig. 11.5. Leukocyte depletion profile for fresh heparinized bovine blood in the presence of a leukocyte depleting arterial line filter at a blood flow rate of 4.5 l/min and a hematocrit of 27%. The data show depletion for total leukocyte count.

the potential of leukodepletion to protect the patient from systemic damage associated with the activation of neutrophils. However, the protection of specific target organs such as the heart and lungs, which undergo long periods of ischemic arrest may require another strategy altogether.

LEUKOCYTE DEPLETION OF CARDIOPLEGIC BLOOD

The cardioplegic delivery line is one of the three points in the perfusion circuit which offers the potential for leukocyte depletion technology. The blood cardioplegia delivery system is that component of the perfusion circuit which facilitates the delivery of cold potassium-rich, hemodiluted, arterialized blood to the myocardium during the period of aortic cross clamping. The source of the blood in this solution is generally the arterial outlet of the blood oxygenator. This blood is typically pumped from the oxygenator and mixed with a potassium-rich saline or Ringers solution in a ratio of between 1:1 and 4:1. This blood saline mixture is then pumped intermittently, normally every 15 to 30 minutes, to the myocardium via the aortic root or cannulated coronary arteries thus cooling and arresting the tissue and reducing tissue oxygen demand. The use of blood cardioplegia solutions has increased in recent years replacing crystalloid solutions as the solution of choice for this technique. Again, this is an area of perfusion practice which includes all of the components required for the generation of reperfusion injury viz intermittent periods of low or no flow followed by periods of perfusion with oxygenated blood. In addition, the blood which passes into the myocardium is in contact with an additional region of foreign materials of relatively large surface area. The source of this blood, the general circulation, may already contain high numbers of contact activated neutrophils which are perfused into a region of tissue which may contain toxic by-products of ischemia. Many studies have been carried out focusing on this particular area of perfusion practice in both rou-

tine perfusion applications and in the organ transplant field. Gu[59] demonstrated the inflammatory response in the later stages of cardiopulmonary bypass associated with the release of the aortic cross clamp and the presence of endotoxins and mediators released from the ischemic heart and lungs. The use of oxygenated blood cardioplegia may reduce the level of ischemia present in the isolated heart and lungs and reduce the magnitude of this late non-contact related inflammatory response. Pearl et al[60] demonstrated that the use of leukocyte depleted cardioplegic blood during the period of aortic cross clamping reduced the evidence of reperfusion injury in human hearts. Trials continue in this exciting new area of myocardial protection which focus on the combination of blood cardioplegia, free radical scavengers and leukocyte depletion. Clearly, if the problems associated with the release of toxins and mediators from the ischemic heart and lungs at the end of the cross clamping period can be overcome by the application of these technologies, the late non-contact inflammatory response so often encountered in routine surgical practice may be moderated or eliminated.

LEUKODEPLETION OF TRANSFUSED BLOOD

Although the volume of donor blood transfused during open heart surgical procedures has reduced substantially over the years, patients undergoing cardiac surgery still require a limited amount of donor blood, particularly in the postoperative phase when hemoglobin levels may remain reduced following hemodilution caused by the relatively large fluid priming volume of the perfusion circuitry. Blood and blood product transfusions may also be required to counteract excessive bleeding associated with inadequate reversal of the heparin load by the administration of protamine and the disturbances in hemostasis due to contact activation. Depletion of leukocytes from whole blood is by no means a new technique, Fleming described just such a technique as long ago as 1928, employing a

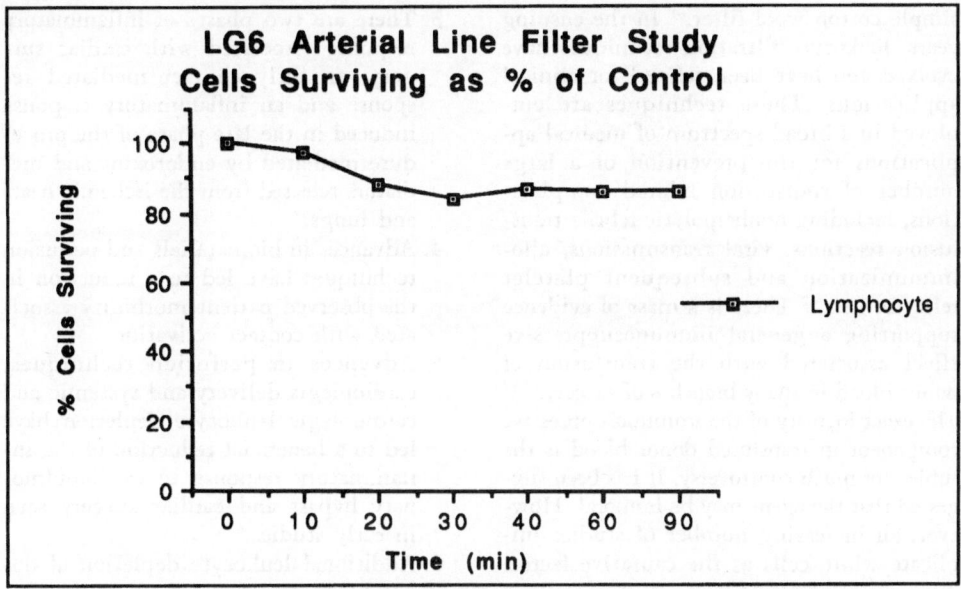

Fig. 11.6. Leukocyte depletion profile for fresh heparinized bovine blood in the presence of a leukocyte depleting arterial line filter at a blood flow rate of 4.5 l/min and a hematocrit of 27%. The data show depletion for lymphocytes.

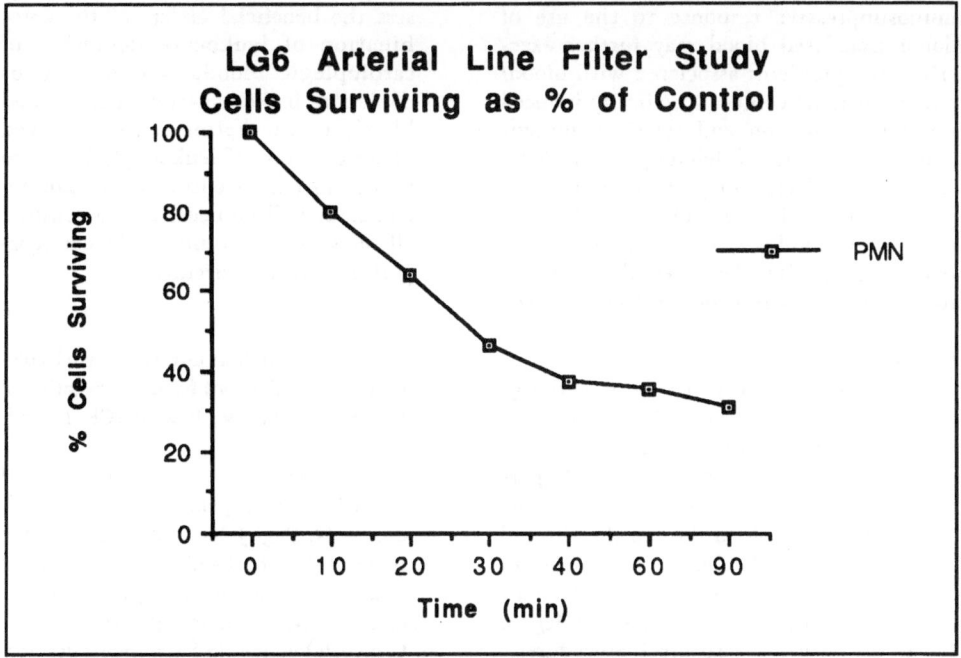

Fig. 11.7. Leukocyte depletion profile for fresh heparinized bovine blood in the presence of a leukocyte depleting arterial line filter at a blood flow rate of 4.5 l/min and a hematocrit of 27%. The data show depletion of polymorphonuclear leukocytes.

simple cotton wool filter.[61] In the ensuing years, leukocyte filtration techniques have evolved and have been refined for clinical applications. These techniques are employed in a broad spectrum of medical applications for the prevention of a large number of transfusion related complications, including nonhemolytic febrile transfusion reactions, viral transmissions, alloimmunization and subsequent platelet refractoriness.[62] There is a mass of evidence supporting a general immunosuppressive effect associated with the transfusion of donor blood in many branches of surgery.[63-67] The exact identity of the immunosuppressive component in transfused donor blood is the subject of much controversy. It has been suggested that the agent may be humoral. However, an increasing number of studies implicate white cells as the causative factor. A recent study by Jensen et al confirmed the reduction in post-operative infection rate in a randomized trial associated with the use of leukocyte depleting filtration techniques.[68] In cardiac patients, the immunosuppressive response to the use of donor transfused blood may further exacerbate the problems associated with blood/foreign material contact specifically induced immunosuppression and systemic inflammation. The use of leukocyte depleting transfusion filters may become routine practice if the benefits of improved biomaterial technology, blood delivery systems, and high flow leukocyte depletion are to be realized in routine clinical practice.

CONCLUSIONS

1. Reperfusion injury has been a recognized causative factor of postoperative morbidity in patients undergoing open heart surgery for some years. Reperfusion injury requires, as the name implies, that blood flow to the affected tissue should be halted and then reinstated for the phenomenon to occur. These conditions occur to some degree in all open heart surgical procedures.

2. Leukocytes, particularly activated neutrophils, have been implicated in reperfusion injury.

3. There are two phases of inflammatory response associated with cardiac surgery; an early contact mediated response and an inflammatory response induced in the late phase of the procedure mediated by endotoxins and mediators released from the ischemic heart and lungs.

4. Advances in biomaterials and perfusion techniques have led to a reduction in the observed patient morbidity associated with contact activation.

5. Advances in perfusion techniques, cardioplegia delivery and systemic and cardioplegic leukocyte depletion have led to a beneficial reduction of the inflammatory response to cardiopulmonary bypass and cardiac surgery seen in early studies.

6. Additional leukocyte depletion of donor blood transfused during and after surgery offers additional suppression of the immunosuppressive effect of blood transfusion.

7. Currently, studies are underway to assess the beneficial effects of the combination of leukocyte depletion of cardioplegic blood, systemic leukodepletion, leukodepletion of transfused blood, normothermia and improved blood delivery. If leukodepletion is to be employed, to ensure its maximum benefit it will be necessary to consider all blood access points of the extracorporeal perfusion circuit.

REFERENCES

1. Gorlick DL, Ortolano GA. Leukocyte Depletion and Implications for the Prevention of Reperfusion Injury. Proc AACP 13:154, 1992.

2. Odeh M. The role of reperfusion induced injury in the pathogenesis of the crush syndrome. N. Engl J Med 324:1417, 1991.

3. Newman S. The incidence and nature of neuropsychological morbidity following cardiac surgery: Perfusion 4:93, 1989.

4. Campbell DE, Raskin SA. Cerebral dysfunction after cardiopulmonary bypass: Aetiology, manifestations and interventions. Perfusion 5:251, 1990.

5. Kirklin JK, Blackstone EH, Kirklin JW. Cardiopulmonary bypass: Studies on its damaging effects: Blood Purif 5:168, 1987.

6. Taylor KM. Pathophysiology of brain damage during open-heart surgery: Tex Heart Inst J 13:91, 1986.

7. Kirklin JK. The postperfusion syndrome: Inflammation and the damaging effects of cardiopulmonary bypass. In: Cardiopulmonary Bypass: Current Concepts and Controversies, Tinkler JH (ed), Philadelphia: WB Saunders Co. 131, 1989.

8. Cleland J, Pluth JR, Tauxe WN, Kirklin JW. Blood volume and body fluid compartment changes soon after closed and open intracardiac surgery. J Thorac Cardiovasc Surg 52:698, 1966.

9. Angell-James JE, de Burgh Daly M. Effects of graded pulsatile pressure on the reflex vasomotor responses elicited by changes of mean pressure in the perfused carotid sinus-aortic arch regions of the dog. J Physiol 214:51, 1971.

10. Bain WH. Measurement and monitoring for cardiopulmonary bypass. In: Cardiopulmonary Bypass, Principals and Management. KM. Taylor ed. Chapman Hall Medical, London 1986.

11. Jacobs LA, Klopp EH, Seamone W, Topaz SR, Gott VL. Improved organ function during cardiac bypass with a roller pump modified to deliver pulsatile flow. J Thorac Cardiovasc Surg 58:703, 1969.

12. Royston D, Fleming JS, Desai JB, Westaby S, Taylor KM. Increased production of peroxidation products associated with cardiac operations. Evidence for free radical generation. J Thorac Cardiovasc Surg; 91:759, 1986.

13. Craddock PR, Fehr J, Brigham KL, et al. Complement and leukocyte-mediated pulmonary dysfunction in hemodialysis. N Engl J Med 296:769, 1977.

14. Colman RW. Platelet and neutrophil activation in cardiopulmonary bypass: Ann Thorac Surg 49:32, 1990.

15. Stahl RF, Fischer CA, Kuchich U, Weinbaum G, Warsaw DS, et al. Effects of simulated extracorporeal circulation on human leukocyte elastase release, superoxide generation, and procoagulant activity: J Thorac Cardio-

16. Herzlinger GA. Activation of complement by polymers in contact with blood. In: Szycher M ed. Blood Compatible Polymers, Metals, and Composites. Lancaster, PA: Technomic, 83:89, 1983.

17. Chenoweth DE. Complement activation produced by biomaterials. Trans Am Soc Artif Intern Organs 32:226, 1986.

18. Leher RI, Ganz T. Antimicrobial polypeptides of human neutrophils. Blood 76:2169, 1990.

19. Lunec J. Free radicals: Their involvement in desease pocesses. Ann Clin Biochem 27:173, 1990.

20. Breda MA, Drinkwater DC, Laks H., et al. Prevention of reperfusion injury in the neonatal heart with leukocyte-depleted blood. J Thorac Cardiovasc Surg 97:654, 1988.

21. Weiss SJ. Tissue destrucion by neutrophils. N Engl J Med 320:365, 1989.

22. Royston D. Blood cell activation. Sem Thorac Cardiovasc Surg 2:341, 1990.

23. Warren JS, Ward PA. Review: Oxidative injury to the vascular endothelium. Am J Med Sci 292:97, 1986.

24. Schmid-Schonbein GW, Skalak R, Simon SI, Engler RL. The interaction between leukocytes and endothelium in vivo. Ann NY Acad Sci 516:348, 1987.

25. Taylor KM. Pulsatile cardiopulmonary bypass. A review. J Cardiovasc Surg 22:561, 1981.

26. Many M, Soroff HS, Birtwell WC, Giron F, Wise H, Detering RA. The physiologic role of pulsatile and non-pulsatile blood flow. II Effects on renal function. Arch Surg 95:762, 1967.

27. Wright G, Sanderson JM. Brain damage and mortality in dogs following pulsatile and non-pulsatile blood flows in extracorporeal circulation. Thorax 27:738, 1972.

28. Shepard RB, Kirklin JW. Relation of pulsatile flow to oxygen consumption and other variables during cardiopulmonary bypass. J Thorac Cardiovasc Surg 58:694, 1969.

29. Taylor KM, Bain WH, Maxted KJ, Hutton MH, Mittra S, Russell M. A comparitive study of pulsatile and non-pulsatile cardiopulmonary bypass in 325 patients. Proc Eur Soc Artif VI:238, 1979.

vasc Surg 101:230, 1991.

30. Fried DW, Wilgus MA, Weiss SJ. The proposed use of a "screening test" to assess oxygenator performance. Perfusion 8:299, 1993.

31. Gourlay T, Aslam M, Fleming J, Taylor KM. Evaluation of the Sorin Monolyth membrane oxygenator. Perfusion 5:209, 1990.

32. Gourlay T, Fleming J, Taylor KM. Evaluation of a range of extracorporeal membrane oxygenators. Perfusion 5:117, 1990.

33. Pradham MJ, Fleming JS, Nkere UU, Arnold J, Wildervuur CRH, Taylor KM. Clinical experience with heparin coated cardiopulmonary bypass circuits. Perfusion 6;235, 1991.

34. Videm V, Svennevig JL, Fosse E, et al. Reduced complement activation with heparin coated oxygenator and tubing in coronary bypass surgery—a clinical study. J Extracorp Technol (in press)

35. Videm V, Mollnes TE, Garred P, Svennevig JL. Biocompatibility of extracorporeal circulation: in vitro comparisons of heparin coated and uncoated oxygenator circuits. J Thorac Cardiovasc Surg 101:654, 1991.

36. Fuller RW, Kelsey CR, Cole PJ, Dollery CT, MacDermot J. Dexamethasone inhibits the production of thromboxane B2 leukotriene B4 by human alveolar and peritoneal macrophanges in culture. Clinical Science 67:653, 1984.

37. Jansen NJG, van Oeveren W, van de Broek L, Oudemans van Straaten HM, et al. Inhibition of the reperfusion phenomena in cardiopulmonary bypass by dexamethasone: J Thorac Cardiovasc Surg; 102:515.

38. Ohtani M, Matsuda H, Shirakura R, Sawa Y, Matsuwaka R, Kuki S, Nakano S, Kawashima Y. Attenuation of pulmonary leukocyte sequestration during extracorporeal circulation by a new c-AMP phosphodiesterase inhibitor. Trans Am Soc Artif Intern Organs 34;761, 1988.

39. Turrens JF, Crapo JD, Freeman BA. Protection against oxygen toxicity by intravenous injection of liposome-entrapped catalase and superoxide dismutase. J Clin Invest 73:87, 1984.

40. Fosse E, Mollnes TE, Osterud A, Aasen AO: Effects of meyhylprednisolone on complement activation and leukocyte counts during cardiopulmonary bypass. Scan J Thor Cardiovasc Surg 21:255, 1987.

41. Jansen NJG, van Oeveren W, Kazatchkine MD, Wildervuur CRH. Methylprednisolone inhibits granulocytopenia induced by infusion of complement activated serum but not complement activated plasma in rabbits. Biomaterials 10:617, 1989.

42. Jansen NJG, van Oeveren W, van Vliet M, Stoutenbeek CP, Eijsman L, Wildervuur CRH. The role of different types of corticosteroids on the cellular and plasmatic systems in cardiopulmonary bypass. Eur J Cardio Thorac Surg 5:211, 1991.

43. Jansen NJG, van Oeveren W, Hoiting BH, Wildervuur CRH. Methylprenisolone prophylaxis protects against endotoxin induced death in rabbits. Inflammation 15:91, 1991.

44. Andersen LW, Baek L, Thomson BS, Rasmussen JP. Effect of methylprednisolone on endotoxiaemia and complement activation during cardiac surgery. J Cardiovasc Anaesth 3:544, 1989.

45. Detterbeck F, Kron E, Paull D, et al. Oxygen free radical scavengers decrease reperfusion injury in lung transplantation. Southern Thoracic Surgical Association. 36th Annual Meeting 1989.

46. Ferriera R, Burgos M, Llesuir S, et al. Reduction of reperfusion injury with mannitol cardioplegia. Ann Thorac Surg 48:77, 1989.

47. Breda M, Drinkwater D, Laks H, et al. Prevention of reperfusion injury in the neonatal heart with leukocyte depleted blood. J Thorac Cardiovasc Surg 97:654, 1989.

48. Hall T, Breda M, Baumgartner W, et al. The role of leukocyte depletion in reducing injury to the lung after hypothermic ischaemia. Current Surgery 44:137, 1990.

49. Schueler S, Hatanaka M, Bando K, et al. Twenty-four hour lung preservation with donor core cooling and leukocyte depletion in a bilateral lung transplantation model. Surgical Forum 41:405, 1990.

50. Bando K, Schueler S, Cameron DE, et al. Twelve hour cardiopulmonary preservation using donor core cooling, leukocyte depletion, and liposomal superoxide dismutase. J. Heart Lung Transplant 10:304, 1991.

51. Bando K, Pillai R, Cameron DE, et al.

Leukocyte depletion ameliorates free radical mediated lung injury after cardiopulmonary bypass. J Thorac Cardiovasc Surg 99:873, 1990.

52. Bando K, Teramoto S, Tago M, et al. Successful extended hypothermic cardiopulmonary preservation for heart lung transplantation. J Thorac Cardiovasc Surg 98:137, 1989.

53. Pillai R, Bando K, Schueler S, et al. Leukocyte depletion results in excellent heart-lung function after 10 hour storage. Ann Thorac Surg 211, 1990.

54. Gourlay T, Fleming J, Taylor KM. Laboratory evaluation of the Pall LG6 leukocyte depleting arterial line filter. Perfusion 7:131, 1992.

55. Gourlay T, Fleming J, Taylor KM. The effects of pulsatile flow on the leukocyte depleting qualities of the Pall LG6 leukocyte depleting arterial line filter: A laboratory investigation. Perfusion 7:227, 1992.

56. Allen SM, Pagano D, Bonser RS. Preliminary clinical evaluation of the Pall Leuko-Guard 6 (LG6) leukocyte depleting filter. Proc Scan Soc Extracorp Tech; Tampere, Finland, 1993.

57. Palanzo DA, Manley NJ, Montesano RM, et al. Clinical evaluation of the LeucoGuard (LG6) arterial line filter in routine open heart surgery. Perfusion 8:489, 1993.

58. Gu YJ, Obster R, Gallandat RCG, Eijgelaar A, van Oeveren W. Leukocyte depletion reduces the postoperative inflammatory response in patients following open heart surgery. Intensive Care Med 18:851, 1992.

59. Gu YJ. Inhibition of the inflammatory response initiated during cardiopulomonary bypass. (PhD Thesis). Gronigen, The Netherlands: University Hospital, 1992.

60. Pearl J, Drinkwater DC, Laks H, Caponya ER, Gates RN. Leukocyte-depleted reperfusion of transplanted human hearts. A randomised, double blind clinical trial. J Heart Lung Transplant 11:1082, 1992.

61. Fleming A. A simple method of removing leukocytes from blood. Br J Exp Path 7:281, 1928.

62. Roe JA. Clinical advantages associated with the use of blood filters. Care Crit III 8:146, 1992.

63. Blumberg N, Triulzi DJ, Heal JM. Transfusion induced immunomodulation and its clinical consequences. Trans Med Rev 4:24, 1990.

64. Dellinger EP, Oreskovich MR, Wertz MJ, Hamasaki V, Lennard ES. Risk of infection following laparotomy for penetrating abdominal injury. Arch Surg 119:20, 1984.

65. Ottino G, De Paulis R, Pasini S, et al. Major sternal wound infection after open heart surgery: a multivariate analysis of risk factors in 2,579 consecutive operative procedures. Ann Thorac Cardiovasc Surg 44:173, 1987.

66. Tartter PI. Blood transfusion and infectious complications following colorectal cancer surgery. Br J Surg 75:789, 1988.

67. Graves TA, Cioffi WG, Mason AD, McManus WF, Pruitt BA. Relationship of transfusion and infection in a burn population. J Trauma 29:948, 1989.

68. Jensen LS, Andersen AJ, Christiansen PM, et al. Postoperative infection and natural killer cell function following blood transfusion in patients undergoing elective colorectal surgery. Br J Surg 79:513, 1992.

CHAPTER 12

THE USE OF LEUKODEPLETED BLOOD COMPONENTS FOR NEONATES AND INFANTS

Naomi L.C. Luban, Louis DePalma

SUMMARY

The indications for the use of leukodepleted blood products in neonates are considerably less clear than for adults. As a result of an immature immune system children are less likely to form red cell antibodies, HLA antibodies or develop febrile reactions post transfusion. However, there is evidence that transfused lymphocytes may persist in the recipient's circulation for long periods of time though the effect of this is unclear. It is at least possible that adult antigen presenting cells could participate in the development of an alloimmune response. Infants are at risk for the development of graft-versus-host disease which may follow infusion of small doses of leukocytes to an immunocompromised recipient. However, current generations of leukodepletion filters cannot consistently achieve the levels of leukodepletion necessary to prevent this and as a result gamma irradiation of blood products is the standard of practice for the situation where the donor and recipient are related. Cytomegalovirus infection in neonatal blood recipients remains a significant risk and studies have increasingly suggested that this may be prevented by pre-storage or blood bank filtration under controlled circumstances. Currently, this remains the only indication for the use of leukodepleted blood products though it is likely that other indications may prevail as more becomes known about the long-term effect of the unwanted passenger leukocytes in conventional blood components.

INTRODUCTION

The neonatal immune response system is both naive as well as functionally immature with respect to that of adult subjects. The neonate's response to blood transfusion differs from that seen in older subjects.[1]

Clinical Benefits of Leukodepleted Blood Products, edited by Joseph Sweeney, M.D. and Andrew Heaton, M.D. © 1995 R.G. Landes Company.

This results in management and therapeutic dilemmas due to a lack of data on the neonatal immune response in these clinical situations. In the context of blood transfusion, it is important to know that many hospitalized neonates require blood transfusion support due to either their underlying disorder or more frequently iatrogenic-induced anemia.[2,3] Yet we do not know what short-term or long-term effects transfusions may have in this patient population. Concerns have been raised in adults regarding the possibility that blood transfusions may be an independent risk factor for greater susceptibility to bacterial infection and cancer recurrence.[4,5] Transfusions may modulate the host immune response with adverse effects on the patient's ability to combat a bacterial challenge or effectively suppress cancer cell growth and spread. Although much has been learned about the adult immune response to blood transfusion, it is unclear how this immunomodulation occurs. Even less is known about the modulation of the neonatal immune system by blood transfusion. Studies are needed to explore the interaction between blood transfusions and the neonatal immune system to better evaluate potential secondary short-term (e.g. febrile transfusion reactions, graft-versus-host disease) and long-term effects (e.g. alloimmunization, transmission of infections to the recipient by white blood cell (WBC) associated organisms).

There is little data that support the utility of WBC-reduced blood products in neonates. Theoretically, certain complications could be either decreased or totally eliminated by the removal of WBCs from blood components prior to transfusion. We will attempt to review what is actually known regarding WBC-mediated effects in neonates and young infants and to establish guidelines regarding the use of leukodepleted blood components in this age group.

IMMUNE MODULATION

Since neonates do not readily synthesize red cell alloantibodies, repeat red cell compatibility testing for infants younger than 4 months of age is routinely omitted, provided that initial antibody screening methods reveal no alloantibodies.[6] One group proposed that neonates do not form red cell alloantibodies due to their immature immune system,[7] while another investigator suggested that transfusion early in life prevented alloimmunization by an acquired tolerance mechanism.[8] Much has been learned about neonatal immunobiology since the appearance of these reports and, clearly, numerous factors may be responsible for this poor alloantibody response. With regards to the acquired tolerance theory, one group has documented long-term survival of transfused lymphocytes from mothers to their babies.[9] In this study, cytogenetic analysis was performed on the peripheral blood of 14 male infants who had received in utero transfusions of maternal blood. As compared to nonrelated sex mismatched transfusions in a control group of neonates, maternal lymphocytes persisted for longer than two years in the peripheral blood of four infants who had received in utero transfusions. Even greater long-term effects from previous transfusion in the neonate were documented in another investigation.[10] In this report a group of women who had been transfused as neonates, showed significantly depressed mixed lymphocyte reaction responses with autologous plasma, as much as 20 years following the transfusion event. One could speculate that the use of leukodepleted blood may not have altered these long-term effects on the basis of what is already known regarding the lymphocyte's role in immune modulation. However, studies are clearly needed to confirm this suspicion.

Using conventional immunohematologic serology, two reports document the lack of alloantibody formation against red cell antigens in neonates and infants.[11,12] Combining the two studies, 143 infants who received multiple (greater than 1900) donor exposures as red cell transfusions, were followed in some cases for up to 30 months of age. In no instances were red cell alloantibodies detected. These studies did not investigate possible mechanisms responsible for the lack of alloantibody formation, nor did they relate the findings to the leukocyte content of the transfused blood. One additional report documented long-term transfusion effects on the CD4/CD8 ratio in infants between 2 and 12 weeks of age.[13] They documented a significant inverse relationship between the number of blood transfusions and the CD4/CD8 ratio. However, no insight into the mechanisms responsible for this influence on the T cell subset distribution were derived from the investigation.

A series of studies, several from our laboratory, delineated several important characteristics of the neonatal early immune response to blood transfusion. A French research group evaluated the expression of Ia-like antigens as well as IL-2R in peripheral blood T lymphocytes from newborns receiving postnatal total blood exchange.[14] Groups were divided according to whether the whole blood was transfused unmanipulated, or irradiated or alternatively leukodepleted. Unfortunately, details regarding irradiation dose, leukodepletion method or final concentration of white cells contained in the various transfused products were not detailed. A significant increase in Ia and IL-2R expressing T cells was seen two days after transfusion in those neonates receiving unmanipulated whole blood exchanges. No significant changes were seen in any other groups except for a modest increase in Ia expressing T cells 5 days after exchange transfusion with leukodepleted blood. Although it is unclear from the study why no lymphocyte activation was seen in the irradiated blood recipients or in most of the group receiving leukodepleted blood, these investigators established that neonates appear to respond immunologically to allogeneic blood transfusion. In fact, they were able to demonstrate that it was the neonatal lymphocyte population that expressed the activated antigens on the basis of sex-matched transfusions and cytogenetic analysis.

We evaluated neonates undergoing extracorporeal membrane oxygenation (ECMO), a modified cardiopulmonary bypass procedure, used for patients requiring cardiac and respiratory support for 3 to 7 days.[15] The ECMO circuit requires a priming volume of two units of packed red blood cells on the day of the procedure, which is equivalent to at least a double-volume exchange transfusion. The packed cell blood prime blood was not leukodepleted. Blood samples obtained on day one after the procedure, and those obtained up to 7 days after the first blood transfusion, failed to show an increase in either IL-2R or HLA-DR expressing T cells or an increase in B cells. A control group of neonates receiving 10 ml/kg aliquot blood transfusions of washed, irradiated red cells also failed to show any increase in lymphocyte activation markers based on cytometric analysis. In fact, no changes were seen in CD3, CD4, CD8, CD19 or natural killer (NK) cell numbers.

In a follow-up study, we evaluated an additional cohort of neonates utilizing flow cytometric analysis of additional lymphocyte subpopulations and serum cytokine determinations.[16] These neonates also received irradiated, washed red blood cell transfusions at a dose of 10 ml/kg with an average white cell concentration of 2×10^7 cells per transfusion. The blood was irradiated with 2500 rads of gamma radiation to the midplane of the bag, and the mean donor exposure was 2 ± 1.5. No changes in T helper cell expressing CD45RA, CD45RO, or UCHL-1 were noted following transfusion. This indicates that a naive to memory shift in lymphocytes did not occur. Mean channel fluorescence intensity was also evaluated for each antigen by overlay-histogram analysis. No shift in fluorescence signal was seen, also indicative of a lack of cellular activation. Post-transfusion gamma interferon and neopterin levels were essentially unchanged with respect to pre-transfusion concentrations in these neonates. The failure to observe lymphocyte activation was in our opinion due to a lack of recipient recognition of the transfused donor allogeneic blood cell antigens.

Our attention focused next on the ability of neonatal and infants' antigen presenting cells (APCs) to effectively prime self

T helper cells. This aspect of the afferent immune arm to alloantigen stimulation is essential for an immune response to T cell dependent antigens such as those expressed both cellularly and extracellularly in transfused blood. We have observed a specific maturative sequence in APCs from birth through infancy and ultimately into childhood and adulthood.[17] Infants' lymphocytes from subjects 24 months of age or less were incapable of responding to irradiated allo-APC depleted adult allogeneic stimulator lymphocytes, indicating an inability to respond via a self-APC pathway. In addition, it was also noted that an infant's T helper lymphocytes could utilize adult allogeneic APCs for an in vitro response in a one way MLC. Therefore, it may be possible to observe a neonate or an older infant synthesize red cell alloantibodies if stimulated by a critical number of allogeneic APCs. It has been established that T helper pathways can utilize both self as well as allo APCs and therefore the presence of immature self APCs does not exclude the possibility of a T helper cell mediated response.[18]

We recently have described the first well-documented case of a massively transfused infant forming an alloantibody.[19] This baby had received a significant exposure to donor APCs as a neonate. This latest investigation documents the presence of the red cell alloantibody anti-E in an 11-week-old infant, in a definitive manner with additional follow-up studies. It still remains to be ascertained whether there is a threshold concentration of allogeneic APCs that may overcome an immature T cell - self-APC priming circuit or if additional co-stimulatory factors are responsible for alloantibody formation. Additional studies are required to more fully evaluate post-transfusion changes in the neonatal immune system. An evaluation of the neonatal immune response to leukodepleted as well as unmanipulated blood components is required to firmly establish whether there are differences. This case study would seem to suggest that a critical number of allogeneic lymphocytes may be an efficient primer of the neonatal immune system.

ALLOIMMUNIZATION TO BLOOD CELL ANTIGENS

Several investigators have followed groups of infants over time to evaluate their ability to mount an alloantibody response to RBC antigens. Two of these studies followed infants specifically to address the issue of RBC alloimmunization while others were more generic. In one study, 0 of 53 infants receiving 683 RBC transfusion[12] and in another 0 of 90 infants receiving 1269 RBC transfusions developed RBC alloantibodies.[11] In an earlier study of 126 infants weighing <2000 grams studied at 12 months of age, specimen from one infant yielded a nonspecific reactive antibody but this infant had not received transfusion.[21]

In another study, 7 of 63 D negative infants born to D positive infants did not demonstrate anti-D in cord blood samples, but had anti-D in specimens obtained between 1 and 9 months of age. The authors propose that these infants had developed anti-D due to prenatal exposure to maternal D-positive RBCs.[22]

Despite the absence of alloimmunization to RBC antigens in larger studies, a few case reports of RBC alloimmunization do exist in the literature. These three case reports include a second case of anti-E in an infant[19,23] and anti-K in another.[24] Each of these infants had been multiply transfused in the postnatal period. Recently, a case of in utero sensitization resulting in a positive DAT with a panagglutinin has been described.[25] This is the second such description of positive DAT in an infant at birth whose mother lacked that antibody[26] and who did not receive in utero transfusion. The etiology of these unusual findings remains elusive, as fetal recognition of RBC antigens resulting in IgG immunoglobulin synthesis goes against conventional wisdom. While removal of donor APCs by leukodepletion might have diminished the production of RBC alloantigens in the infants in the case reports, it certainly would have no effect on the rare case of fetal RBC alloimmunization.

Alloimmunization to WBCs has similarly been studied rarely. In three instances, the same studies evaluating RBC alloimmunization also assessed WBC alloimmunization. In one study, 0/13 multiply transfused infants produced either lymphocyte or granulocyte antibodies.[12] In another study, 3 of 126 infants had HLA antibodies, but in two instances the infant had never received transfusion. One infant had been transfused; the donor was HLA-A1 negative, mother was positive and infant had anti-HLA A1, suggesting that the infant's antibody was directed against maternal lymphocytes.[21]

Maternal immunization to anti-HLA and antigranulocyte antibody has been reported in up to 40% of pregnant women.[27] The role of these antibodies in the pathogenesis of neonatal neutropenia and thrombocytopenia is still questionable. There are rare reports of fetal immunization to lymphocyte,[28] lymphocyte and granulocyte[29] and platelet glycoprotein IIIa[30] antigens with subsequent production of antibody by the infant. Each of these studies attempted to confirm that the antibody was produced by the infant. In one study, the antibody was removed by absorption with maternal but not paternal antigens.[28] In the second study, the authors concluded that the antibodies were of fetal origin by comparing the titer of antibody in maternal, umbilical artery, and umbilical vein samples.[29] In the third case of an infant with Glansmann's thrombasthenia without platelet glycoprotein IIIa whose mother had IIIa on her platelets, the presence of IgG alloantibody to IIIa at one month of age was thought to be due to in utero sensitization with subsequent alloantibody production. However, the infant had received transfusions during the first week of life, raising the possibility that the antibody was passive.[30]

One recent study suggests that infants can become WBC alloimmunized and that this can be prevented.[31] In this study, preterm infants <37 weeks gestation with no evidence of anti-HLA antibody on maternal sample were randomized to receive RBCs transfused using a standard filter or an in-line leukocytedepletion filter adapted from a Sepacell filter. Babies were recruited if they were likely to receive two or more blood transfusions; they were studied pretransfusion and monthly. Fifty-seven babies were entered into the study of whom 42 were evaluable. Seven out of 23 (30%) infants developed anti-HLA antibody using standard microlymphocytotoxicity assays, while none of the 19 infants in the filtered blood group developed antibody. One infant received only two transfusions prior to development of the antibody; this infant who received 17 transfusions had the most strongly positive antibody. Of interest, of the seven infants with anti-HLA antibody, only two had positive results on more than one sample. The disappearance of the antibodies is not discussed by the authors. In addition, no clinically adverse effects were reported in either group. This is the only study that supports leukodepletion to abrogate anti-HLA sensitization, but clinical benefit remains elusive.

GRAFT VERSUS HOST DISEASE

Post-transfusion graft-versus-host disease (PT-GVHD) was first recognized in individuals with hematological malignancies and in infants with congenital immunodeficiency. Since these early reports in the 1960s, much has been learned regarding the types of infants and children who are susceptible, the blood components implicated in the disorder, its pathogenesis, and prevention. PT-GVHD occurs when an immunosuppressed or immunodeficient transfusion recipient receives immunologically competent donor lymphocytes. The transfused histoincompatible T lymphocytes proliferate and engraft in the immunocompromised host who is incapable of rejecting these foreign cells. Although the disparity in HLA phenotype between donor and recipient is a necessary component of the pathogenesis of PT-GVHD, recent reports have focused on the importance of similarities in HLA which encourages initial engraftment of the foreign transfused lymphocytes. Recently, a growing number of reports of fatal PT-GVHD occurring in nonimmunocompromised patients have been published.[32,34a] One explanation for this phenomenon is the transfusion of viable lymphocytes expressing two identical HLA haplotypes (homozygosity) into a recipient possessing only one of the haplotypes (heterozygosity). The recipient does not recognize a non-self haplotype because of donor homozygosity. However, donor lymphocytes "attack" the non-shared HLA haplotype of the recipient. Although this is an infrequent occurrence between two unrelated donor recipient pairs in the US, it is much more frequent in more homogeneous ethnic groups and when family members are the transfusion donors and recipients.[34a-34b] Any infant who receives blood or blood products from a donor who is a first degree (mother, father) or second degree relative is at risk for PT-GVHD based on this concept.[35]

PT-GVHD may occur following blood transfusions in fetuses and neonates because of their immature and inexperienced immune system (reviewed in ref. 36). Although the fetus and neonate are not immunocompromised in the conventional sense of the term, they may not be able to reject transfused allogeneic lymphocytes. The actual incidence of PT-GVHD in the perinatal period is not known.[32] Most likely, only fatal or very severe cases are recognized and reported. Fatal PT-GVHD has been reported in neonates with severe combined immunodeficiency syndrome, those receiving intrauterine transfusion followed by exchange transfusions and in neonates who received exchange transfusion soon after birth. The outcome is frequently fatal with documented histopathologic changes of GVHD. There are also rare case reports of GVHD in premature infants,[37] and in infants with neonatal alloimmune thrombocytopenia who receive nonirradiated maternal platelets (reviewed in ref. 32).

The single most important characteristic of a blood component's ability to cause PT-GVHD is its white blood cell content, specifically, its lymphocyte number. Based on animal studies, an estimated 1×10^7

white blood cells per kilogram of body weight is needed to initiate GVHD. The average white blood cell content of different blood components varies, but a quantity sufficient to elicit PT-GVHD may be present in all but fresh frozen plasma, and cryoprecipitase. Red blood cells, white blood cells, platelets and fresh plasma have all been implicated in PT-GVHD. Fresh frozen plasma (FFP), cryoprecipitate and frozen deglycerolized red blood cells have not been reported to cause GVHD. However, sufficient white blood cells may be present in frozen deglycerolized blood cells to cause PT-GVHD and 8×10^4 cells per kg in fresh plasma has been reported to produce PT-GVHD.

Gamma radiation of blood components is the only method documented to abrogate PT-GVHD by reducing mitogen responsiveness and inhibiting in vitro proliferation of T-lymphocytes. Doses of irradiation used to abrogate PT-GVHD range from 1500 to 5000 cGy; cesium, linear acceleration and cobalt sources have been used. Irradiation of red blood cells up to 4000 cGy was thought to be innocuous to the red blood cells[38] but when irradiation is followed by long-term, 4°C storage, there are significantly increased levels of potassium and decreased in vivo RBC survival.[39] The function and survival of random platelet pools appear to be unaffected by irradiation,[40] but pheresis collected platelets have not been studied to date.

Three cases of post-transfusion GVHD in patients receiving blood irradiated with 1500 to 2000 cGy have recently appeared.[41-43] They raise issues as to the adequacy of the irradiation with currently available equipment due to the dosimetry of the radiation dose to the blood bag.[44] In addition, the adequacy of the lower doses of 1500 cGy is in question. A recent study has shown that 2500 cGy to the midplane of the bag is necessary to assure that lymphocyte reactivity is abrogated; this study used limiting dilution analysis, a far more sensitive test of lymphocyte responsiveness than MLR used in some studies.[45]

Filtration with third generation leuko-depletion filters will not uniformly remove sufficient white blood cells to prevent GVHD. Recently, experimental filters have been shown to remove 10^6 white blood cells from red blood cell units, but these are as yet unlicensed in the United States. Leukodepletion could theoretically reduce the number of WBC to less than 10^6 per blood unit, well below the threshold. However the efficacy of removal of WBCs from blood/blood products is variable particularly if bedside filters are used.[46] One adult case of PT-GVHD has been reported in a patient with non-Hodgkin's lymphoma who received an estimated 15.4×10^7 total WBCs in 28 units of leukocyte reduced blood and blood products.[47] Gamma irradiation, therefore, remains as the only technique to abrogate PT-GVHD in at risk patients, and a dose of 2500 cGy is recommended by FDA.[48]

CYTOMEGALOVIRUS

Cytomegalovirus (CMV) is an ubiqui-tous virus of the herpes class that causes infection in all age groups. CMV is likely harbored in leukocytes, most likely lym-phocytes, and thus may be transmitted via saliva, semen, urine, cervical secretions and blood. Three types of CMV infection are known to occur. These include primary in-fection, reactivation and secondary infection.

There are no well-established patient characteristics that predispose to activation or secondary infection, nor are there ad-equate estimates of their frequencies. Esti-mates for the risk of primary infection range from 2.5-12% per transfused unit in older studies.[49-51]

These data were obtained prior to the use of more stringent donor deferral guide-lines and additional serological testing for HIV-1/2, HTLV-I/II, HCV and two sur-rogate tests for non-A/non-B hepatitis. Despite these high estimates, clinically sig-nificant CMV disease occurs infrequently, suggesting that both blood components and patient characteristics play an impor-tant role in acquisition of post-transfusion CMV. In all three types of infection, immunoincompetent individuals are more likely to have clinical sequelae of post-transfusion infection. The greater the con-centration of white blood cells in the trans-fused product, the greater the likelihood that the CMV infection will occur if the unit is infectious. Granulocyte concentrates, for example, transmit CMV readily, pro-ducing significant disease while fresh fro-zen plasma (FFP) does not.[52]

The issue of whether to provide blood products with low risk of transmitting CMV to neonatal patients has become in-creasingly controversial. Studies conducted during the 1970s and early 1980s found a high incidence of transfusion-transmitted CMV, with some infants dying of the in-fection.[53] However, several studies per-formed more recently failed to confirm these high rates of infection and there was no mortality or morbidity in infants receiv-ing CMV seropositive blood and blood products.[49,51] Of note, CMV seropositive infants of any weight are not at risk for clinically significant CMV, presumably because maternal antibody is protective.[53] Hence, the need to supply blood with low risk of transmitting CMV to neonatal pa-tients has been questioned. The AABB rec-ommends that all cellular components be provided in a form known to have low risk of transmitting CMV to neonatal patients with birth weights <1200 g who fulfill two criteria: (1) they (or their mother) must be CMV seronegative or of unknown serologic status and (2) their treatment is being conducted in a geographical region where post-transfusion CMV is a signifi-cant clinical problem.[6] Fetuses and preg-nant women who require transfusion are also at risk for post-transfusion CMV and should be placed on similar restrictions.

Several different maneuvers have been used to decrease post-transfusion CMV in infants. These include the use of sero-negative blood,[53] frozen deglycerolized seronegative blood,[54] frozen deglycerolized blood of unknown or seropositive status,[55] leukocyte depletion by washing,[56,57] by us-ing third generation leukocyte depletion filters[58,59] or the use of blood from donors screened for IgM anti-CMV.[60] Cellular blood components that have been frozen (e.g., deglycerolized RBCs, FFP, cryoprecipitate) from any donor, regardless of serologic status, are so leukodepleted that they fail to infect the susceptible recipient.

There are two studies which specifically address leukofiltration in neonates as a method to ameliorate CMV. In the first study, 9 out of 42 infants (21%) who received unfiltered, untested red blood cells either seroconverted or shed virus in their urine at 6-month follow-up as compared to 0 of 30 who received blood filtered using an Imugard IG 500 filter designed to remove 93-99% of WBC.[59] In this study, filtration was done by the blood center. As in other studies, the clinical condition of the infants precluded attributing the clinical signs and symptoms seen exclusively to CMV infection. In another study from the U.S.,[60] infants received either a spin-cool-filter RBC product (26 infants) or blood filtered by one of two leukodepletion filters (22 infants). The two filters (the Erypur or Sepacell) were used to leukodeplete the blood in the hospital blood bank prior to issue. Forty-seven of 48 infants neither seroconverted nor shed CMV virus. One infant had a transient seroconversion thought to be due to passive antibody. There was no control group in this study, so it is impossible to know what the background CMV seroconversion rate might be in this population, an especially important point in view of the decreasing incidence of TA-CMV transmission and morbidity.[49,51] By combining these studies with others in the literature on adults with malignancy receiving leukodepleted products,[61-63] it appears that the use of these filters may be a viable alternative to the use of seronegative products. Granulocyte transfusion should still be provided from CMV seronegative donors. Three caveats however, must be added. First, no study comparing CMV seronegative to leukodepleted products has yet been published to enable a head-on comparison. Secondly, bedside filters may not be used according to manufacturers' instructions,[46] so that under certain circumstances residual WBC

could well escape filtration and fail to consistently produce a product that is sufficiently leukodepleted to ensure no infection. Lastly, using leukodepleted products with plasma that is CMV antibody positive, one may not be able to accurately assess a neonate for seroconversion; shell viral or viral culture of urine, buffy coat saliva, or PCR analysis may become necessary to confirm infection.

ACTIVATION OF LEUKOCYTES IN CARDIOPULMONARY BYPASS

When leukocytes in blood are exposed to nonbiological surfaces in mechanical devices like cardiopulmonary bypass (CPB), oxygen free radicals are released that result in activation of the complement system and contact activation of the kinin, fibrinolytic and coagulation systems. Platelet dysfunction, fibrinolysis and disseminated intravascular coagulation may ensue. The cytokines tumor necrosis factor (TNF), interleukin-1 (IL-1), interleukin-6 (IL-6) and interleukin-8 (IL-8) are likely involved as well as leukotrienes, prostaglandins and neutrophil elastase. If one could ameliorate free radical production, then at least some of the complications of CPB could be avoided. In one study, 10 mongrel dogs were subjected to CPB with bubble oxygenation and hypothermia. One group of five animals had a leukocyte filter incorporated into the bypass circuit. A Pall RC100 filter was incorporated in the circuit before the arterial filter. There was less generation of free radicals as assessed by quantifying conjugated dienes as well as less intravascular leukocyte aggregation on post mortem in those animals who underwent bypass with the filter; pulmonary function as assessed by arterial oxygenation was also improved 60 to 90 minutes post bypass in the leukodepleted blood group. Complement activation, as evidenced by increased CH50 and C5 was however seen in both groups.[64] Ischemic preservation of hearts for transplantation was studied by another group of investigators who worked with neonatal piglet hearts. In one group of eight piglet hearts reperfused with leukocyte depleted blood, there was a significantly better stroke work index than in the group of eight piglets reperfused with whole blood. A Sepacell filter was used with a mean post filtration count of .15 x 10^3 cells/mm. Pathological and electron microscopic examination confirmed normal ultrastructure in the leukodepleted group as compared to myofibrillar disarray, with swelling of mitochondria and nuclear chromatin clumping in the whole blood model.[65]

One study in 10 human neonates has recently been published and has attempted to better describe the elements of the inflammatory response. A large number of parameters were measured over time including in part tissue plasminogen activator, factor XIIa-CI esterase complex, thrombin-antithrombin III and C3a. In those infants supported with extracorporeal life support using ECMO, there was a biphasic development of contact and complement activation. The first phase developed immediately upon surface contact while the second occurred 72 hours after ECMO had begun; increases in intravascular coagulation and fibrinolysis only were increased. The purpose of the study was to ascertain what interventions might decrease the leukocyte activation that contributes to increased capillary permeability, resulting in compromised pulmonary gas exchange. While aprotinin might assist in reducing thrombin formation and antithrombin III consumption, a pharmacological approach to decreasing complement activation has not yet been developed.[66] No mention is made of utilizing leukodepletion of the prime or blood products used during the procedure as a way to decrease the interactions of plasma coagulation, fibrinolysis and complement activation in that study.

Schleuming et al have demonstrated that third generation leukodepletion was effective in reducing the concentration of C4a in CPD A1 blood units collected and stored under standard blood bank conditions.[67] Of note, increase in C3a des Arg concentrations over storage time were not altered by leukocyte reduction and was

thought to be due to activation of the alternative pathway of complement by contact of plasma with plastic surfaces. Although still theoretical, it might be possible to decrease blood/plastic activation by utilizing leukodepleted blood/blood products for selected patients requiring extracorporeal life support (ELS) and cardiopulmonary bypass, but definitive recommendations cannot be made at this time, due to the complexity and timing of the bypass induced activation.[68] Studies in ECMO are ongoing to determine whether routine leukodepletion is helpful in moderating neutrophil activation and cytokine release,[69,70] but have as yet resulted in no peer review publication.

FEBRILE TRANSFUSION REACTIONS

In older children, especially those who have been previously transfused, febrile transfusion reactions may occur. However, transfusion reactions in infants are thought to occur only very rarely. It is unclear whether this is due to the peculiar nature of the neonate or infant's immune response system or the fact that diagnostic signs and symptoms are difficult to appreciate in this age group. Unlike febrile transfusion reactions in older children and adults, it appears that those in neonates are more likely to be caused by passively acquired antibodies. Transplacentally acquired anti-A has been reported to react with transfused group A red blood cells from adult donors.[71] In addition, a near-fatal reaction was reported during a granulocyte transfusion in a neonate.[72] The plasma contained in the granulocyte concentrate contained WBC antibody from a female donor who had recently been pregnant. A theoretical risk for a passive antibody-mediated febrile transfusion reaction could be the transfusion of paternal WBC containing blood components. In this setting maternally derived antibodies (anti-neutrophil specific as well as anti-HLA) directed to paternal antigenic specificities may cause a febrile reaction.

No recommendations can be made for the routine use of leukodepleted blood components for the prevention of febrile transfusion reactions in this age group. The evidence to date appears to indicate that such reactions are indeed rare.

Leukoreduced blood products using third generation filters have limited usefulness in the neonate.[73] Until such time as additional clinical trials are performed, the following recommendations are offered for review and discussion by neonatologists, hematologists and others caring for neonates.

CONCLUSIONS

1. Leukodepletion may be indicated for prevention of CMV in a subpopulation of at risk infants if one can assure adequency of the leukodepletion.
2. Leukodepletion is not indicated to abrogate RBC, WBC or HLA alloimmunization, as these are likely isolated and rare events. Febrile transfusion reactions, similarly, are rare in infants.
3. Leukodepletion is not indicated to ameliorate the immunomodulatory effects of transfusion, as data has not yet been generated to support that infants are placed at risk for increased number or severity of infections, immunological aberration or cancer from transfusions.
4. Leukodepletion is not indicated to abrogate transfusion-induced graft-versushost disease. Gamma irradiation is the only currently acceptable method.

REFERENCES

1. DePalma L. Red cell alloantibody formation in the neonate and infant: Considerations for current immunohematologic practice. Immunohematology 8:33, 1992.
2. DePalma L, Luban NLC. Blood component therapy in the perinatal period: Guidelines and recommendations. Semin Perinat 14:403, 1990.
3. DePalma L, Ness PM, Luban NLC. "Red blood cell transfusion." In: Transfusion Therapy in Infants and Children, Luban NLC (ed.), Johns Hopkins University Press, Baltimore, MD p.1, 1991.
4. Blumberg N, Heal JM. Transfusion and host

defenses against cancer recurrence and infection. Transfusion 29:236, 1989.
5. Brunson ME, Alexander JW. Mechanisms of transfusion-induced immunosuppression. Transfusion 30:651, 1990.
6. Wideman F, ed. Standards for Blood Banks and Transfusion Services, 15th ed. Bethesda, MD; American Association of Blood Banks, 1993.
7. Lucivero G, Osso AD, Iannone A, et al. Phenotypic immaturity of T and B lymphocytes in cord blood of full-term normal neonates. Biol Neonate 44:303, 1983.
8. Diamond LK, Allen DM, Magill FB. Congenital (erythroid) hypoplastic anemia. Am J Dis Child 102:403, 1961.
9. Hutchinson DL, Turner JH, Schlesinger ER. Persistence of donor cells in neonates after fetal and exchange transfusion. Am J Obstet Gynec 109:281, 1971.
10. Beck I, Scott JS, Pepper M, Speck EH. The effect of neonatal exchange and later blood transfusion on lymphocyte cultures. Am J Reprod Immunol 1:224, 1981.
11. Ludvigsen CW, Swanson JL, Thompson TR, McCullough J. The failure of neonates to form red blood cell alloantibodies in response to multiple transfusions. Am J Clin Pathol 87:250, 1987.
12. Floss AM, Strauss RG, Gocken N, Knox L. Multiple transfusions fail to provoke antibodies against blood cell antigens in human infants. Transfusion 26:419, 1986.
13. Pahwa S, Sia C, Harper R, Pahwa R. T lymphocyte subpopulations in high-risk infants influence of age and blood transfusions. Pediatrics 76:914, 1985.
14. Romano M, El Marsafy A, Marseglia GL, Rigal D, Salle B, Touraine JL. Increased percentage of activated Ia+ T lymphocytes in peripheral blood of neonates following exchange blood transfusion. Clin Immunol Immunopathol 43:301, 1987.
15. DePalma L, Short BL, Van Meurs K, Luban NLC. A flow cytometric analysis of lymphocyte subpopulations in neonates undergoing extracorporeal membrane oxygenation. J Pediatr 118:117, 1991.
16. DePalma L, Duncan B, Chan MM, Luban NLC. The neonatal immune response to washed and irradiated red blood cells: Lack

of evidence of lymphocyte activation. Transfusion 31:737, 1991.

17. Clerici M, DePalma L, Roilides E, Baker R, Shearer GM. Analysis of T helper and antigen presenting cell functions in cord blood and peripheral blood leukocytes from healthy children of different ages. J Clin Invest 91:2829, 1993.

18. Via CS, Tsokos GC, Stocks NI, Clerici M, Shearer GM. Human in vitro allogeneic responses. Demonstrations of three pathways of T helper cell activation. J Immunol 144:2524, 1990.

19. DePalma L, Criss VR, Roseff S, Luban NLC. Presence of the red cell alloantibody anti-E in an 11-week old infant. Transfusion 32:177, 1992.

20. Pass MA, Johnson JD, Schulman IA, et al. Evaluation of a walking-donor blood transfusion program in an intensive care nursery. J Pediatr 89:646, 1976.

21. Rawls WE, Wong CL, Blajchman M, et al. Neonatal cytomegalovirus infections: the relative role of neonatal blood transfusion and maternal exposure. Clin Invest Med 7:13, 1984.

22. Bowen FW Jr, Renfield M. The detection of anti-D in Rh_o (D)-negative infant born of Rh_o (D)-positive mothers. Pediatr Res 10:213, 1976.

23. Maniatis A, Theodoris H, Aravani K. Neonatal immune response to red cell antigens (letter). Transfusion 33:90, 1993.

24. Smith MR, Storey CG. Allo-anti-E in an 18-day-old infant (letter). Transfusion 24:540, 1984.

25. Erler BX, Smith L, McQuiston D, et al. Red cell auto antibody production in utero: a case report. Transfusion 34:72, 1994.

26. Marsh WL, Mawby LJ, Mueller KA, Hall JW, Colucci J. Positive direct antiglobulin tests at birth without demonstrative maternal antibody. Transfusion 24:19, 1984.

27. Skacel PO, Stacey TE, Tidmarsh EF, Contreras M. Maternal alloimmunization to HLA, platelet and granulocyte-specific antigens during pregnancy: its influence on cord blood granulocyte and platelet counts. Br J Haematol 71:119, 1989.

28. Chardonnens X, Jeannet M. Immunobiology of pregnancy: evidence for a fetal immune response against the mother. Tissue Antigens 15:401, 1980.

29. Mathur S, Keane M, Williamson HO, et al. Antibodies to sperm, ovary, B and T lymphocytes, and granulocytes in the umbilical circulation and in newborn infants. Clin Immunol Immunopathol 20:116, 1981.

30. Bierling P, Fromont P, Elbez A, Duedari N, Kieffer N. Early immunization against platelet glycoprotein IIIa in a newborn Glanzmann type I patient. Vox Sang 55:109, 1988.

31. Russell ARB, Rivers RPA, Davey N. The development of anti-HLA antibodies in multiply transfused preterm infants. Arch Dis Child 68:49, 1993.

32. Anderson KC, Goodnough LT, Sayers M, et al. Variation in blood component irradiated practice: Implications for prevention of transfusion-associated graft-versus-host disease. Blood 77:2096, 1991.

33. Thaler M, Shamiss A, Orgad S, et al. The role of blood from HLA-homozygous donors in fatal transfusion-associated graft-versus-host disease after open heart surgery. N Engl J Med 321:25, 1989.

34a. Hatley RM, Reynolds M, Pather AS, Chou S. Graft versus host disease following ECMO. J Pediatr Surg 26:317, 1991.

34b. Otsuka S, Kunieda K, Kitamura F, et al. The critical role of blood from HLA homozygous donors in fatal transfusion-associated graft-versus-host disease in immunocompetent patients. Transfusion 31:260, 1991.

35. Kanter MH. Transfusion-associated graft-versus-host disease: Do transfusions from second degree relatives pose a greater risk than those from first degree relatives? Transfusion 32:323, 1992.

36. Sanders MR and Graeber JE. Post-transfusion graft-versus-host disease in infancy. J Pediatr 117:159, 1990.

37. Funkhouse AW, Vogelsang G, Zehnbauser SM, et al. Graft-versus-host disease after blood transfusions in a premature infant. Pediatrics 87:247, 1991.

38. Moore GL, Ledford ME. Effects of 4000 rad irradiation on the in vitro storage properties of packed cells. Transfusion 25:583, 1985.

39. Davey RJ, McCoy MC, Yu N, Sullivan JA, Spiegal DM, Leitman SF. The effect of prestorage irradiation post-transfusion red cell survival. Transfusion 32:525, 1992.

40. Read EF, Kodis C, Carter CS, Leitman SF. Viability of platelets following storage in the irradiated state. Transfusion 28:446, 1988.

41. Dobryski W, Thibodeau S, Truitt RL, et al. Third party mediated graft rejection and graft versus host disease after T cell depleted bone marrow transplantation. Blood 74: 2285, 1989.

42. Sproul AM, Chalmers EA, Mills KI, Burnett AK, Simpson E. Third party mediated graft rejection despite irradiation of blood products. Br J Haematol 80:261, 1992.

43. Lowenthal RM, Challis DR, Griffiths AE, Chappell RA, Goulder PJR. Transfusion-associated graft-versus-host disease: Report of a case following administration of irradiated blood. Transfusion 133:524, 1993.

44. Pelszynski M, Moroff G, Luban NLC, et al. Dose dependent lymphocyte activation in red blood cell units with gamma irradiation. Blood 83: 1994. (In press).

45. Masterson ME and Febo R. Pre-transfusion blood irradiation: Clinical rationale and dosimetric considerations. Med Phys 19:649, 1992.

46. Sirchia G, Rebulla P, Parravicini A, Marangoni F, Cortelezzi A, Stefania A. Quality control of red cell filtration at the patient's bedside. Transfusion 34:26, 1994.

47. Akahoshi M, Takanashi M, Masuda M, et al. A case of transfusion-associated graft-versus-host-disease not prevented by white cell reduction filters. Transfusion 32:169, 1992.

48. FDA Draft Memoranda. License amendments and procedures for gamma irradiation of blood products, June 22, 1993.

49. Preiksaitis JK. Indicators for the use of cytomegalovirus seronegative blood products. Trans Med Rev 5:1, 1991.

50. Sayers MH, Anderson KC, Goodnough LT, et al. Reducing the risk for transfusion-transmitted cytomegalovirus. Ann Intern Med 116:55, 1992.

51. Tegtmeier GE. The use of cytomegalovirus-screened blood in neonates (Editorial). Transfusion 28:201, 1988.

52. Adler, SP. Data that suggest that FFP does not transmit CMV. Transfusion 28:604, 1988 (letter).

53. Yeager AS, Grumet FC, Hafleight EB, et al. Prevention of transfusion-acquired cytomegalovirus infections in premature infants. J Pediatr 102:918, 1983.

54. Adler SP, Lawrence LT, Baggett J, Biro V, Sharp DE. Prevention of transfusion-associated cytomegalovirus infection in very low birthweight infants using frozen blood and donors seronegative for cytomegalovirus. Transfusion 24:333, 1985.

55. Brady MT, Milam JD, Anderson DC, Hawkins EP, Speer ME, Seavy D, Bijou H, Yow MD. Use of deglycerolized red blood cells to prevent post-transfusion infection with cytomegalovirus in neonates. J Infec Dis 150:334, 1984.

56. Demmler GJ, Brady MT, Bijou H, et al. Post-transfusion cytomegalovirus infection in neonates: Role of saline-washed red blood cells. J Pediatr 108:762, 1986.

57. Luban NLC, Williams AE, MacDonald MG, Mikesell GT, Williams KM, Sacher RA. Low incidence of acquired cytomegalovirus infection in neonates transfused with washed red blood cells. Am J Dis Child 141:416, 1987.

58. Eisenfeld L, Silver H, McClaughlan J, et al. Prevention of transfusion-associated cytomegalovirus infection in neonatal patients by the removal of white cells from blood. Transfusion 32:205, 1992.

59. Gilbert GL, Hayes K, Hudson IL, James J. Prevention of transfusion-acquired cytomegalovirus infection in infants by blood filtration to remove leukocytes. Lancet II:1228, 1989.

60. Lamberson HV, McMillan JA, Weiner LB, et al. Prevention of transfusion-associated cytomegalovirus (CMV) infection in neonates by screening donors for IgM to CMV. J Infec Dis 157:820, 1988.

61. Bowden RA, Sayers MH, Cays M, Slichter SJ. The role of blood product filtration in the prevention of transfusion-associated cytomegalovirus infection after marrow transplant. Transfusion 29(Suppl):57S, 1989.

62. Bowden RA, Slichter SJ, Sayers MH, et al. Use of leukocyte-depleted platelets and cy-

tomegalovirus seronegative red blood cells for prevention of primary cytomegalovirus infection after marrow transplant. Blood 78:246, 1991.

63. DeGraan-Hentzen YCE, Gratama JW, Mudd GL, et al. Prevention of primary cytomegalovirus infection during induction treatment of acute leukemia using random leukocyte poor blood products. Br J Haematol 66:421, 1987.

64. Bando K, Pillai R, Cameron DE, et al. Leukocyte depletion ameliorates free radical-mediated injury after cardiopulmonary bypass. J Thorac Cardiovasc Surg 99:873, 1990.

65. Breda NA, Drinkwater DC, Laks H, Bhuta, et al. Prevention of reperfusion injury in the neonatal heart with leukocyte-depleted blood. J Thorac Cardiovasc Surg 97:654, 1989.

66. Plotz FB, van Oeveren W, Bartlett RN, Wildevuur CRH. Blood activation during neonatal extracorporeal life support. J Thorac Cardiovasc Surg 105:823, 1993.

67. Schleuming N, Schmid-Haslbeck N, Utz H, Jochum M, Heim M, Mempel W, Wilmanns W, Complement activation during storage of blood under normal blood bank conditions. Effect of proteinase inhibi-

tors and leukocyte depletion. Blood 79:3071, 1992.

68. Verdonck LF, DeGraan-Hentzen YC, Dekker AW, et al. Cytomegalovirus seronegative platelets and leukocyte poor red blood cells can present primary cytomegalovirus infection after bone marrow transplantation. Bone Marrow Transplant 2:73, 1987.

69. Finn A, Naik S, Klein N, et al. Interleukin-8 release and neutrophil degranulation after pediatric cardiopulmonary bypass. J Thorac Cardiovasc Surg 105:234, 1993.

70. Fortenberry JD, Bhardwaj V, Bland L, Cornish D, Niemer P, Wright J. Effect of neonatal extracorporeal membrane oxygenation in neutrophil activation and cytokine levels. Clin Res 41:783A, 1993.

71. Falterman CG, Richardson CJ. Transfusion reaction due to unrecognized ABO hemolytic disease of the newborn infant. J Pediatr 97:812, 1980.

72. O'Connor JC, Strauss RG, Goeken NE, Knox LB. A near-fatal reaction during granulocyte transfusion of a neonate. Transfusion 28:173, 1988.

73. Strauss RG, Selection of white cell-reduced blood components for transfusion during early infancy. Transfusion 33:352, 1993.

CHAPTER 13

LEUKOCYTE DEPLETED BLOOD TRANSFUSION IN HEMATOPOIETIC STEM CELL RECONSTITUTION THERAPY

John P. Miller, Paul D. Mintz

SUMMARY

The transfusion of red blood cells and platelets is an essential element in the treatment of patients undergoing hematopoietic stem cell transplantation. While blood component therapy has enabled patients to survive the cytopenic period of stem cell therapy, it has been accompanied by the risks and discomforts of transfusion. Although it has been known for almost 30 years that leukocyte depletion is an effective means of preventing many febrile reactions to red blood cell transfusions, only in the last few years has it become apparent that the present technical capability for leukocyte depletion of red blood cell and platelet concentrates affords the opportunity potentially to prevent alloimmunization to HLA antigens and also reduce cytomegalovirus (CMV) transmission as effectively as CMV-seronegative components. Additionally, it is possible that leukocyte depleted components do not cause the immunosuppressive effects noted after allogeneic blood transfusion. Further, there is evidence that there is no clinical disadvantage to providing leukocyte depleted red blood cells and platelets.

There is strong circumstantial evidence that the use of leukocyte depleted red blood cell and platelet components from the time of diagnosis in individuals who may undergo stem cell transplantation and their continued use during transplant therapy is a cost effective strategy for improving patient care.

Clinical Benefits of Leukodepleted Blood Products, edited by Joseph Sweeney, M.D. and Andrew Heaton, M.D. © 1995 R.G. Landes Company.

INTRODUCTION

The advent of transplantation of hematopoietic stem cells from bone marrow or peripheral blood for patients with hematologic and solid tumor malignancies has created a demand for customized blood products in these multiply transfused, immunocompromised individuals. Patients receiving stem cell transplantation are at risk for many of the adverse effects associated with donor leukocytes (Table 13.1) infused during red blood cell (RBC) or platelet transfusion.[1,2] Repeated transfusion of passenger leukocytes may stimulate the patient to develop alloantibodies to human leukocyte antigens (HLA). The predominant clinical effects of this alloimmunization include febrile nonhemolytic transfusion reactions and refractoriness to platelet transfusions with associated risk of thrombocytopenic bleeding. Donor lymphocytes are the cause of transfusion associated graft versus host disease (GVHD) and may have an independent immunosuppressive effect. Patients with hematologic malignancies who receive chemotherapy to induce remission or myeloablative therapy in the course of hematopoietic stem cell transplantation are also at risk for developing leukocyte-associated viral diseases such as EBV and potentially devastating infection with CMV. Recent reports suggest pre-storage leukocyte depletion may prevent the proliferation of contaminating bacteria in stored RBCs. This chapter will focus on the evidence to support the use of leukocyte depleted RBC and platelet components in the prevention of these adverse effects of passenger leukocyte transfusion in patients undergoing hematopoietic stem cell reconstitution and will also briefly address the cost effectiveness of the use of leukocyte depleted blood in this patient population.

Table 13.1. Potential adverse effects of donor leukocytes in patients undergoing hematopoietic stem cell transplantation

Immunologically-mediated Effects
- Alloimmunization to human leukocyte antigens (HLA)
  - Febrile nonhemolytic transfusion reactions (FNTRs)
  - Platelet refractoriness
  - Transplant rejection
- Graft versus host disease (GVHD)
- Immunosuppression
- Viral disease reactivation

Infectious Disease Transmission
- Viruses (e.g. CMV, HTLV I/II, EBV)
- Bacteria (e.g. Yersinia enterocolitica)

Table 13.2. Differential diagnosis of transfusion related fever

Nonhemolytic, febrile transfusion reaction
Hemolytic transfusion reaction
Septic transfusion reaction
Not caused by transfusion
  (e.g. infection, drug malignancy)

PREVENTION OF FEBRILE REACTIONS (FNTRs)

Fever has long been recognized as a consequence of transfusion of donor leukocytes,[3-5] occurring in about 1% of all transfusions, usually in association with previous pregnancy or prior transfusion.[6] A febrile, nonhemolytic transfusion reaction (FNTR) is usually defined as a rise in patient temperature of 1°C associated with a transfusion, with or without chills and rigors, provided other sources of fever (Table 13.2) have been excluded.[7] While the fever of a FNTR may not be life-threatening, frequently associated chills and rigors can cause considerable patient discomfort. The cost of a transfusion reaction workup and/or "septic workup" may be incurred in order to exclude other sources of fever including a hemolytic transfusion reaction, a septic transfusion reaction and other etiologies of infection; particularly in the neutropenic leukemic patient. Furthermore, the transfusion may be discontinued delaying the benefit of transfusion and adding the cost and additional disease exposure of a replacement unit.[8] Clearly, it would be desirable to prevent such febrile reactions to avoid this discomfort, risk and expense.

Recipient antibodies directed against HLA and non-HLA antigens on donor leukocytes or platelets are the cause of most, but not all, FNTRs.[8-10] Decary et al[9] and deRie et al[10] found the majority of these antibodies were directed against HLA antigens. In contrast, Brubaker[11] recently reported that granulocyte antibodies were as frequent as HLA antibodies in patients with FNTRs, and in addition, the granulocyte antibodies were associated with the most severe reactions. Traditionally, fever is thought to result from recipient antibody binding to donor antigen causing release of endogenous pyrogens such as interleukin-1 (IL-1) from donor leukocytes.[10] IL-1 stimulates PGE_2 production in the hypothalamus producing fever.[12] Alternately, antigen-antibody binding may cause complement activation, with $C5_a$ stimulating IL-1 release from recipient monocytes.[8,13,14] Recent studies support the suggestion of Dzik[13] that another source of fever may be the accumulation of donor cytokine released during the storage of blood products, especially in platelet products which are stored at room temperature.[15-18]

Muylle and colleagues[15] demonstrated increasing IL-1, tumor necrosis factor (TNF) and IL-6 concentrations with increasing platelet storage time and also noted febrile transfusion reactions correlated with high levels of these cytokines. Aye[16] also showed increasing IL-1, TNF IL-6 and IL-8 levels with platelet storage. Stack and Snyder[17] found elevated levels of IL-8 in stored platelet concentrates. Leukocyte depletion prevented this from happening. Increases in IL-1 and IL-8 have also been documented in stored packed RBCs, but not in pre-storage leukocyte depleted RBCs.[19] Accumulation of these soluble donor cytokines during storage might explain some of the FNTRs which occur in spite of the use of leukocyte depleted blood components.

FNTRs associated with RBC transfusion often may be avoided by reducing the number of donor leukocytes transfused. Each unit of RBCs contains approximately $2-5 \times 10^9$ contaminating leukocytes. Most FNTRs can be prevented by a 1-2 log (90-99%) depletion in the leukocyte count of the donor unit to less than 5×10^8. This degree of depletion can be accomplished through the use of saline washed RBCs, frozen deglycerolized RBCs or through the use of microaggregate ("second generation") filters.[20] Leukodepletion filters capable of removing 2-3 logs (99.0-99.9%) of leukocytes from a unit of RBCs have been shown by Sirchia and colleagues[21,22] to reduce the patient rate of febrile transfusion reactions in transfusion dependent thalassemia patients from 13% to between 0.4 and 0.5% depending upon the filter employed. While febrile reactions due to the accumulation of soluble cytokines will not be prevented by post-storage leukocyte depletion, it is possible that pre-storage removal of these leukocytes will prevent these reactions since cytokine accumulation is avoided.[18] Although the third generation filters are more expensive than other methods of leukodepletion of RBCs, they may provide added benefits such as depleted refractoriness to platelet transfusion and prevention of viral and bacterial transmission (discussed below).

Evidence for the effectiveness of WBC-poor platelets in the prevention of FNTRs is more controversial. Six studies published between 1986 and 1990 report a reduced incidence of febrile reactions with platelets that had approximately 1 log (76-95%) of the leukocytes removed.[23-28] These studies are limited by the small number of patients and transfusions examined, the largest study involving 10 patients.[25] Mangano and colleagues[29] reported a limited, but statistically significant, drop in the incidence of FNTRs following the use of leukocyte depleted platelets. However, the majority of patients continued to experience FNTRs. In addition, all but two patients failed to

Table 13.3. Differential diagnosis of platelet refractoriness

Fever
Infection
Hypersplenism
Disseminated intravascular coagulation (DIC)
ABO incompatibility
Alloimmunization
Bleeding
Veno-occlusive disease
Drug-induced thrombocytopenia
Immune thrombocytopenic purpura

demonstrate a significant decrease in their individual reaction rate, but this may have been due to the small number of transfusions per patient. Goodnough and colleagues[30] recently reported no difference in the rate of FNTRs in 12 intensely transfused patients before and after the use of Pall PL 50 filtration to reduce leukocytes. Thus, even leukocyte depleted platelet concentrates can cause FNTRs, albeit at a lower rate. The limited efficacy of leukocyte depletion in the prevention of FNTRs associated with platelet transfusions may be due to soluble cytokines as discussed previously or it may depend upon the nature of the offending alloantibodies. Filtration of WBCs will remove leukocyte-specific antigens and prevent febrile reactions due to antibodies with anti-leukocyte specificity. On the other hand, it is less likely that a febrile response will be prevented if the fever is the result of alloimmunization against platelet specific or class I HLA antigens expressed on platelets. Even so, it is possible that patients with HLA antibodies may benefit from leukocyte poor platelet products since HLA class I antigens are expressed less strongly on platelets than leukocytes.[8] As in the case of RBC transfusion, pre-storage removal of leukocytes prevents cytokine accumulation and may be helpful in reducing the incidence of febrile transfusion reactions to platelets.[15-18] For further discussion on this topic, the reader is referred to chapter 6.

Taken together, the above studies suggest use of leukocyte depleted platelets may diminish the incidence of FNTRs, but can not eliminate them entirely. For most patients, the clinician must decide which patients will benefit from leukocyte depleted platelets given their increased cost. In patients with hematologic malignancies, especially those who are candidates for stem cell therapy, the amelioration of FNTRs may be viewed as a fringe benefit of the more important reasons for providing leukocyte depleted RBC and platelet concentrates.

PREVENTION OF PLATELET REFRACTORINESS

Refractoriness to platelet transfusion represents one of the most difficult problems in the transfusion therapy of patients undergoing hematopoietic stem cell transplantation. Lack of response to platelet transfusion increases the risk of thrombocytopenic bleeding and may be the result of alloimmunization or a variety of clinical conditions,[31,32] (Table 13.3). Alloimmunization occurs in up to 50% of patients with hematologic malignancies or solid tumors,[33-35] although it may be reversible in some patients.[33] A poor 1 hour platelet increment often indicates the alloimmunized state,[36,37] but this may also be due to fever, infection, hypersplenism, DIC or amphotericin antifungal therapy.[38] Antibody mediated platelet refractoriness may be confirmed by lymphocytotoxicity testing for HLA antibodies and/or demonstration of platelet specific antibodies.[39] The management of platelet refractoriness resulting from alloimmunization can be a significant clinical challenge, especially in patients with broadly reactive antibodies. Approaches to overcome platelet refractoriness include the use of HLA-matched platelets, crossmatched platelets, high dose intravenous immune globulin[40] and Rh immunoglobulin.[41] These interventions are not universally available or effective. Therefore, the prudent goal in platelet transfusion therapy of stem cell transplant patients is the prevention of alloimmunization rather than management of future platelet refractoriness.

Strategies to prevent the development of alloimmunization and platelet refractoriness include the use of single donor[41,42] or HLA matched apheresis platelets,[43] as well as ultraviolet (UV) irradiation[44] or leukocyte reduction[45-55] of platelet products. By restricting exposure to a single donor at a time, transfusion of apheresis platelets minimizes recipient exposure to alloantigens, but evidence for the efficacy of this approach is limited.[41,42] In addition, using a canine model, Slichter et al demonstrated that single donor platelets may delay, but not prevent alloimmunization.[56] Leukocyte depletion and UV irradiation of platelet products minimize stimulation of the recipient immune response which results in alloimmunization by reducing, respectively, the number or immunogenicity of donor leukocytes.

Functional leukocytes bearing class II HLA antigens are essential for development of antibodies to class I HLA antigens.[2] In fact, platelets which express only class I HLA antigens are poorly immunogenic.[57] Furthermore, the class I and class II HLA antigens need to be expressed on the same cell, as third party leukocytes fail to stimulate alloimmunization to platelets[57] or cause skin graft rejection.[58] Initiation of the host immune response to foreign antigens involves processing of these proteins by antigen presenting cells (monocytes, macrophages, B lymphocytes and dendritic cells) bearing class II HLA antigens. These antigen presenting cells then present fragments of the antigenic proteins to helper/inducer (CD4+) lymphocytes via their class II molecules.[31] Interruption of this process by removing or UV-inactivating class II bearing leukocytes interferes with the development of alloimmunization. Clinical studies to support the use of UV irradiated platelets are few, but preliminary reports have demonstrated a decrease in alloimmunization[59-61] while platelet function[62,63] and in vivo recovery[63,64] have remained intact.

Numerous clinical studies[45-55] have examined the effect of leukocyte depletion on the rate of alloimmunization and development of platelet refractoriness (Table 13.4). Variation in the statistical and experimental design of these studies make interpretation and comparison of the results difficult.[31,43] First, the eligibility requirements used to determine the population studied varied with respect to hematologic diagnosis, myelosuppressive therapy and history of prior pregnancy or transfusion. Second, some investigations were cohort studies,[45,48] others were randomized, but none were double blind. The largest study by Brand and colleagues[30] lacked a control group and the latest study of Saarinen et al only had a small reference group.[55] Third, the methods and efficacy of leukocyte removal varied widely. Earlier studies achieved leukocyte depletion by centrifugation,[45,46,48] while later studies[47,49-55] accomplished more efficient WBC removal with third generation filters. The ongoing Trial to Reduce Alloimmunization to Platelets (TRAP) sponsored by the National Heart, Lung, and Blood Institute, is a multicenter, double blind, prospective clinical study of patients with acute myelogenous leukemia which overcomes the statistical limitations of the earlier investigations.[31] The results should provide more definitive data on the use of leukocyte filtration and UV irradiation in the prevention of alloimmunization.

In spite of their individual limitations, these studies taken together provide strong evidence that use of leukocyte depleted blood products prevents alloimmunization and platelet refractoriness in patients with hematologic malignancies. All but two of the earlier studies,[46,48] which employed less effective methods of leukocyte removal, demonstrated decreased refractoriness as a result the use of leukocyte depleted platelets and RBCs. The development of refractoriness appears to be dose dependent with a lower incidence seen in the studies with more efficient[47,52-55] compared to less efficient[45,46,48-51] leukocyte removal. The threshold for prevention of refractoriness appears to be approximately $1-5 \times 10^6$ leukocytes/transfusion. The magnitude of this threshold is consistent with that obtained from extrapolated data from mice.[31] Currently available filters which remove 3 logs (99.9%) of donor leukocytes from RBC and platelet products are capable of achieving this degree of WBC reduction.[31] The role the number of transfusions and, hence, total WBC exposure from different donors plays in alloimmunization and the potential need for greater WBC depletion in heavily transfused patients is uncertain at present. Blajchman et al[65] demonstrated in an animal model that prestorage leukocyte depletion is associated with a lower incidence of refractoriness and better platelet survival than post-storage leukocyte depletion.

Although the evidence that use of leukocyte depleted products in patients with hematologic malignancies prevents allo-immunization is strong, the cost effectiveness of the strategy of providing these customized blood products has been challenged.[43,66,67] Factors increasing the cost of leukocyte depleted blood components include not only the cost of the filter, but the extra labor involved in its use by blood bank or nursing staff. In addition, many patients who are at risk of becoming alloimmunized will not, but would require leukocyte depleted blood products since it is not possible to predict the fraction of this population that is susceptible. Heddle[43] also raises the issue that the refractory state needs to be correlated with the risk of clinically significant thrombocytopenic bleeding rather than with laboratory evidence of HLA antibodies or a poor post-transfusion platelet increment.

Table 13.4. Prevention of alloimmunization by leukocyte removal

Study (ref)		Patients (n)	Residual WBC (x10⁶µL)		HLA Alloimmunity (%)		Platelet Refractoriness (%)	
			RBC	PLT	Control	LD	Control	LD
Eernisse (45)	1981	96‡	100	1.25	10/16 (63)	19/68 (28)	26/28 (94)	16/68 (24)
Schiffer (46)	1983	56	NA	12	13/31 (42)	5/25* (20)	6/31 (19)	4/25* (16)
Fisher (47)	1985	24	NA	<5	5/12 (42)	0/12 (0)	NA	NA
Murphy (48)	1986	50	<8	90-220	13/31 (48)	3/19 (16)	7/31 (23)	1/19* (5)
Sniecinski (49)	1988	40	50	6	10/20 (50)	3/20 (15)	10/20 (50)	3/20 (15)
Andreu (50)	1988	69	61	50-150	11/35 (31)	4/34 (12)	14/30 (47)	6/28 (21)
Brand (51)	1988	335	<0.5	<20	NA	69/335 (21)	NA	31/335 (9)
Saarinen (52)	1990	47‡	0.1	.04	NA	NA	11/21 (52)	0/26 (0)
Oksanen (53)	1991	31	0.1	.04	3/15 (20)	2/16 (13)	1/15 (7)	0/16 (0)
van Marwijk Kooy (54)	1991	53	<5	5	11/26 (42)	2/27 (7)	12/26 (46)	3/27 (11)
Saarinen (55)	1993	60‡,†	0.1	0.04	3/10 (30)	0/50¶ (0)	1/10 (10)	0/50¶ (0)

LD: Leukodepleted   PLT: Platelet   NA: Not available
(*): P>0.05, ¶ P not determined, otherwise P<0.05 (‡): Not randomized
(†): Reference group received partially leuko-depleted components

Contrary to these objections, several reports demonstrated cost savings with use of leukocyte depleted blood in patients with leukemia[68-70] and lymphoma.[71] Savings were due to decreased platelet usage, utilization of fewer HLA or crossmatched platelets and shortened length of hospital stay. The more rapid hematopoietic recovery and lower infection rate seen in bone marrow transplant patients receiving filtered blood recently reported by Oksanen and colleagues[72] may yield additional cost savings. While the results of these studies should not be generalized to all multiply transfused patients, they suggest that use of leukocyte depletion in patients who are candidates for stem cell transplantation is cost effective. Pending the results of the TRAP study, use of leukocyte reduction filters for all RBC and platelet transfusions in stem cell transplant patients and candidates is not only cost effective, but clinically prudent. For further information, the reader is referred to chapter 7.

PREVENTION OF CYTOMEGALOVIRUS BY TRANSFUSION

Cytomegalovirus (CMV) is a leukotropic herpes virus which may be transmitted by transfusion resulting in a heterophil-antibody negative mononucleosis syndrome in immunocompetent patients.[73,74] In contrast, primary or reactivation CMV infection occurs in 40-70% of hematopoietic stem cell transplant patients and may be manifested by a combination of pneumonia, gastroenteritis, hepatitis, retinitis and disseminated disease.[75] CMV pneumonitis may be seen in up to 20% of bone marrow transplantation patients and is associated with a case fatality rate of approximately 85%.[73] CMV infection may cause delayed engraftment,[76-77] although this has not been confirmed by a recent study by Reusser and colleagues.[78] Risk factors for CMV infection following transplantation include older age, granulocyte transfusion, graft-versus host disease and pretransplant seropositivity.[73]

Transfusion associated CMV infection has been prevented through the use of CMV seronegative blood products for patients at risk including seronegative transplant patients receiving seronegative hematopoietic stem cells[78,79] or solid organ grafts.[75] Other patient populations at risk include pregnant women, neonates who weigh less than 1200 g and seronegative AIDS patients.[75] Transmission of CMV by transfusion may also be diminished through the use of leukocyte depleted RBCs prepared by centrifugation,[80] washing,[81] or frozen deglycerolization[82-86] and by filtration of blood components.[87-95] Lang and colleagues[80] demonstrated that a 60% depletion of leukocytes by centrifugation diminished, but did not eliminate, CMV transmission by whole blood in cardiopulmonary bypass patients. Similarly, washing of RBCs has been shown to reduce the transmission of CMV in neonates.[81] No cases of CMV infection were seen in several studies of hemodialysis patients[82,83] and neonates[84-86] receiving frozen, deglycerolized RBCs, although this cumbersome procedure is not practical for routine use. Leukocyte depletion by filtration as a possible alternative to CMV seronegative blood is enticing since the prevalence of CMV seropositivity in the donor population is high (40-60%),[92] although, at most only about 10% of units from these donors are actually capable of transmitting CMV infection.[75] In addition, use of leukocyte depletion would eliminate the cost of screening units for CMV antibody in hematopoietic stem cell patients who already receive leukocyte depleted blood for other purposes. Furthermore, units from donors who are infected, but in the window period before becoming seropositive are not identified by serotesting but would be rendered safe by leukoreduction.

There have been numerous studies that have examined the effect of leukocyte depletion on the transmission of CMV by blood transfusion,[87-95] (Table 13.5). With the exception of the most recent study by Bowden et al (ref. 95, discussed below), the cumulative use of leukocyte depleted blood prevented transmission of CMV by transfusion in all patients studied (0/257, 0%).

The incidence of CMV infection in patients receiving unscreened, nonleukocyte depleted blood was much higher (28/167, 17%). These studies are limited in that many lack a control group[87,91,92,94] and only two are prospective.[91,95] Nevertheless, taken together, these studies provide strong evidence that leukocyte filtration is an effective means of preventing CMV transmission by blood products.

Bowden et al[95] conducted a prospective study comparing CMV-seronegative to leukocyte depleted (at the bedside) blood components in 487 patients undergoing allogeneic or autologous bone marrow

transplantation. They reported (in abstract form) that the incidence of CMV infection was comparable in the two groups but CMV disease occurred more frequently in the group receiving leukocyte depleted blood components. Nevertheless, when infections that occurred within 21 days of entry into the study were excluded because these infections presumably were acquired prior to enrollment, the two groups were not significantly different (oral presentation[95]). Definitive interpretation of these data await final publication of the results. In the meantime, use of leukocyte depleted blood components for seronegative recipi-

---

Table 13.5. Prevention of CMV transmission by leukocyte depletion

Study	Patients	Diagnosis	Post Transfusion CMV (%)		
(ref)	(n)		Control	L.D.	Seroneg.
Verndonck (87) 1987	29	Bone marrow transplant	NA	0/29 (0)	NA
Murphy (88) 1988	20	Acute leukemia	2/9 (22)	0/11 (0)	NA
Gilbert (89) 1989	72	Neonates	9/42 (21)	0/30 (0)	NA
De Graan-Hentzen (90) 1989	145	Leukemia, lymphoma	10/86 (12)	0/59 (0)	NA
Bowden (91) 1989	17	Bone marrow transplant	NA	0/17 (0)	NA
Dewitte (92) 1990	28	Bone marrow transplant	NA	0/28 (0)	NA
Bowden (93) 1991	65	Bone marrow transplant	7/30 (23)	0/35 (0)	NA
Eisenfeld (94) 1992	48	Neonates	NA	0/48 (0)	NA
Bowden (95) 1993	487	Bone marrow transplant	NA	5/241	0/246
Total	911		28/167 (17)	5/498 (1)	0/246 (0)

L.D. = Leukocyte depleted. Seroneg. = Seronegative. NA = Not applicable.

ents of seronegative hematopoietic stem cell transplants should be reserved only for situations where CMV seronegative blood is unavailable. For further information, the reader is referred to chapter 8.

PREVENTION OF BACTERIAL GROWTH AND TRANSFUSION BY PRE-STORAGE FILTRATION

Septic transfusion reactions owing to the transfusion of blood components contaminated with bacteria are rare, occurring in approximately 1 in 4000 platelet[96-97] and 1 in 31,000 RBC transfusions.[97] These septic reactions are usually associated with endotoxin producing organisms (e.g. *Yersinia enterocolitica*) and the clinical manifestations in hematopoietic stem cell reconstitution patients can be quite severe consisting of a combination of high fever, hemoglobinuria, shock, DIC and/or renal failure.[7] Current strategies employed to prevent bacterial contamination include: meticulous attention to sterile technique during phlebotomy and component preparation, exclusion of donors at risk for transient bacteremia and refrigeration of RBCs.[7]

Several recent in vitro studies have evaluated the potential role of leukocyte depletion in the prevention of bacteremia resulting from contaminated units.[98-102] These studies employed fresh blood (RBCs or whole blood) that had been inoculated with *Yersinia entercolitica* following donation. Following several hours of storage, an aliquot of blood was leukocyte depleted and another control aliquot remained unfiltered.[103] Bacterial cultures were obtained during subsequent storage. In all the studies, the development of culture positivity with extended storage was lower in the aliquot that had been leukocyte depleted. Högman et al have suggested that this effect may be due to the removal of leukocytes containing ingested bacteria as inoculated units containing leukocytes show less bacterial growth than leukocyte depleted units.[104] In addition, units containing leukocytes initially appear sterile but grow Yersinia with storage, presumably resulting from release of viable bacteria from

disintegrated leukocytes.[97] On the other hand, Ali and Blajchman[105] have reported preliminary results that show leukocyte reduction filters can directly remove bacteria (*Staphylococcus xylosus*) from units that had already been leukocyte depleted.

These initial reports support the efficacy of leukocyte depletion in the removal of bacteria from contaminated blood components in vitro. The prevention of transfusion-associated sepsis may be an added benefit of pre-storage leukocyte depleted blood components in hematopoietic stem cell transplant patients (see also chapter 6).

PREVENTION OF GRAFT-VERSUS-HOST DISEASE

Graft-versus-host disease (GVHD) is a complication seen following allogenic bone marrow transplantation when immunocompetent donor T lymphocytes engraft and attack the recipient's tissues as "foreign". Clinical features of GVHD include immunosuppression, fever, skin rash, hepatic disease and GI distress which can include nausea, vomiting, and diarrhea. Transfusion associated graft-versus-host disease (TA-GVHD) is an extremely severe form characterized by pancytopenia secondary to bone marrow aplasia, with most cases being fatal.[106] Gamma irradiation of cellular products with a dose of at least 2500 Gy is effective in inactivating T lymphocytes and preventing TA-GVHD.[7] Ultraviolet irradiation has been shown to prevent TA-GVHD in dogs, but not humans.[107]

As few as 10^4 viable lymphocytes per kg may be capable of producing TA-GVHD[108] although this has been questioned.[109] This suggests current leukocyte depletion filter technology may be able to reduce the risk of TA-GVHD.[109] Using the mixed lymphocyte reaction (MLR) as a model of TA-GVHD, Dzik and colleagues[109] demonstrated that WBC depletion caused a dose dependent exponential decrease in the MLR. However, the clinical utility of leukocyte depletion in the prevention of TA-GVHD has not been determined.[106] In fact, a case of TA-GVHD has been reported in a patient with non-Hodgkin's lymphoma who received exclusively leukocyte depleted components.[110] Thus, gamma irradiation of blood components remains the standard of practice for the prophylaxis of TA-GVHD and leukocyte depletion must not be employed as a substitute[7] (also see chapter 6).

OTHER POTENTIAL EFFECTS OF ALLOGENEIC LEUKOCYTES

Allogeneic blood transfusion has been demonstrated to be immunosuppressive.[111] There is circumstantial evidence that allogeneic transfusions are associated with increased infections and increased recurrence of solid tumor malignancy in humans. There is strong experimental evidence in animals that infections and malignant cell proliferation are enhanced by allogeneic transfusion.[112] Recent data show that leukocyte depletion eliminated the effect of promoting malignant growth by blood transfusion.[112] There is no evidence that hematologic malignancy has been enhanced by allogeneic transfusion.

It has been suggested that the leukocytes in blood transfusions may contribute to the well-known graft-versus-leukemia effect seen in allogeneic bone marrow transplantation and therefore, removing the WBCs from blood transfused to patients receiving hematopoietic stem cell transplantation may be harmful. However, three studies have failed to demonstrate a graft-versus-leukemia effect, as the median survival was similar in leukemia patients whether or not they had received leukocyte depleted blood components.[113-115] Furthermore, Oksanen and colleagues[72] found a favorable effect of leukocyte depleted blood transfusion on median disease free survival, hematopoietic recovery and incidence of post-transplant infection in patients who received bone marrow transplantation for acute myelogenous leukemia.

As stem cell transplantation from non-HLA identical donors increases, the potential value of avoiding HLA alloimmunization is enhanced. Pretransplant alloimmunization to HLA antigens present in a prospective donor could potentially delay or prevent engraftment. Thus, avoiding alloimmunization could provide a substantial benefit in addition to avoiding refractoriness to platelet transfusion (see also chapter 9).

CONCLUSION

1. Considering the potential benefits of leukocyte depletion, it is preferable to provide leukocyte depleted RBCs and platelet concentrates from the time of diagnosis for patients who may undergo stem cell transplantation and to continue their use during transplant therapy.

2. Although leukocyte depletion may be performed during storage or at the time of transfusion, pre-storage depletion offers the advantages of preventing cytokine accumulation and reducing the likelihood of bacterial proliferation.

3. Leukocyte depletion offers a cost-effective approach for increasing the safety and reducing the discomfort and risks of blood transfusion for patients undergoing hematopoietic stem cell reconstitution.

REFERENCES

1. Freedman JJ, Blajchman MA, McCombie N. Canadian Red Cross Society Symposium on Leukodepletion: report of proceedings. Transf Med Rev 8:1, 1994.

2. Lane TA, Anderson KC, Goodnough LT, et al. Leukocyte reduction in blood component therapy. Ann Int Med 117:151, 1992.

3. Doan CA. The recognition of a biologic differentiation in the white blood cell with especial reference to blood transfusion. JAMA 86:1593, 1926.

4. Brittingham TC, Chaplin H Jr. Febrile transfusion reactions caused by sensitivity to donor leukocytes and platelets. JAMA 165:819, 1957.

5. Perkins HA, Payne R, Ferguson J, Wood M. Nonhemolytic febrile transfusion reactions. Quantitative effects of blood components with emphasis on isoantigenic incompatibility of leukocytes. Vox Sang 11:578, 1966.

6. Menitove JE, McElligott MC, Aster RH.

Febrile transfusion reaction: what component should be given next? Vox Sang 42:318, 1982.

7. Walker RH, ed. Technical Manual. 11th ed. Bethesda, MD. American Association of Blood Banks, 1993.

8. Mintz PD. Febrile reactions to platelet transfusions. Am J Clin Pathol 95:609, 1991.

9. Decary F, Ferner P, Giavedoni L, et al. An investigation of non-hemolytic transfusion reactions. Vox Sang 46:277, 1984.

10. de Rie MA, van der Plas-van Dalen CM, Engelfriet CP, von dem Borne AEGK: The serology of febrile transfusion reactions. Vox Sang 49:126, 1985.

11. Brubaker DB. Clinical significance of white cell antibodies in febrile nonhemolytic transfusion reactions. Transfusion 30:733, 1990.

12. Dinarello CA, Wolff SM. Molecular basis of fever in humans. Am J Med 72:799, 1982.

13. Dzik WH. Is the febrile response to transfusion due to donor or recipient cytokine? Transfusion 32:594, 1992.

14. Okusawa S, Dianrello CA, Endres S, et al.: C5a induction of human interleukin-1: synergistic effect with endotoxin or interferon-α. J Immunol 139:2635, 1987.

15. Muylle L, Joos M, Wouters E, De Bock R, Peetermans ME. Increased tumor necrosis factor α (TNFα), interleukin 1, and interleukin 6 (IL-6) levels in the plasma of stored platelet concentrates: relationship between TNFα and IL-6 levels and febrile transfusion reactions. Transfusion 33:195, 1993.

16. See Aye as referenced in Freedman JJ, Blajchman MA, McCombie N. Canadian Red Cross Society Symposium on Leukodepletion: Report of Proceedings. Transf Med Rev 8:1, 1994.

17. Stack G, Snyder EL. Cytokine generation in stored platelet concentrates. Transfusion 34:20, 1994.

18. Smith KJ, Sierra ER, Nelson EJ. Plasma 1L-8 and 1L-6 increase in platelet concentrates (PC) stored for 5 days but not in PC leukodepleted pre-storage. Transfusion 33:53S, 1993.

19. Smith KJ, Sierra ER, Nelson EJ. Histamine, IL-1ß, and IL-8 increase in packed RBCs

stored for 42 days but not in RBCs leukodepleted pre-storage. Transfusion 33:53S, 1993.

20. Meryman HT, Hornblower M. The preparation of red cells depleted of leukocytes: review and evaluation. Transfusion 26:101, 1986.

21. Sirchia G, Rebulla P, Parravicini A, Carnelli V, Gianotti AG, Bertolini F. Leukocyte depletion of red cell units at the bedside by transfusion through a new filter. Transfusion 27:402, 1987.

22. Sirchia G, Wenz B, Rebulla P, Parravicini A, Carnelli V, Bertolini, F. Removal of white cells from red cells by transfusion through a new filter. Transfusion 30:30, 1990.

23. Dan ME, Stewart S. Prevention of recurrent febrile transfusion reactions using leukocyte poor platelet concentrates prepared by the "leukotrap" centrifugation method. Transfusion 26:569, 1986.

24. Stec N, Kickler TS, Ness PM, Braine HG. Effectiveness of leukocyte (WBC) depleted platelets in preventing febrile reactions in multi-transfused oncology patients. Transfusion 26:569, 1986.

25. Schiffer CA, Patten E, Reilly J, Patel S. Effective leukocyte removal from platelet preparations by centrifugation in a new pooling bag. Transfusion 27:162, 1987.

26. Kalmin ND, Orell JE, Villarreal IG. An effective method for the preparation of leukocyte-poor platelets. Transfusion 27:281, 1987.

27. Sternbach M, Champagne J, Rybka W, Paquin M. Leukotrap, a device for white cell poor platelets. Quality control studies in vitro and in vivo. Trans Science 10:57, 1989.

28. Slichter SJ. Mechanisms and management of platelet refractoriness. In: Nance SJ, ed. Transfusion Medicine in the 1990s. Arlington, VA. American Association of Blood Banks, 95, 1990.

29. Mangano MM, Chambers LA, Kruskall MS. Limited efficacy of leukopoor platelets for prevention of febrile transfusion reactions. Am J Clin Pathol. 95:733, 1991.

30. Goodnough LT, Riddell J, Lazarus H, Chafel TL, Prince G, Hendrix D, Yomtovian R. Prevalence of platelet transfusion reactions

before and after implementation of leukocyte-depleted platelet concentrates by filtration. Vox Sang 65:103, 1993.

31. Confer DL. The prevention of HLA
alloimmunization. In: Clinical Decisions in
Platelet Therapy 1992.

32. Rio B, Nichol AG, et al. Thrombocytopenia
in venoocclusive disease after bone marrow
transplantation or chemotherapy. Blood
67:1773, 1986.

33. Lee EJ, Schiffer CA. Serial measurement of
lymphocytotoxic antibody and response to
non-matched platelet transfusions in
alloimmunization patients. Blood 70:1727,
1987.

34. Schiffer CA, Lichtenfeld JL, Wiernik PH,
Mardiney MR, Joseph JM. Antibody response in patients with acute non-lymphocytic leukemia. Cancer 37:2177, 1976.

35. Dutcher JP, Schiffer CA, Aisner J, Wiernik
PH. Long-term follow-up of patients with
leukemia receiving platelet transfusions:
Identification of a large group of patients
who do not become alloimmunized. Blood
58:1007, 1981.

36. Daly PA, Schiffer CA, Aisner J, Wiernik
PA. Platelet transfusion therapy—One hour
post-transfusion increments are valuable in
predicting the need for HLA-matched preparations. JAMA 243:435, 1980.

37. O'Connell B, Lee EJ, Schiffer CA. The value
of 10-minute posttransfusion platelet counts.
Transfusion 28:66, 1988.

38. Bishop JF, McGrath K, Wolf MM, et al.
Clinical factors influencing the efficacy of
pooled platelet transfusions. Blood 71:383,
1988.

39. Kickler TS. The challenge of platelet
alloimmunization: management and prevention. Trans Med Rev 4:8, 1990.

40. Kickler T, Braine HG, Piantodosi S, et al.
A randomized, placebo-controlled trial of
intravenous gammaglobulin in alloimmunized thrombocytopenic patients. Blood
75:313, 1990.

41. Sintnicolaas K, Sizoo W, Haije WG, et al.
Delayed alloimmunisation by random single
donor platelet transfusions. A randomised
study to compare single donor and multiple donor platelet transfusions in cancer
patients with severe thrombocytopenia. Lan-

cet 1:750, 1981.

42. Gmür J, von Felten A, Osterwalder B, et
al. Delayed alloimmunization using random
single donor platelet transfusions: A prospective study in thrombocytopenic patients
with acute leukemia. Blood 62:473, 1983.

43. Heddle NM. The efficacy of leukodepletion
to improve platelet transfusion response: a
critical appraisal of clinical studies. Trans
Med Rev. 8:15, 1994.

44. Andreu G, Boccaccio C, Klaren J, et al.
The role of UV radiation in the prevention
of human leukocyte antigen alloimmunization. Trans Med Rev 6:212, 1992.

45. Eernisse JG, Brand A. Prevention of platelet refractoriness due to HLA antibodies by
administration of leukocyte-poor blood components. Exp Hematol 9:77, 1981.

46. Schiffer CA, Dutcher JP, Aisner J, et al. A
randomized trial of leukocyte-depleted platelet transfusion to modify alloimmunization
in patients with leukemia. Blood 62:815,
1983.

47. Fisher M, Chapman JR, Ting A, Morris PJ.
Alloimmunisation to HLA antigens following transfusion with leucocyte-poor and
purified platelet suspensions. Vox Sang
49:331, 1985.

48. Murphy ME, Metcalfe P, Thomas H, et al.
Use of leucocyte-poor blood components and
HLA-matched-platelet donors to prevent
HLA alloimmunization. Br J Haematol
62:529, 1986.

49. Sniecinski I, O'Donnell MR, Nowicki B, et
al. Prevention of refractoriness and HLA-
alloimmunization using filtered blood products. Blood 71:1402, 1988.

50. Andreu G, Dewailly J, Leberre C, et al.
Prevention of HLA immunization with leukocyte-poor packed red cells and platelet
concentrates obtained by filtration. Blood
72:964, 1988.

51. Brand A, Claas FHJ, Voogt PJ, et al.
Alloimmunization after leukocyte-depleted
multiple random donor platelet transfusions.
Vox Sang 54:160, 1988.

52. Saarinen UM, Kekomäki R, Siimes MA, et
al. Effective prophylaxis against platelet
refractoriness in multitransfused patients by
use of leukocyte-free blood components.
Blood 75:512, 1990.

53. Oksanen K, Kekomäki R, Ruutu T, et al. Prevention of alloimmunization in patients with acute leukemia by use of white cell-reduced blood components—A randomized trial. Transfusion 31:588, 1991.

54. van Marwijk Kooy M, van Prooijen HC, Moes M, et al. Use of leukocyte-depleted platelet concentrates for the prevention of refractoriness and primary HLA alloimmunization: A prospective, randomized trial. Blood 77:201, 1991.

55. Saarinen UM, Koskimies S, Myllylä G. Systematic use of leukocyte-free blood components to prevent alloimmunization and platelet refractoriness in multitransfused children with cancer. Vox Sang 65:286, 1993.

56. Slichter SJ, O'Donnell MR, Weiden PL, et al. Canine platelet alloimmunization: the role of donor selection. Br J Hematol 63:713, 1986.

57. Welsh KI, Burgos H, Batchelor JR. The immune response to allogeneic rat platelets: Ag-B antigens in matrix form lacking 1a. Eur J Immunol 7:267, 1977.

58. Dausset J, Rapaport FT. Transplantation antigen activity of human blood platelets. Transplantation 4:182, 1966.

59. Buchholz DH, Miripol J, Aster RH, et al. Ultraviolet irradiation of platelets to prevent recipient alloimmunization. Transfusion 28:S91, 1988.

60. Menitove JE, Kagen LR, Aster RH, et al. Alloimmunization is decreased in patients receiving UV-B irradiated platelet concentrates and leukocyte-depleted red cells. Blood 76:1607, 1990.

61. Pamphilon DH, Blundell EL. Ultraviolet B irradiation of platelet transfusions: A strategy to reduce recipient alloimmunization. Semin Hematol 29:118, 1992.

62. Kahn RA, Duffy BF, Rodey GG. Ultraviolet irradiation of platelet concentrate abrogates lymphocyte activation without affecting platelet function in vitro. Transfusion 25:547, 1985.

63. Snyder EL, Beardsly D, Smith B, et al. Storage of platelet concentrates after UV-B irradiation. Blood 74:179a (abstr), 1989.

64. Pamphilon DH, Potter M, Cutts M, et al. Platelet concentrates irradiated with ultra-violet light retain satisfactory in vitro storage characteristics and in vivo survival. Br J Haematol 75:240, 1990.

65. Blajchman MA, Bardossy L, Carmen RA, Goldman M, Heddle NM, Singal DP. An animal model of allogeneic donor platelet refractoriness: the effect of the time of leukodepletion. Blood 79:1371, 1992.

66. Schiffer CA. Prevention of alloimmunization against platelets. Blood 77:1, 1991.

67. Perkins HA. Is white cell reduction cost-effective? Transfusion 33:626, 1993.

68. Balducci L, Benson K, Lyman GH, Sanderson R, Fields K, Ballester OF, Elfenbein GJ. Cost-effectiveness of white cell-reduction filters in treatment of adult acute myelogenous leukemia. Transfusion 33:665, 1993.

69. Blumberg N, Heal J, Kirkley S, Panzer R, Rowe J. Cost effectiveness of leukodepleted (LD) transfusions during induction therapy for acute leukemia. Transfusion 33:84S, 1993.

70. Sniecinski I. Prevention of immunologic and infectious complications of transfusion by leukocyte depletion. In: Clinical Application of Leukocyte Depletion. Sekiguchi S, ed, Blackwell Scientific Publication, Osney Mead Oxford, 1993.

71. Blumberg N, Heal J, Rapoport A, DiPersio J, Rowe J, Panzer R. Effect of ABO-identical platelets and leukodepletion (LD) on blood utilization and costs of autologous marrow transplantation (BMT). Transfusion 33:83S, 1993.

72. Oksanen K, Elonen E. Impact of leucocyte-depleted blood components on the haematological recovery and prognosis of patients with acute myeloid leukaemia. Br J Haem 84:639, 1993.

73. Hirsch MS. Ctyomegalovirus infection. In: Harrison's Principles of Internal Medicine. 12th ed. Wilson JD, et al, eds., McGraw-Hill, Inc. 1991.

74. Kaariainen L, Klemola E, Paloheimo J. Rise of cytomegalovirus antibodies in an infectious mononucleosis-like syndrome after transfusion. Br Med J 1:1270, 1966.

75. Sayers MH, Anderson KC, Goodnough LT. Reducing the risk for transfusion-transmitted cytomegalovirus infection. Ann Int Med 116:55, 1992.

76. Verdonck LF, van Heugten H, de Gast GC. Delay in platelet recovery after bone marrow transplantation: impact of cytomegalovirus infection. Blood 66:921, 1985.

77. Wingard JR, Ghen DY, Burns WH, Fuller DJ, Braine HG, Yeager AM, et al. Cytomegalovirus infection after autolgous bone marrow transplantation with comparison to infection after allogeneic bone marrow transplantation. Blood 71:1432, 1988.

78. Reusser P, Fisher LD, Buckner CD, Thomas ED, Meyers JD. Cytomegalovirus infection after autologous bone marrow transplantation: occurrence of cytomegalovirus disease and effect on engraftment. Blood 75:1888, 1990.

79. Bowden RA, Sayers M, Flournoy N, Newton B, Banaji M, Thomas ED, et al. Cytomegalovirus immune globulin and seronegative blood products to prevent primary cytomegalovirus infection after marrow transplantation. N Engl J Med 314:1006, 1986.

80. Lang DJ, Ebert PA, Rodgers BM, Boggess HP, Rixse RS. Reduction of postperfusion cytomegalovirus infections following the use of leukocyte depleted blood. Transfusion 17:391, 1977.

81. Luban NL, Williams AE, McDonald MG, Mikesell GT, Williams KM, Sacher RA. Low incidence of cytomegalovirus infection in neonates transfused with washed red blood cells. Am J Dis Child 141:416, 1987.

82. Tolkoff-Rubin NA, Rubin RH, Keller EE, Baker GP, Stewart JA, Hirsch MS. Cytomegalovirus infection in dialysis patients and personnel. Ann Intern Med 89:625, 1978.

83. Betts RF, Cestero RV, Freeman RB, Douglas RG Jr. Epidemiology of cytomegalovirus infection in end stage renal disease. J Med Virol 4:89, 1979.

84. Adler SP, Lawrence LT, Baggett J, Biro V, Sharp DE. Prevention of transfusion-associated cytomegalovirus infection in very low-birth-weight infants using frozen blood and donors seronegative for cytomegalovirus. Transfusion 24:333, 1984.

85. Brady MT, Milam JD, Anderson DC, Hawkins EP, Speer ME, Seavy D, et al. Use of deglycerolized red blood cells to prevent posttransfusion infection with cytomegalovirus in neonates. J Infect Dis 150:334, 1984.

86. Taylor BJ, Jacobs RF, Baker RL, Moses EB, McSwain BE, Shulman G. Frozen deglycerolyzed blood prevents transfusion-acquired cytomegalovirus infections in neonates. Pediatr Infect Dis 5:188, 1986.

87. Verdonck LF, de Graan-Hentzen YC, Dekker AW, Mudde GC, de Gast GC. Cytomegalovirus seronegative platelets and leukocyte-poor red blood cells from random donors can prevent primary cytomegalovirus infection after bone marrow transplantation. Bone Marrow Transplant 2:73, 1987.

88. Murphy MF, Grint PC, Hardiman AE, Lister TA, Waters AH. Use of leukocyte-poor blood components to prevent primary cytomegalovirus (CMV) infection in patients with acute leukemia. Br J Haematol 70:253, 1988.

89. Gilbert GL, Hayes K, Hudson IL, James J. Prevention of transfusion-acquired cytomegalovirus infection in infants by blood filtration to remove leucocytes. Neonatal Cytomegalovirus Infection Study Group. Lancet 1:1228, 1989.

90. De Graan-Hentzen YCE, Gratama JW, Mudde GC, et al. Prevention of primary cytomegalovirus infection in patients with hematologic malignancies by intensive white cell depletion of blood products. Transfusion 29:757, 1989.

91. Bowden RA, Sayers MH, Cays M< Slichter SJ. The role of blood product filtration in the prevention of transfusion associated cytomegalovirus (CMV) infection after marrow transplant (Abstract). Transfusion 29:57S, 1989.

92. DeWitte T, Schattenberg A, van Dijk BA, Galama J, Olthuis H, Van der Meer JW, Kunst VA. Prevention of primary cytomegalovirus infection after allogeneic bone marrow transplantation by using leukocyte-poor random blood products from cytomegalovirus-unscreened blood-bank donors. Transplantation 50:964, 1990.

93. Bowden RA, Slichter SJ, Sayers MH, Mori M, Cays MJ, Meyers JD. Use of leukocyte-depleted platelets and cytomegalovirus-seronegative red blood cells for prevention of primary cytomegalovirus infection after marrow transplant. Blood 78:246, 1991.

94. Eisenfield L, Silver H, McLaughlin J, et al. Prevention of transfusion-associated cytomegalovirus infection in neonatal patients by the removal of white cells from blood. Transfusion 32:205, 1992.

95. Bowden RA, Cays M, Schoch G, et al. Comparison of filtered blood (FB) to seronegative blood products (SB) for prevention of cytomegalovirus (CMV) infection after marrow transplant. Blood 82:204a, 1993.

96. Morrow JF, Braine HG, Kickler TS, et al. Septic reactions to platelet transfusions. A persistent problem. JAMA 266:555, 1991.

97. Barrett BB, Andersen JW, Anderson KC. Strategies for the avoidance of bacterial contamination of blood components. Transfusion 33:228, 1993.

98. Pietersz RNI, Reesink HW, Pauw W, Dekker WJA, Buisman L. Prevention of *Yersinia enterocolitica* growth in red-blood-cell concentrates. Lancet 340:755, 1992.

99. Högman CF, Gong J, Hambraeus A, Johansson CS, Eriksson L. The role of white cells in the transmission of *Yersinia enterocolitica* in blood components. Transfusion 32:654, 1992.

100. Kim DM, Brecher ME, Bland LA, Estes TJ, McAllister SK, Aguero SM, Carmen RA, Nelson EJ. Prestorage removal of *Yersinia enterocolitica* from red cells with white cell-reduction filters. Transfusion 32:658, 1992.

101. Wenz B, Burns ER, Freundlich LF. Prevention of growth of *Yersinia enterocolitica* in blood by polyester fiber filtration. Transfusion 32:663, 1992.

102. Buchholz DH, AuBuchon JP, Snyder EL, et al. Removal of *Yersinia enterocolitica* from AS-1 red cells. Transfusion 32:667, 1992.

103. Nusbacher J. *Yersinia enterocolitica* and white cell filtration. Transfusion 32:597, 1992.

104. Högman CF, Gong J, Eriksson L, Hambraeus A, Johansson CS. White cells protect donor blood against bacterial contamination. Transfusion 31:620, 1991.

105. See Ali and Blajchman as referenced in Freedman JJ, Blajchman MA, McCombie N. Canadian Red Cross Society Symposium on Leukodepletion: report on proceedings. Transf Med Rev 8:1, 1994.

106. Anderson KC, Weinstein HJ. Transfusion-associated graft-versus-host disease. N Engl J Med 323:315, 1990.

107. Deeg HJ, Graham TC, Gerhard-Miller L, et al. Prevention of transfusion-induced graft-versus-host disease in dogs by ultraviolet irradiation. Blood 74:2592, 1989.

108. Rubinstein A, Radl J, Cottier H, Rossi E, Gugler E. Unusual combined immunodeficiency syndrome exhibiting kappa-IgD paraproteinemia, residual gut immunity and graft-versus-host reaction after plasma infusion. Acta Paediatr Scand 62:365, 1973.

109. Dzik WH, Jones KS. The effects of gamma irradiation versus white cell reduction on the mixed lymphocyte reaction. Transfusion 33:493, 1993.

110. Akahoshi M, Takanashi M, Masuda, M, et al. A case of transfusion-associated graft-versus-host disease not prevented by white cell-reduction filters. Transfusion 32:169, 1992.

111. Klein HG. Transfusion in transplant patients: the good, the bad, and the ugly. J Heart Lung Transplant 12:S7, 1993.

112. Blajchman MA, Bardossy L, Carmen R, Sastry A, Singai DP. Allogeneic blood transfusion-induced enhancement of tumor growth: two animal models showing amelioration by leukodepletion and passive transfer using spleen cells. Blood 81:1880, 1993.

113. Lopez J, Fernandez-Villalta MJ, Gomez-Reino F, Fernandez-Ranada JM. Absence of graft-versus-leukemia effect of standard hemotherapy in patients with acute myeloblastic leukemia. Transfusion 30:191, 1990.

114. Norol F, Parquet N, Kuentz M, et al. Absence of graft-versus-leukaemia (GVL) effect by leucocytes transfused: a prospective randomized trial in acute myeloid leukaemia (AML) patients. Br J Haem 78:591, 1991.

115. Rebulla P, Pappalettera M, Barbui T, et al. Duration of first remission in leukaemic recipients of leucocyte-poor blood components. Br J Haem 75:441, 1990.

CHAPTER 14

COST-EFFECTIVENESS OF LEUKODEPLETION

John M. Forbes, Maren A. Anderson, Steven A. Gould

SUMMARY

The use of leukodepleted blood components has grown dramatically in recent years. This growth has been fueled by the demand to minimize risks and optimize the quality of cellular blood components used in transfusion practice. Blood filtration, using high performance filters, is effective in removing significant numbers of donor leukocytes. However, filtration increases the cost of red cell transfusions by 25% and platelet transfusions by 17% over standard blood components. The important issue in determining the cost-effectiveness of leukodepletion is whether any added benefit attributable to a reduced leukocyte load is worth this increased cost.

Recent reports suggest that the use of leukodepleted blood components may be cost-effective in patients with hematologic malignancies who require long-term transfusion support. The precise clinical indications and cost-effectiveness in other patient groups have not been defined. If the preliminary results for hematologic indications are applicable to other diseases, it would appear that wider use of leukodepletion may be both inevitable and desirable.

INTRODUCTION

Today, a growing number of clinicians are using leukodepleted blood components to enhance the safety and quality of transfusion therapy. Using a variety of techniques, it is possible to remove donor leukocytes, which have been associated with a host of deleterious effects in transfusion recipients.[1] Industry sources estimate that use has grown annually by 20 to 25% since the late 1980s. Currently, between 15 to 20% of red cell transfusions and 25 to 30% of platelet transfusions in the United States are leukodepleted.

Clinical Benefits of Leukodepleted Blood Products, edited by Joseph Sweeney, M.D. and Andrew Heaton, M.D. © 1995 R.G. Landes Company.

Leukodepletion has grown dramatically in the absence of cost-effectiveness data, suggesting that blood quality and risk avoidance have been more important than cost. Only recently, has attention been focused on the cost-effectiveness of this emerging transfusion practice.[2-6] This is not surprising given the rigorous cost scrutiny taking place in all areas of health care. What is surprising is the length of time it has taken to address this important question. Today, cost-effectiveness analysis is becoming an integral and important aspect of medical practice. Determining the cost-effectiveness of a medical procedure is a strategy for comparing treatment alternatives by their relative costs per unit of output, where output is an outcome such as lives saved, years of life extended, utility, or additional cases of newly detected disease.[7] The critical question with leukodepletion is whether its costs are justifiable in terms of improved health outcomes.

It is widely acknowledged that leukodepleted blood is more expensive than standard blood on a per-unit basis because of the high performance filters and sophisticated apheresis technologies that are used. But the literature on leukodepletion uses various techniques for estimating costs, leading to highly variable results. In any cost-effectiveness analysis it is essential to calculate costs with precision and accuracy. This chapter provides information on how to determine the costs of leukodepleted blood components and reviews the cost-effectiveness literature related to leukodepletion.

DEFINING TRANSFUSION COSTS

The first step in cost-effectiveness analysis is to define the true costs associated with the technology. Unfortunately, none of the cost-effectiveness studies on leukodepleted blood components have used the same approach to determining these costs.[3-6] Presumably, this is because there is no industry standard or norm for calculating transfusion costs.

THE DIFFERENCE BETWEEN COSTS AND CHARGES

A review of the transfusion cost literature indicates that researchers usually present charge data rather than cost data, most likely because such data are more readily available. Charges are the fees charged to patients for care, which are generally passed on to the patient's health insurance plan.[8] Charges are retail prices, which reflect desired margins and such factors as cost shifting to compensate for reimbursement shortfalls from Medicare, Medicaid, and other fixed price payers. These charges have been a major focus of the debate over health care reform. Today, few hospitals collect their full charges from more than 25 to 40% of their customers. As a result, clinicians, administrators and policymakers are more interested in costs, which reflect the actual expenses incurred by health care providers when delivering patient care.

THE COMPONENTS OF TRANSFUSION COST

Blood transfusion costs, regardless of the type of blood component, are comprised of six elements: acquisition, handling, laboratory, administration, waste, and adverse effects. These costs are defined in Table 14.1.

It is clear from this table that using acquisition cost alone, as most published studies do, seriously understates the total costs associated with blood transfusion.

METHODS OF DERIVING COSTS

Transfusion costs can be calculated using several costing methods. These include the application of standard cost accounting principles, the use of the College of American Pathology (CAP) Workload Recording Method,[9] and the use of the cost-to-charge ratio provided in the Medicare Cost Reports.[10]

The use of standard cost accounting principles is the most precise but requires microcosting analyses that are expensive and time-consuming, subject to hospital-to-hospital variability, and dependent on the type of cost being considered (e.g., standard cost versus actual cost). The CAP Workload Recording Method captures the labor component of the laboratory department by quantifying the units of labor required to perform a certain task. However, the cost of materials and the allocation of overhead costs must be derived by other means. Finally, the cost-to-charge ratio method, which has been developed by the Health Care Financing Administration (HCFA), is widely used by hospital accounting personnel to derive costs from patient charges. Costs generated by this technique provide an important dimension of consistency in multi-hospital cost analyses. Each of these methods has its strengths and limitations and may be selected depending on the degree of precision required, the resources available, and the time element involved to accomplish a specific goal.

THE COSTS
OF LEUKODEPLETED BLOOD
COMPONENTS

There are a number of techniques for achieving leukodepletion and they each have different costs. The most common technique is filtration using a white blood cell removal device. Many researchers have expressed concern that filtration of blood components is significantly more costly than conventional transfusions. The main concerns are that leukodepletion involves expensive filters, increases production and administrative costs in blood banks, and is associated with product losses ranging from 5-10% of red cells and from 5-15% of platelets.[6,11-14]

THE COST
OF LEUKODEPLETED RED CELLS

The costs of a red cell transfusion were examined in a multicenter study conducted in 1989.[15] The cost-to-charge ratio method of deriving costs from charges was used. In this study, the weighted average total cost of a red cell transfusion was $155.25. This total cost included the acquisition cost (37%), handling cost (13%), laboratory cost (43%), and blood administration cost (7%), but did not include the cost of waste or adverse effects. Leukodepleted red cells cost 25% more than standard red cells in this study.

THE COST
OF LEUKODEPLETED PLATELETS

Available cost data on leukodepleted platelets routinely distort the true costs of

---

Table 14.1. Components of blood transfusion costs

Type of Cost	Description
Acquisition cost	The cost to purchase blood or collect blood in-house.
Handling cost	The cost to verify blood type, label product, and establish inventory controls.
Laboratory testing	The cost to insure unit-to-patient compatibility and transfusion-readiness.
Blood administration	The cost to administer the blood component.
Waste	The cost associated with shelf life expiration, loss or damage.
Adverse effects	The direct and indirect costs incurred as a consequence of transfusion-associated morbidity and mortality.

platelet therapy. Some investigators consider only the acquisition cost of platelets or blood filters while others only consider charges. In view of this inadequacy, we conducted an original study in 1993 documenting platelet costs in five tertiary care hospitals which participated in the 1989 red cell cost study referenced above.[15] The same methodology was used to derive costs and the results of this study are summarized in Tables 14.2 and 14.3.

Table 14.2 compares the utilization of pooled (6 random units per pool) platelet concentrates (PCs) and single donor platelets (SDPs). SDPs accounted for 88% of total platelet products transfused. This differs dramatically from platelet usage figures reported in a 1989 study by Wallace

et al.[16] In this study, SDPs represented only 29% of total platelets. Today, SDPs may be more commonplace, especially in hospitals with cancer treatment centers which have a transfusion-intensive patient mix. Filtered platelet products accounted for 35% of total units transfused in our study.

The total costs of platelet transfusion are summarized in Table 14.3. These costs include acquisition, handling, laboratory and administration but exclude waste and adverse affects. The weighted average total cost of a PC and SDP unit was $526.46 and $591.35 respectively. When combined, the weighted average total cost was $584.03. At a cost of $635.46, filtered units cost 17% more than standard units, which cost $543.36. It is interesting to

---

Table 14.2. Platelet utilization in five tertiary care hospitals in 1993

| Type of Product | Units Transfused | | | |
	PCs	SDPs	Total	Percent
Standard units	4,152	12,440	16,592	40.4%
Washed units	117	921	1,038	2.5%
Filtered units	25	14,218	14,243	34.6%
CMV negative units	45	2,220	2,265	5.5%
Resuspended units	299	1,764	2,063	5.0%
HLA-matched units	0	3,822	3,822	9.3%
Pediatric units	0	1,093	1,093	2.7%
Total	4,638	36,478	41,116	

Table 14.3. Weighted average total cost per platelet product transfused in five tertiary care hospitals in 1993

| Type of Product | Weighted Average Cost ($) | | |
	PCs	SDPs	Total
Standard units	487.35	561.91	543.36
Washed units	708.95	660.97	666.37
Filtered units	911.71	634.98	635.46
CMV negative units	685.26	585.00	586.99
Resuspended units	718.87	545.02	571.22
HLA-matched units		644.97	644.97
Pediatric units		264.01	264.01
Total	526.46	591.35	584.03

note that filtered PCs were very costly ($911.70). The data, however, were limited to only one hospital and are unlikely to be representative in a larger survey.

THE COST OF WASTE

Blood products represent a relatively scarce, highly perishable and extremely valuable resource to any health care system. Unfortunately, waste is a problem of significant proportions. The literature has recently reported that 10.5% (1.5 million units) of the national supply of red cells in 1989 were outdated or lost (7%), or unaccounted for by subtraction (3.5%).[16] No data were available for platelet waste. In our study of platelet utilization and costs, 8.3% of PCs and 2.1% of SDPs were outdated. These data suggest that the economic impact of blood product waste can be significant and renewed efforts must be focused on eliminating this waste. As the use of leukodepleted products expands, even greater vigilance will be necessary to avoid wasting expensive filtered blood components particularly if prestorage leukodepletion techniques become more popular.

THE COST OF ADVERSE EFFECTS

A complete cost analysis would incorporate the economic consequences of adverse transfusion events, including transfusion reactions, infectious disease transmission, and postoperative wound infections. Several authors have examined this important subject by calculating direct and indirect costs resulting from these adverse events.[17-20] Each of these studies demonstrate the difficulty in assigning costs to diseases that occur rarely and are not always directly attributable to a blood transfusion. In recent years, the safety of the national blood supply has improved to the point where the potential risks of transfusion have been reduced substantially.[21] Although the incidence and costs of adverse effects may be lower as a result, a thorough study should include the economic consequences of adverse transfusion events.

QUANTIFYING THE BENEFITS OF LEUKODEPLETION

The next step in cost-effectiveness analysis is comparing the outcomes associated with various treatment alternatives. There are a number of studies, particularly in patients with hematologic malignancies, that support the therapeutic benefit of leukodepletion. (Table 14.4)

In these studies, the incidence of alloimmunization is significantly reduced in patients receiving only leukodepleted blood components compared to patients receiving only standard blood components. While these data are useful and imply that a strategy of only using leukodepleted blood components in patients with hematologic malignancies is cost-effective, they do not adequately document the economic impact that reduced alloimmunization has on patient health and survival. Three recent studies, using different methods for calculating benefits, provide useful data that begin to examine this important outcome question.

COST-EFFECTIVENESS IN ACUTE MYELOID LEUKEMIA (AML)

In Oksanen et al,[6] clinical outcomes and resource consumption data were examined retrospectively in 115 patients. The patients were assigned to one of two groups according to the policy adopted by the participating hospitals. One group used only standard components and the second only leukodepleted (filtered) components. The data are summarized in Table 14.5.

In this study, patients who received filtered blood components required substantially fewer units of red cells (20%) and platelets (30%) than patients receiving standard blood components. In addition, patients in the filtered group had better outcomes. They recovered faster from hematopoiesis, experienced fewer serious infections, stayed fewer days in the hospital, and survived longer. Building on the persuasive results of this study, one would assume that the increased cost of filtered blood components is more than offset by the reduced consumption of health care resources in patients who received only leukodepleted blood, thereby producing a net savings. However, the retrospective nature of this study, the variability in clinical practice between participating hospitals, and the absence of financial data make it difficult to conclude that leukodepletion is cost-effective in this patient group.

In another study, Balducci et al,[3] used decision analysis to measure the cost-effectiveness of three transfusion strategies in the treatment of AML. One strategy used unfiltered pooled platelets until allo-immunization developed and crossmatch-compatible SDPs thereafter. The second strategy used filtered blood components until alloimmunization developed and crossmatch-compatible SDPs thereafter. The third strategy used SDPs from the beginning. The authors established a decision tree framework to show the outcomes that may occur at each node of the tree using each of these strategies. They used their own experience and the literature to determine the probability that a particular outcome (e.g., death, complete remission, refractoriness, etc.) would occur among the various patient groups. They used the same

Table 14.4. Impact of leukocyte reduction on the incidence of alloimmunization in patients with hematologic malignancies

| Author (Year) | Patients alloimmunized | |
	Using Standard Components	Using Filtered Components
Eernisse (1981)[22]	26/28	16/68
Schiffer (1983)[23]	4/12	4/15
Murphy (1986)[24]	15/21	3/19
Andreu (1988)[25]	11/35	4/34
Sniecinski (1988)[13]	10/20	3/20
Saarinen (1990)[26]	12/17	0/18
van Marwijk Kooy (1991)[27]	12/26	3/27
Total	90/169	33/201
	53%	16%

Table 14.5. Comparison of clinical outcomes and resources consumed in patients with AML

Description	Standard blood components	Filtered blood components
Number of patients (n)	50	65
Mean number of platelets	48.8	34.1
Mean number of red cells	8.3	6.6
Mean days of neutropenia	30.5	26.8
Mean days of granulocytopenia	30.6	26.7
Serious infections	59%	44%
Mean days in hospital	34.7	27.6
Rate of remission	80%	78.5%
Median survival (months)	17	45

Adapted from: Oksanen et al, Br J of Haematol 84:639,1993.

sources for projecting the clinical course of care. The results are expressed as the cost per added month of survival.

The authors found that the use of leukodepleted blood is the most cost-effective approach to delaying or preventing platelet alloimmunization. They concluded that cost considerations should not be a factor in the decision to use leukodepleted blood components because filtered components prevent or delay alloimmunization by reducing or eliminating the need for more costly HLA-matched or ABO-identical platelets.

There have been some criticisms about the clinical assumptions used in this study.[3] In addition, when assigning costs, they used blood acquisition cost and some testing charges. These costs are incomplete as they do not factor in handling cost, or the cost of laboratory testing and administration. Using a similar decision model and more reliable data, it should be possible to replicate Balducci's work to confirm or deny the cost-effectiveness of leukodepletion in AML.

EVIDENCE OF COST SAVINGS IN BONE MARROW TRANSPLANT (BMT)

In another recent study, Blumberg et al[4] present an economic analysis comparing resources consumed by 49 adult patients with relapsed Hodgkin's disease or lymphoma undergoing autologous bone marrow transplant. In this retrospective study, patients were separated into two groups, one group received only ABO-unmatched platelets, the other only ABO-identical platelets leukodepleted by bedside filtration. Data on patient charges, length of stay, and blood component usage are summarized in Table 14.6.

Dramatic differences in health care resources consumed between the two groups were found. The ABO-identical and leukodepleted group incurred significantly lower charges, spent fewer days in the hospital, and required fewer blood components compared to the ABO-unmatched group. On average, total charges for the ABO-identical and leukodepleted group were $31,048 lower than the ABO-unmatched group. Further analysis of the total charge data, in terms of average charge per hospital day, reveals that patients receiving only leukodepleted blood had average daily charges of $2,109 compared to $1,951 for the ABO-unmatched group. This analysis suggests that the difference in total charges between the two groups may be attributable to the difference in length of stay.

Although this study was not designed as a cost-effectiveness analysis the data show significant savings in resource consumption. The authors conclude that the use of only filtered ABO-identical platelets was associated with dramatic reductions in both cost and transfusion requirements.

Table 14.6. Comparison of resource utilization in bone marrow transplant patients

Category	ABO unmatched platelets (n=20)	ABO identical filtered platelets (n=29)	p value
Total charges	$85,886	$54,838	p=0.003
Ancillary charges	$42,600	$24,700	p=0.002
Blood bank charges	$11,533	$5,810	p=0.008
Pharmacy charges	$13,359	$8,173	p=0.006
Hospital days	44	26	p=0.002
Red cell units	15	8.9	p=0.02
Platelet units	143	72	p=0.005

Adapted from: Blumberg et al., Transfusion 33:83S,1993.

Unfortunately, however, this study is not methodologically rigorous and uses charge data rather than costs.

The data from these three studies provide preliminary evidence that the clinical and economic benefits of leukodepletion outweigh the increased costs of filtration in patients with hematologic malignancies. No cost-effectiveness data exist, however, to support the use of leukodepletion in other patient groups. In spite of this, there is pressure to increase the number of clinical indications across a wider range of clinical settings. Ongoing research, using the cost methods described in this chapter in conjunction with an assessment of the benefits of leukodepletion, are necessary to justify expanded use of this emerging clinical practice especially in today's cost-conscious environment.

New filters, able to reduce the leukocyte content by several logs more than current filters, are under development and prestorage filtration techniques are becoming available. Filter cost, loss of product during filtration, and documentation of benefits are the major issues that need to be resolved with these improved filtration technologies. If these filters are safe and effective, if they are priced reasonably and easy to use, and if their use contributes measurably to improved health outcome, leukodepletion has the potential of becoming standard practice in transfusion therapy.

CONCLUSIONS

1. There is evidence of rapid growth in the use of leukodepleted blood products.
2. This growth has been fueled by pressures to improve the safety and quality of transfusion practice.
3. The growth of leukodepletion is contributing to increased costs of red cell and platelet products.
4. Cost-effectiveness analyses have not been adequately conducted although preliminary data are available in the care of patients with AML and undergoing bone marrow transplant.
5. Capturing all the components of cost

and health outcomes is essential to the conduct of such analyses.
6. Although growth in the use of leukodepleted products is likely to continue, and increased volume may reduce cost-per-unit, analysis of cost-effectiveness should be encouraged in other clinical situations.

REFERENCES

1. Lane TA, Anderson KC, Goodnough LT, et al. Leukocyte reduction in blood component therapy. Annals of Internal Medicine 117:151, 1992.
2. Perkins HA. Is white cell reduction cost-effective? Transfusion 33:626, 1993.
3. Balducci L, Benson K, Lyman GH, et al. Cost-effectiveness of white-cell reduction filters in treatment of adult acute myeloid leukemia. Transfusion 33:665, 1993.
4. Blumberg N, Heal J, Rapoport A, et al. Effect of ABO-identical platelets and leuko-depletion (LD) on blood utilization and costs of autologous marrow transplantation (BMT). Transfusion 33:A16;83S, 1993.
5. Blumberg N, Heal J, Kirkley S, et al. Cost-effectiveness of leukodepleted transfusions during induction therapy for acute leukemia. Transfusion 33:83S, 1993.
6. Oksanen K, Elonen E. Impact of leukocyte-depleted blood components on the haematological recovery and prognosis of patients with acute myeloid leukaemia. Br J of Haematol 84:639, 1993.
7. Sox HC, Blatt MA, Higgins MC, Marton KI. Medical Decision Making. Boston: Butterworth, 1988.
8. Finkler SA. The distinction between costs and charges. Annals of Internal Medicine 96:102, 1982.
9. Conn RB, ed. Manual for laboratory workload recording method. Chicago: College of American Pathologists, 1989.
10. Provider Specific file. US Dept of Health and Human Services, Health Care Financing Administration, Office of Statistics and Data Management, Bureau of Data Management and Strategy, Baltimore: 1990.
11. Schiffer CA. Prevention of alloimmunization against platelets. Blood 77:1, 1991.
12. Masse M, Andreu G, Angue M, et al. A

multicenter study on the efficiency of white cell reduction by filtration of red cells. Transfusion 31:792, 1991.

13. Sniecinski I, O'Donnell MR, Nowicki B, et al. Prevention of refractoriness and HLA-alloimmunization using filtered blood products. Blood 71:1402, 1988.

14. Rebulla P, Porretti L, Bertolini F, et al. White cell-reduced red cells prepared by filtration: a critical evaluation of current filters and methods for counting residual white cells. Transfusion 33:128, 1993.

15. Forbes JM, Anderson MD, Anderson GF, et al. Blood transfusion costs: a multicenter study. Transfusion 31:318, 1991.

16. Wallace EL, Surgenor DM, Hao HS, et al. Collection and transfusion of blood components in the United States, 1989. Transfusion 33:139, 1993.

17. Hornbrook MC, Dodd RY, Jacobs P, et al. Reducing the incidence of non-A, non-B post-transfusion hepatitis by testing donor blood for alanine aminotransferase. NEJM 307:1315, 1982.

18. Eisenstaedt RS, Getzen TE. Screening blood donors for human immunodeficiency virus antibody: cost-benefit analysis. Am J Public Health 78:450, 1988.

19. Scitovsky AA, Rice DP. Estimates of the direct and indirect costs of acquired immunodeficiency syndrome in the United States, 1985, 1986, 1991. Public Health Reports 102:5, 1987.

20. Birkmeyer JD, Goodnough LT, AuBuchon JP, et al. The cost-effectiveness of preoperative autologous blood donation for total hip and knee replacement. Transfusion 33:544, 1993.

21. Dodd RY. The risk of transfusion-transmitted infection. N Engl J Med 327:419, 1992.

22. Eernisse JG, Brand A. Prevention of platelet refractoriness due to HLA antibodies by administration of leukocyte-poor blood components. Exp Hematol 9:77, 1981.

23. Schiffer CA, Dutcher JP, Aisner J, et al. A randomized trial of leukocyte-depleted platelet transfusion to modify alloimmunization in patients with leukemia. Blood 61:815, 1983.

24. Murphy MF, Metcalfe P, Thomas H, et al. Use of leukocyte-poor components and HLA-matched-platelet donors to prevent HLA alloimmunization. Br J Haematol 62:529, 1986.

25. Andreu G, Dewailly J, Leberre C, et al. Prevention of HLA immunization with leukocyte-poor packed red cells and platelet concentrates obtained by filtration. Blood 71:964, 1988.

26. Saarinen UM, Kekomaki R, Siimes MA et al. Effective prophylaxis against platelet refractoriness in multitransfused patients by use of leukocyte-free blood components. Blood 75:512, 1990.

27. van Marwijk Kooy M, van Prooijen HC, Moes M. Use of leukocyte-depleted platelet concentrates for the prevention of refractoriness and primary HLA alloimmunization: A prospective, randomized trial. Blood 77:201, 1991.

INDEX

Page numbers in italics denote figures (f) and tables (t).

A

Acute myeloid leukemia (AML)
  cost-effectiveness of leukodepletion, 187-189, *188f*
Adams PT, 100
Adenine, 45
Adult respiratory distress syndrome (ARDS), 6, 130
AIDS. See *Human immunodeficiency virus (HIV)*.
Akahoshi M, 74
Ali (initial not given), 175
Allen SM, 145
Allergic transfusion reactions, 69-71
Alloimmunization, 81-92
  clinical consequences, 83-84, *83f*
  hematopoietic stem cell transplantation, 168
  maternal, 157
  mechanisms, 82-83
  prevention, 84-85
    HLA matching, 85
    leukodepletion, 85-87, *86t*
      leukocyte dose, 90
      randomized, prospective clinical trials, 87-90, *89t*
      unrandomized clinical trials, 87
    UVB irradiation, 90-92, *91t, 92t*
Alpha-1-protease, 141
Ammonium chloride, 45
Anaphylactoxin, 68, 70
Andreu G, 88, 92
Angue M, 47
Antigen-presenting cells (APC), 82, 156
Apheresis, 12
Aprotinin, 161
AS-3, 45
Aye (initial not given), 169

B

B7-CD28, 82
B cell, 82
Balducci L, 188
Basophils, 70
Beaujean F, 38
Bedside filtration, 11
Berg WN, 18
Berkson J, 18
BEST (Biomedical Excellence for Safer Transfusion), 24
Bg antibodies, 69
Billingham RE, 114
Blajchman MA, 7, 8, 86, 119, 172, 175

Blood cell properties, *31t*, 34
Blumberg N, 7, 189
Bock M, 55
Bodensteiner DC, 36
Bone marrow transplantation. *See also* Hematopoietic stem cell transplantation.
  cost-effectiveness, 189-190, *189t*
Bowden RA, 8, 173, 174
Brand A, 87, 171
Brecher M, 48
Brittingham TE, 132
Brubaker DB, 169
Buffy coat layer, 46
Buffy coat platelets (BC-PC), 54-55
Bürker chamber, 22
Burrows L, 114, 118
Busch ORC, 116

C

Ca^{2+}, 37
Callaberts AJ, 11
Cancer recurrence
  transfusion-induced immunomodulation, 117-121, *119f, 120f*
Cardiac transplantation, 115
  cytomegalovirus (CMV), 108, *109t*
Cardiopulmonary bypass (CPB)
  hemodynamics, 138-139, *139f, 140f*
  leukocyte activation, 139-141, 160-161
Catalase (CAT), 143
CD4, 82, 155
CD8, 82, 155
Cell-cell interactions, 36
Cell counting, 8, 17-20, *19t, 20f*
  methods, 20-21, *21t*
    flow cytometry, 22
    microscopic chamber, 21-22
    PCR (polymerase chain reaction), 22-23
    radioimmunoassays, 22
  quality control (QC), 23-24, *24f*
Cellulose acetate, 10, 11
Centrifugation, 9
Cheung K-S, 101
Claas FHJ, 86
Cleland J, 138
CLX®, 45
Colorectal cancer
  transfusion-induced immunomodulation, 118, *119f*

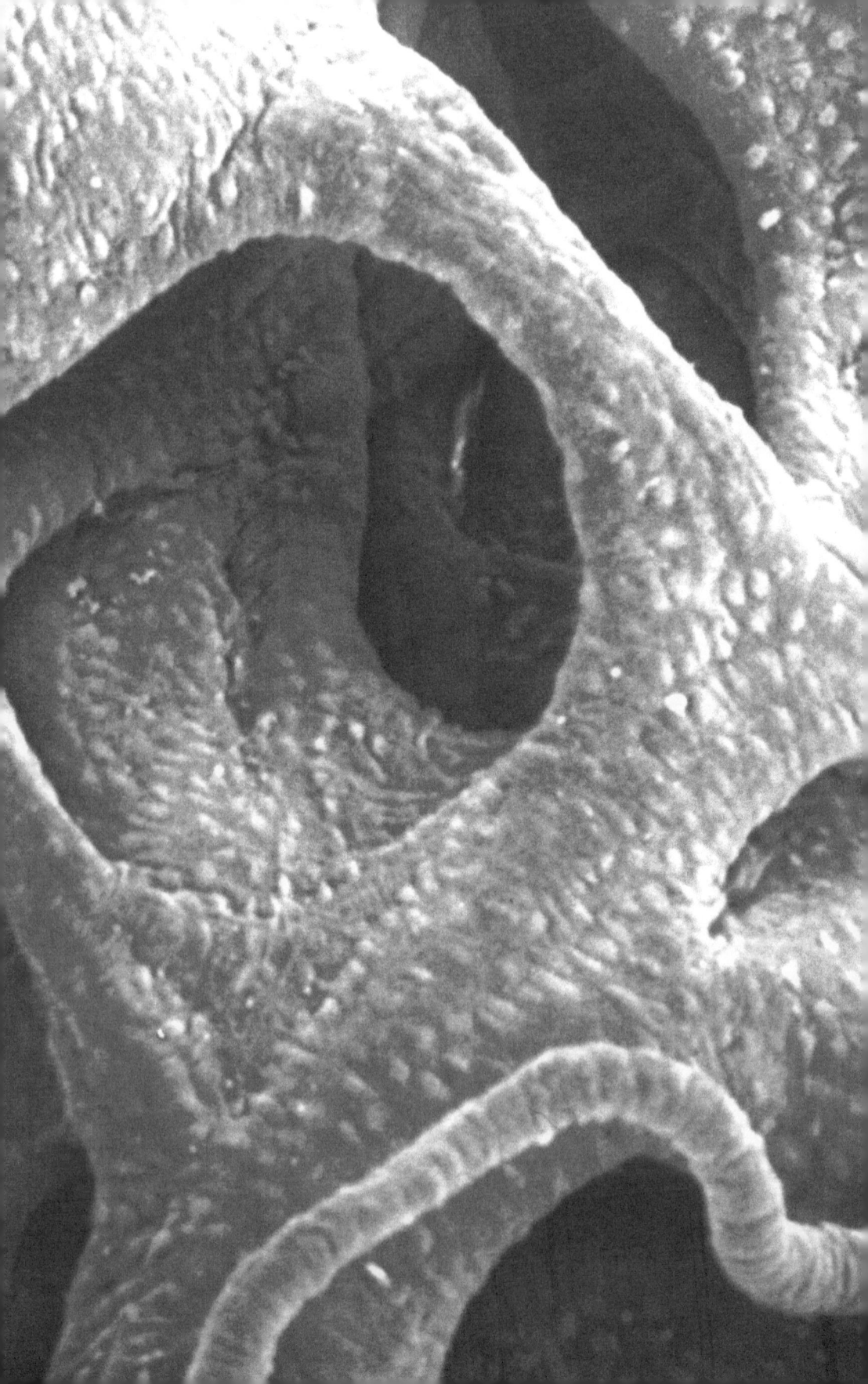

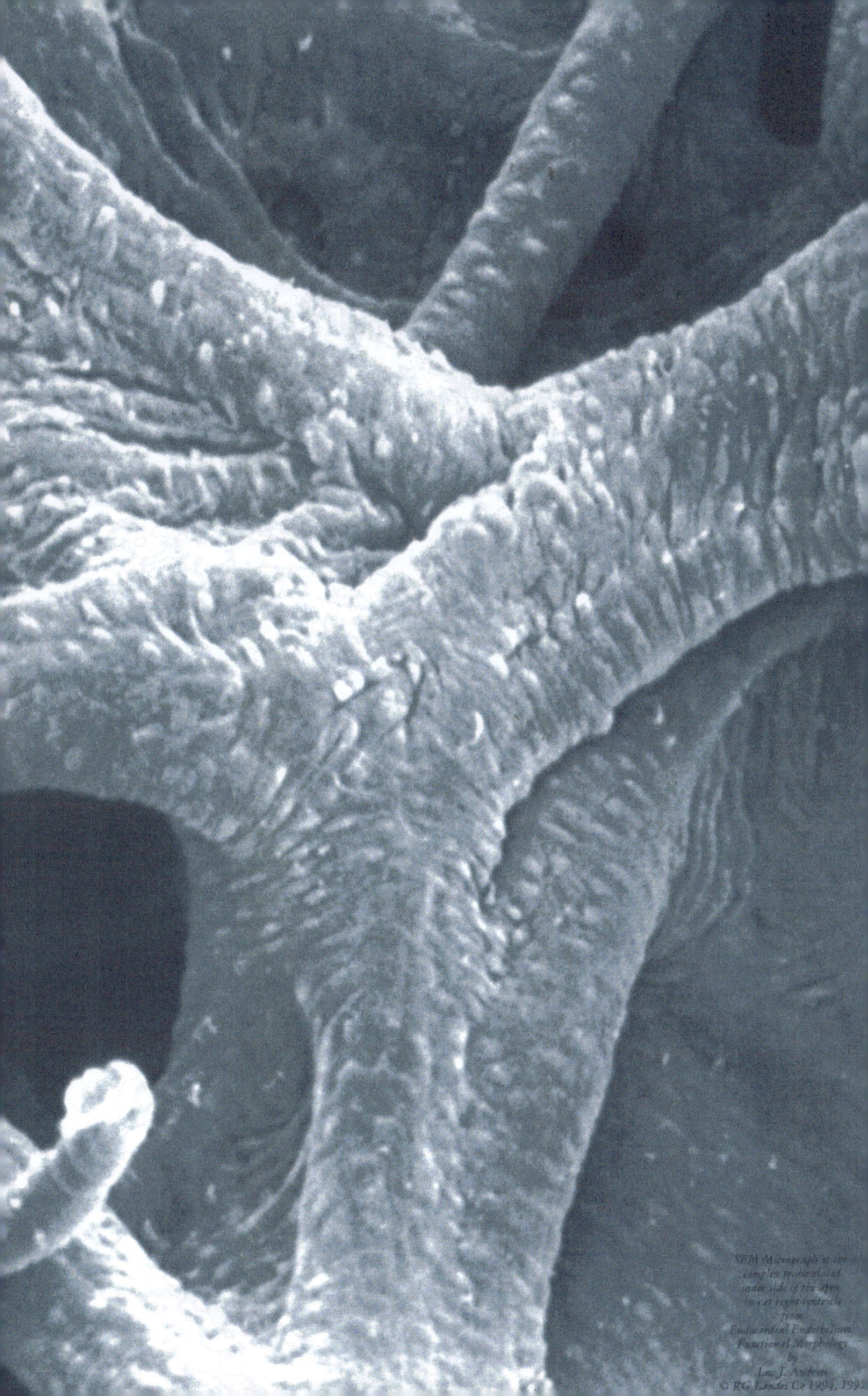

SEM Micrograph of the
complex trabeculated
inner side of rat apex
in rat right ventricle
from
Endocardial Endothelium
Functional Morphology
by
Lou J. Andries
© R.G. Landes Co 1993, 199